COMPREHENSIVE GYNECOLOGY REVIEW

SYNTEX LABORATORIES, INC.
3401 HILLVIEW AVENUE, P.O. BOX 10850
PALO ALTO, CALIFORNIA 94303

(415) 855-5545
TELEX 4997273 SYNTEX PLA

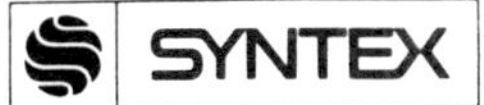

LOUIS HAGLER, M.D., DIRECTOR
RONALD H. LEWIS, M.D., SR. ASSOC. DIR.
MEDICAL SERVICES DEPARTMENT

Dear Doctor:

Preparation for specialty boards is an intimidating experience. We at Syntex would like to make the process a little less traumatic by providing you with a copy of *Comprehensive Gynecology Review* that can help to organize and facilitate your preparation.

The *Review* has been written to complement Herbst and Droegemueller's *Comprehensive Gynecology*, a standard and respected textbook. As you work through the broad collection of board-type questions and answers, you can identify areas in which your knowledge is adequate and others in which additional study might be required. Each answer is explained in a detailed comment which reinforces the learning process. Even if you are not planning to take the board exam this year, the *Review* can still serve as a valuable tool for self assessment.

We at Syntex look forward to continuing our close relationship with you throughout your career, by keeping you updated on support services, and providing product information on and samples of our OB/GYN products: TRI-NORINYL® (norethindrone and ethinyl estradiol), ANAPROX® DS (naproxen sodium), ANAPROX® (naproxen sodium), FEMSTAT® Prefill (butoconzole nitrate), TORADOL® ORAL (ketorolac tromethamine), TORADOL® IM (ketorolac tromethamine), and SYNAREL® (nafarelin acetate). Please consult enclosed full prescribing information before using any of these products.

We hope you find the *Review* useful. Good luck at examination time.

Sincerely,

Louis Hagler, M.D.
Director
Medical Services Department

COMPREHENSIVE GYNECOLOGY REVIEW

Gerald B. Holzman, M.D.
Professor and Vice-Chairman
Department of Obstetrics and Gynecology
Medical College of Georgia
Augusta, Georgia

Frank W. Ling, M.D.
Associate Professor and Director
Division of Gynecology
Department of Obstetrics and Gynecology
University of Tennessee College of Medicine
Memphis, Tennessee

Douglas W. Laube, M.D.
Professor
Department of Obstetrics and Gynecology
University of Iowa
Iowa City, Iowa

Louis A. Vontver, M.D., M.Ed.
Professor and Director of Education
Department of Obstetrics and Gynecology
University of Washington
Seattle, Washington

SECOND EDITION

with 114 illustrations

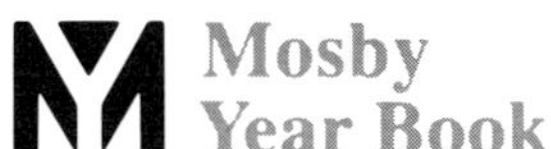

St. Louis Baltimore Boston Chicago London Philadelphia Sydney Toronto

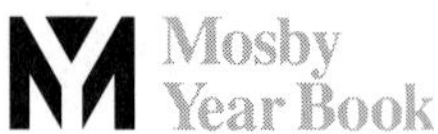

Editor: Stephanie Manning
Editorial Assistant: Colleen Boyd
Project Manager: Gayle May Morris
Production Editor: Deborah Vogel

SECOND EDITION

Printed in the United States of America

Mosby–Year Book, Inc.
11830 Westline Industrial Drive
St. Louis, Missouri 63146

Library of Congress Cataloging-in-Publication Data

Comprehensive gynecology review / Gerald B. Holzman . . . [et al.].
2nd ed.
p. cm.
Intended to complement: Comprehensive gynecology / Arthur L. Herbst . . . [et al.]. 2nd ed. 1991.
ISBN 0-8016-2279-4 : $23.95
1. Gynecology--Examinations, questions, etc. I. Holzman, Gerald B., 1933- , II. Comprehensive gynecology.
[DNLM: 1. Genital Diseases, Female. 2. Gynecology—methods. WP 140 C737 Suppl.]
RG101.C726 1991 Suppl.
818.1'0076--dc20
DNLM/DLC
for Library of Congress

92-5943
CIP

92 93 94 95 96 CL/CL/MY 9 8 7 6 5 4 3 2 1

Preface

This second edition of *Comprehensive Gynecology Review* has been written to complement the second edition of *Comprehensive Gynecology*. Its intended audience is practicing physicians, residents, and students interested in gynecology. It can be used to identify areas of weakness, to reinforce new information obtained by reading the textbook, or to reassure oneself that the subject matter is understood. The format should be familiar: it is the standard testing format used by the Educational Testing Service. *Comprehensive Gynecology Review* chapters follow the textbook chapters exactly. The questions within the chapters have been scrambled, and the answers appear in a separate section. Each answer includes a page reference in *Comprehensive Gynecology*, second edition, occasionally an additional reference, and a comment. Questions were chosen for a variety of reasons. Since the book is to help the learner, the questions are not always of the same difficulty that a final, summative, or certifying examination would accept. The purpose of these examinations is to assure an agency or school that the examinee has attained a requisite amount of knowledge. The examination must discriminate between those who know and those who do not know. Questions that everyone should be able to answer are not included. Since the *Review* is not written with a specific "level" of physician in mind, it was not possible to eliminate a question that everyone might know. Besides, one purpose of the *Review* is to reinforce knowledge. Thus, there are easy questions. Likewise, in a final, or certifying examination one must avoid the controversial; such questions are not avoided in the *Review*. In practice, one has to treat the controversial. For this reason, some readers will disagree with some of our answers, but this is a self-assessment instrument.

An attempt has been made to put the subject in a clinical perspective and to clarify. There are many illustrations that require interpretation. There is a certain amount of cueing in each chapter that would not exist in a final, or certifying examination. In organizing the book by chapters, this could **not** be avoided, as the most conceivable answer for a question in the chapter on endometriosis is likely to be endometriosis.

To simulate test conditions, an examinee should take 45 to 60 seconds to answer each question. Answer all the questions in a chapter before verifying the answers. To reinforce the material, read all the comments.

In this second edition 30% to 40% of the questions have been modified. Questions have been written on new material; there are fewer multiple answer, multiple choice questions; and those that remain conform to the Educational Testing Service format.

We wish to thank the authors of *Comprehensive Gynecology*, Arthur L. Herbst, Daniel Mishell, Jr., Morton Stenchever, and William Droegemueller, for suggesting the *Review* and inviting us to write it. Our thanks to our families for their patience and support, and our gratitude to our editor, Stephanie Manning, for her encouragement.

Gerald B. Holzman
Frank W. Ling
Douglas W. Laube
Louis A. Vontver

Contents

PART FOUR
GYNECOLOGIC ONCOLOGY

PART FIVE
ENDOCRINOLOGY AND INFERTILITY

PART ONE BASIC SCIENCES

CHAPTER 1 Embryology

DIRECTIONS for questions 1 - 4: Select the one best answer or completion.

1. Human chorionic gonadotrophin reaches its peak at which week of pregnancy?
   A. 3-4
   B. 9-10
   C. 20-21
   D. 28-30
   E. 38-40
2. Germ cells are derived from the
   A. Primitive coelomic epithelium
   B. Yolk sac
   C. Bone marrow
   D. Germinal epithelium
   E. Ovarian stroma
3. The first functioning organ system in the embryo is the
   A. nervous
   B. digestive
   C. cardiovascular
   D. genitourinary
   E. skeletal
4. Blood formation in the embryo first occurs in the
   A. liver
   B. spleen
   C. bone marrow
   D. lymph nodes
   E. heart

DIRECTIONS for questions 5 - 18: For each numbered item, select the one heading most closely associated with it. Each lettered heading may be used once, more than once, or not at all.

5-8. Match the stages of the first meiotic division with the appropriate description.
   (A) Chromosome pairs in contact
   (B) Condensation of chromatin as thread-like material
   (C) Development of chiasmata
   (D) Migration of chromosomes to equatorial plate

5. Leptotene
6. Zygotene
7. Pachytene
8. Diplotene

9-10. Match the postovulatory day with the appropriate event.
   (A) 3-4
   (B) 6-7
   (C) 9-11
   (D) 12-13
   (E) 15-16

9. Implantation
10. Trophoblastic venous sinuses formed

11-15. Match the male and female homologous structures.
   (A) Vagina
   (B) Labia majora
   (C) Ovarian follicles
   (D) Clitoris
   (E) Round ligament

11. Scrotum
12. Penis
13. Prostatic utricle
14. Seminiferous tubules
15. Gubernaculum testis

16-18. Match the congenital abnormality with the embryonic developmental failure.
   (A) Sinovaginal bulb fails to canalize
   (B) Paramesonephric duct does not develop
   (C) Paramesonephric duct does not fuse
   (D) Failure of rupture of anal membrane

16. Absence of uterus
17. Uterus didelphys
18. Transverse vaginal septum

DIRECTIONS for questions 19 - 26: For each of the questions below, ONE or MORE of the responses is correct. Select the best answer based on the following

A if 1, 2, and 3 are correct
B if only 1 and 2 are correct
C if only 2 and 3 are correct

D if only 1 is correct
E if only 3 is correct

19. Arrest of oocyte meiosis occurs at the
    1. metaphase of the first meiotic division
    2. prophase of the first meiotic division
    3. metaphase of the second meiotic division
20. Which of the following events occur during or concurrent with meiosis?
    1. pairing of homologous chromosomes
    2. ovulation
    3. fertilization
21. True statements regarding fertilization include:
    1. capacitation occurs in the sperm as they are transported up the female genital tract
    2. fertilization usually occurs in the ampulla of the fallopian tube
    3. a significant proportion of fertilized ova do not complete cleavage
22. Effects of a teratogen depend on
    1. duration of exposure of teratogen
    2. stage of embryonic development
    3. dose of teratogen
23. True statements concerning development of the excretory system include: The
    1. pronephros and its ducts serve as the first fetal kidney
    2. mesonephros produces urine for several weeks
    3. metanephros begins as a pelvic organ
24. True statements concerning the development of the genital duct system include:
    1. leydig cells of the fetal testes produce testosterone while Sertoli cells produce MIF (mullerian inhibiting factor)
    2. the paramesonephric duct develops if no gonads are present
    3. structures developing from both mesonephric and paramesonephric ducts occur in some adult females
25. True statements about sex differentiation include:
    1. if testes are to develop, H-Y antigen must be activated.
    2. the ovary differentiates at approximately the 11th week.
    3. a Y chromosome is required for the development of the testes.
26. It is currently believed the suppression of meiosis in the dictyate stage is due to a substance produced in the
    1. granulosa
    2. theca
    3. rete cords

ANSWERS

1. **B,** Page 9. Human chorionic gonadotrophin doubles every 1.2 to 2 days in early pregnancy with its peak being reached at 7 to 9 weeks of pregnancy.
2. **B,** Page 4. Germ cells are derived from the endoderm in the wall of the yolk sac, and migrate to the germinal ridge which later forms the gonads. The "germinal" epithelium is derived from the primitive coelomic epithelium and invests the ovary but does not produce germ cells.
3. **C,** Page 9. Blood vessel formation (angiogenesis) is seen in the extraembryonic mesoderm by day 15 or 16. By the 21st day, the primitive heart is connected with blood vessels of the embryo to become the first functioning organ system.
4. **A,** Page 9. In the embryo, blood formation does not begin until the second month of gestation, occurring first in the developing liver. Blood vessel formation begins in the extraembryonic mesoderm of the yolk sac by day 15 or 16. Embryonic vessels are seen approximately 2 days later.

5-8. 5, **B;** 6, **D;** 7, **A;** 8, **C;** Page 4. In the earliest stage, the leptotene stage, chromatin material condenses into threadlike structures. During zygotene, migration to the equatorial plate occurs and homologous chromosomes pair up to form bivalents. At the end of this phase, tight pairing of the chromosomes along their entire length, synapsis, takes place. During the subsequent pachytene stage, each chromosome splits into two chromatids united at the centromere. The bivalent is thus transformed into tetrads. There are 23 tetrads in the human ovum. During diplotene, the chromosomes of the bivalents are held together at points called chiasmata, where crossing over of genetic material occurs between chromatids of homologous chromosomes.

9-10. 9, **B;** 10, **C;** Pages 6-7. Subsequent to the first mitotic division, the cells continue to divide as the embryo passes along the fallopian tube and into the uterus. This takes 3 to 4 days after fertilization, and the embryo enters the uterus in any form, from 32 cells to the early blastula stage. Implantation typically occurs 3 days after the embryo enters the uterus. Invading syncytiotrophoblast comes in intimate contact with endometrial capillaries to form venous sinuses at 7 1/2 to 9 days after con-

TABLE 1-1. Events of Implantation

Event	Days After Ovulation
Zona pellucida disappears	4-5
Blastocyst attaches to epithelial surface of endometrium	6
Trophoblast erodes into endometrial stroma	7
Trophoblast differentiates into cytotrophoblastic and syncytial trophoblastic layers	7-8
Lacunae appear around trophoblast	8-9
Blastocyst burrows beneath endometrial surface	9-10
Lacunar network forms	10-11
Trophoblast invades endometrial sinusoids, establishing a uteroplacental circulation	11-12
Endometrial epithelium completely covers blastocyst	12-13
Strong decidual reaction occurs in stroma	13-14

ception which would be 9-11 days after ovulation.

11-15. 11, **B**; 12, **D**; 13, **A**; 14, **C**; 15, **E**; Table 1-2, Page 14. There are homologous male and female derivatives for each embryonic structure. Paired structures include scrotum/labia majora, penis/clitoris, prostatic utricle/vagina, seminiferous tubules/ovarian follicles, and gubernaculum testis/round ligaments.

16-18. 6, **B**; 17, **C**; 18, **A**; Page 13. Abnormalities in specific developmental processes can result in discrete congenital abnormalities. If the paramesonephric duct does not develop, absence of the uterus occurs. Uterus didelphys is a result of lack of fusion of the paramesonephric duct. A transverse vaginal septum results from failure of the sinovaginal bulb to canalize.

19. **C** (2, 3); Page 4. At approximately 5 months gestation, oocytes of the fetus enter the process of meiosis and progress to the prophase of the first meiotic division before entering the first arrest, which lasts for several years. After puberty maturation of selected follicles continues to the second meiotic metaphase, when the second arrest occurs. This arrest lasts until the oocyte is activated by fertilization.

20. **A** (All); Page 4. One of the first events in meiosis is the tight pairing of homologous chromosomes. This is followed by the formation of a tetrad, as each chromosome of the pair splits longitudinally forming 2 chromatids. Meiosis is arrested at this point until after puberty. In each cycle a few follicles ripen and in those follicles the oocyte resumes meiosis. Ovulation begins during the 2nd meiotic division, and the final steps of the 2nd meiotic division are completed after fertilization.

21. **A** (All); Page 6. As the spermatozoa are transported through the cervical mucus, uterus, and fallopian tubes, they undergo capacitation and acrosome reaction, thus activating enzyme systems to make it possible for the sperm to penetrate the barrier of the zona pellucida. Once the sperm enters the cytoplasm of the egg, the sperm head swells and gives rise to the male pronucleus. The egg casts off the second polar body and the female pronucleus is formed. The pronuclei contain the haploid sets of chromosomes of maternal and paternal origin. Although the two do not fuse, the nuclear membranes surrounding them disappear, and this establishes the diploid complement of chromosomes. Cleavage gives rise to the two-cell embryo while still in the fallopian tube. Due to failure of chromosome arrangement on the spindle, gene defects, and environmental factors, a significant number of fertilized ova do not complete cleavage.

22. **A** (All); Page 10. All organ systems are usually formed from the fourth to the seventh week of gestation. A teratogenic event occurring during this time will result in a malformation related to the organ systems developing at the time of insult. In addition, the effects of a teratogen depend on dose and duration of exposure to the teratogen, as well as the genetic makeup of the individual. Therefore, cardiovascular abnormalities are expected if ateratogen is to take effect early in the embryonic period. Teratogens may be chemical substances, their by-products, or physical conditions such as temperature elevation and irradiation. After the 49th day teratogens usually will not cause specific malformations. They may kill the embryo or injure cells leading to cellular malfunction or growth retardation.

23. **C** (2, 3), Pages 10-11. Three sets of excretory ducts and tubules develop bilaterally in the fetus. First, the pronephros forms at about the fourth week after conception.

The associated tubules probably have no excretory function. Late in the fourth week, the mesonephric tubules develop. The mesonephros functions as a fetal kidney, producing urine for 2 or 3 weeks. The permanent kidney, the metanephros, originally a pelvic organ, begins development in the fifth week and by differential growth it ultimately relocates in the lumbar region. The fetus produces urine throughout gestation, but the placenta handles the excretory functions of the fetus.

24. **A** (All), Pages 11, 13. The mesonephric duct development precedes the paramesonephric duct development with the latter set developing on each side from evaginations of the coelomic epithelium. The mesonephric duct differentiates into the vas deferens, epididymis, and seminal vesicles. Leydig cells produce testosterone and the Sertoli cells of the testes produce mullerian inhibiting factor. In the presence of ovaries or if no gonads are present at all, the mesonephric ducts regress and the paramesonephric ducts develop. Structures developing from both mesonephric (Gartner's duct and paraovarian cysts) and paramesonephric (tubes and uterus) duct systems occur in some adult females.
25. **A** (All), Pages 17, 19. In general a Y chromosome is required for the development of the testes. Genes on the Y chromosome are either responsible for the development of the H-Y antigen or for activator genes that will induce production of the H-Y antigen. In some rare instances, the H-Y antigen may express itself in the absence of the Y chromosome. In such cases, the gene for H-Y antigen expression is expected to be found on another chromosome, probably the X chromosome. Another theory proposes an interaction of 2 genes, a testes determining gene on the Y chromosome and an ovary determining gene on the X or an autosome. Their presence and timing of their expression initiatesthe formation of the gonad. In order for testes to be formed, however, the H-Y antigen must be activated. For normal male development, the testes must differentiate and function normally. The ovary, which develops at the 11th or 12th week, requires two functional X chromosomes. In cases where one X chromosome is missing, ovaries almost invariably lack oocytes. Conversely, germ cells in testes develop best when only one X chromosome is present.
26. **D** (1 only), Pages 4, 6. Meiosis is stimulated by a meiotic inducing substance produced in the rete cords. As the ovary develops the granulosa cells surround the ova and separate them from the rete. The granulosa produces an inhibiting substance. Loss of contact with the rete and the granulosa produced inhibiting substance act to suppress meiosis in the dictyate stage. Meiosis will resume after puberty when each set of follicles begins to grow. The theca is not known to participate.

CHAPTER 2

Genetics

DIRECTIONS for questions 1 - 14: Select the one best answer or completion.

1. The pedigree in Figure 2-1 suggests the inheritance of a trait that is
   A. autosomal dominant
   B. autosomal recessive
   C. X-linked recessive
   D. X-linked dominant
   E. male-limited autosomal dominant
2. Assume the trait is fully penetrant. The pedigree in Figure 2-2 is most consistent with a gene that is a(n)
   A. autosomal dominant
   B. autosomal recessive
   C. X-linked recessive
   D. X-linked dominant
   E. male-limited autosomal dominant
3. A couple who had a barren marriage for 10 years now have had two spontaneous abortions at 6 and 8 weeks. A karyotype was done on both the husband and wife. He is 46 XY, and her karyotype is reproduced in Figure 2-3. She is 30 and he is 32. Which of the following statements are correct and should be mentioned during counseling?
   A. patients with her karyotype do not carry to term
   B. patients with her karyotype do not give birth to a chromosomally normal neonate

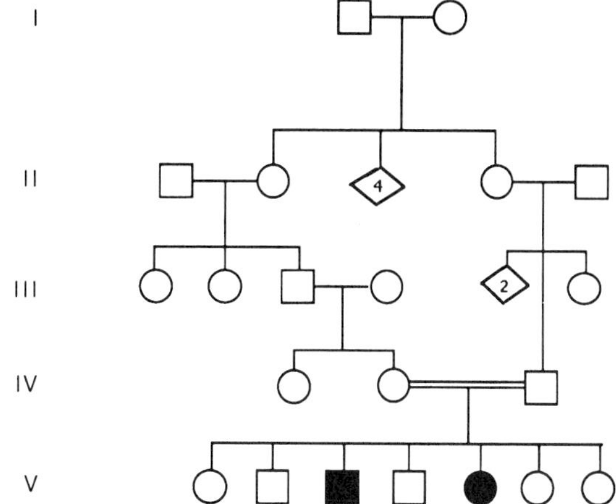

FIGURE 2-2.

   C. they might have a chromosomally abnormal neonate, but it would be identical to that of its mother
   D. there is an increased risk of having a child with a trisomy
   E. there is no chromosomal explanation for their poor reproductive history
4. A couple who has had recurrent abortions had a karyotype done on the last abortus. The karyotype was 47 XX, +16. Given this information, you would tell the couple

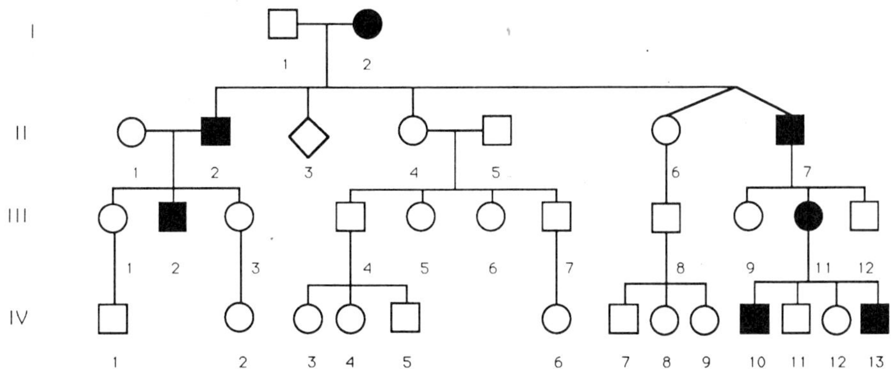

FIGURE 2-1.

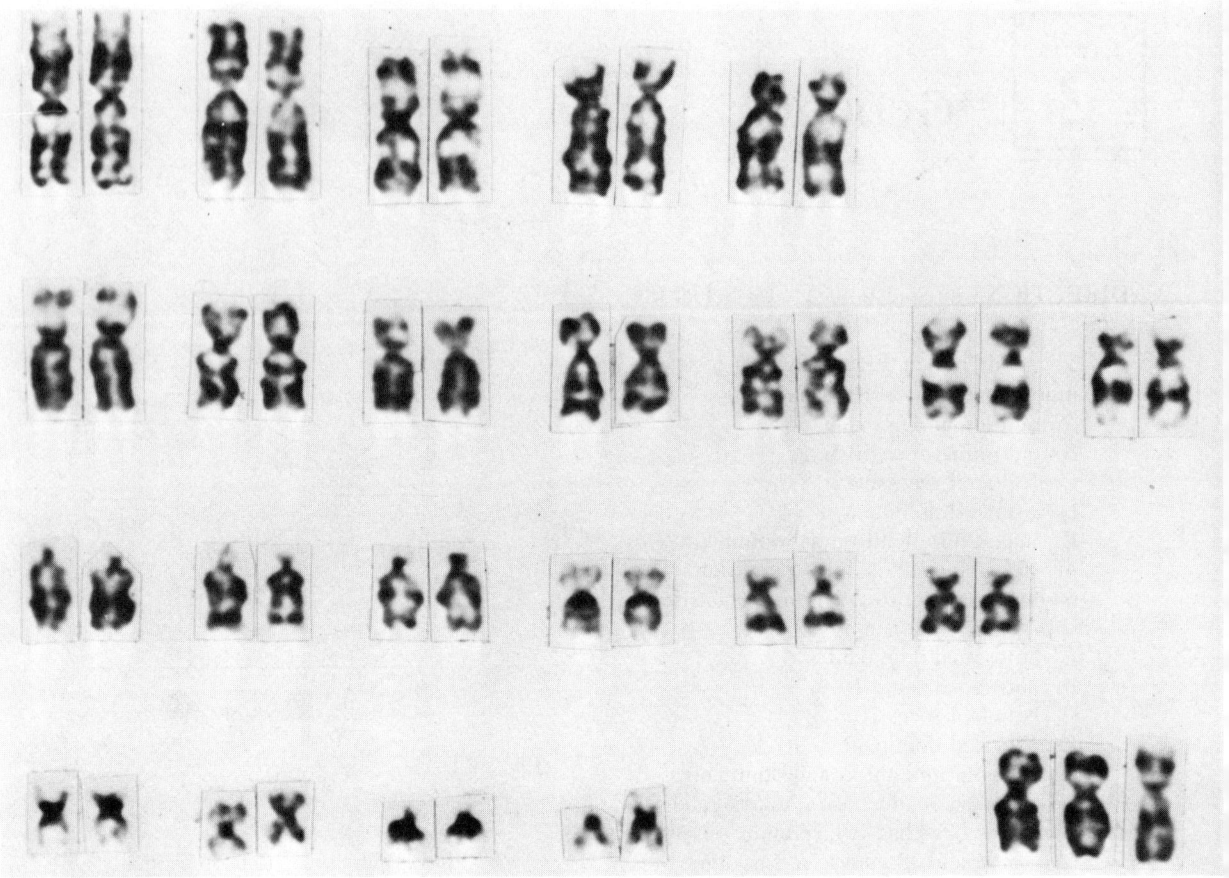

FIGURE 2-3.

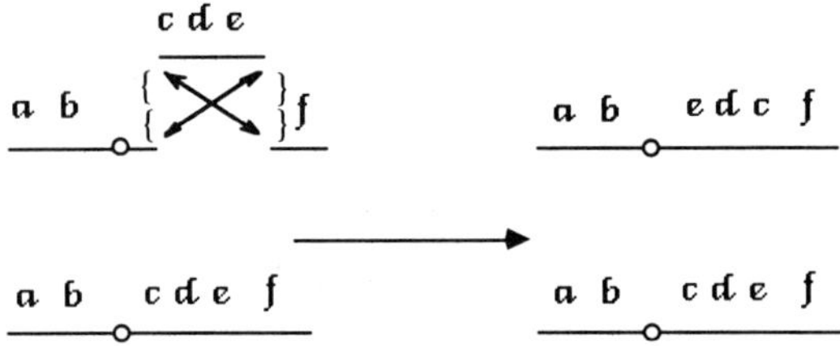

FIGURE 2-4.

that the chance of delivering a live-born infant with a trisomy is approximately

A. 0.1%
B. 1%
C. 5%
D. 10%
E. 25%

5. Figure 2-4 represents a(n)
   A. Robertsonian fusion (translocation)
   B. isochromosome
   C. reciprocal translocation
   D. pericentric inversion
   E. paracentric inversion
6. A prenatal patient has had her karyotype reported as containing a Robertsonian fusion involving chromosome 21.

   Theoretically, the likelihood of her having a live-born with a trisomy is
   A. none
   B. 25%
   C. 33%
   D. 50%
   E. 100%
7. The actual risk of giving birth to a trisomic infant in the situation mentioned in question 6 is
   A. 1%
   B. 5%
   C. 10%
   D. 25%
   E. 33%
8. The spontaneous abortion figure quoted in most textbooks is 10% to 20%. If this number includes all embryos that do not result in live-born infants, the number
   A. is correct
   B. should be 20%-30%
   C. should be 31%-40%

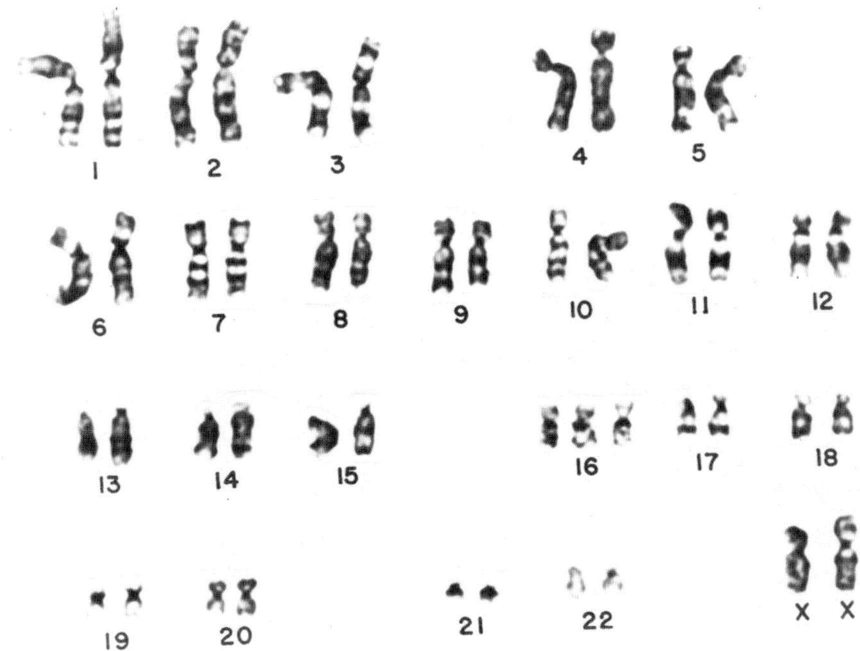

FIGURE 2-5.

D. should be 41%-50%
E. should be greater than 50%

9. A sonogram is obtained because the uterine fundus of a patient thought to be 24 weeks pregnant measures 21 cm. In addition to what appears to be cerebral ventriculomegaly, there is oligohydramnios, and a hydropic appearing placenta. This sonogram should suggest that the karyotype of the fetus is
   A. 45, X
   B. 47, XX, 21
   C. 47, XYY
   D. 45, X /46,XY
   E. 69, XXX
10. A couple, both of whom have neurofibromatosis, seek genetic counseling. You should tell this couple that
    A. 100% of the offsprings will either have the disease or be a carrier
    B. 75% of the offsprings will have the disease
    C. 50% of the offsprings will be homozygous for the gene
    D. 25% of the males will have the more severe form of the disease
    E. the abnormal gene is found on the Y chromosome
11. An Israeli couple seeks information about Tay-Sachs disease. A comment that you might make includes:
    A. it is an X-linked autosomal recessive condition
    B. it is most common in Jews of African descent
    C. a carrier can be detected by determining the concentration of serum hexosaminidase A
    D. death usually occurs in the fourth decade
    E. the best time to determine carrier state is during pregnancy
12. A true statement about the karyotype depicted in Figure 2-5 includes:
    A. it is associated with severe mental retardation
    B. it is usually but not always lethal
    C. it is the most common karyotype associated with a stillborn
    D. it is noted in about one third of trisomic abortus material
    E. affected individuals have a 50% chance of having a congenital heart defect
13. A 23 year-old gravida 3 para 0-0-3-0 is married to a 27 year-old gentleman who has never fathered a pregnancy that went to term. This couple seeks your advice. Before you recommend that each have a karyotype, you would explain that
    A. if either of them has a 21-21 translocation, it is incompatible with a normal gestation

B. recurrent abortions occur in one out of every 500 couples attempting pregnancy
C. each has an equal chance of having an abnormal karyotype
D. the percentage of men with chromosomal abnormalities in this group is 5%
E. the most frequent parental chromosomal abnormality seen in a group of patients who have had recurrent abortions is a sex chromosome trisomy

14. Identification of a fetus who carries the genes for cystic fibrosis can
    A. be accomplished by amniocentesis and determining the fetal karyotype
    B. be accomplished by chorionic villus sampling and using restriction endonucleases to isolate the gene sequence
    C. not be achieved at this time although there have been several preliminary reports that suggest this is theoretically possible
    D. be identified by determining the NaCl content of the amniotic fluid between 16 and 20 weeks of gestation
    E. be accomplished by performing a Southern Blot directly on material obtained from a chorionic villus biopsy

DIRECTIONS for questions 15 - 21: For each numbered item, select the one heading most closely associated with it. Each lettered heading may be used once, more than once, or not at all.

Questions 15-16.

(A) nondisjunctional event identified in abortus material
(B) nondisjunctional event not identified in living or abortus material
(C) Patau syndrome
(D) Edwards syndrome
(E) Down syndrome

15. Trisomy 13
16. Trisomy 17

17-18. **Partial Deletions of Chromosome**

(A) 4
(B) 5
(C) 18
(D) Short arm X
(E) Long arm X

17. Wolf syndrome
18. Cri-du-chat syndrome

19-21. Match the specific chromosomal abnormality with its frequency of occurrence in chromosomally abnormal abortus material.

(A) 50%
(B) 20%
(C) 15%
(D) 5%
(E) 1%

19. Turner's syndrome
20. Triploidy
21. Trisomy

DIRECTIONS For each numbered item 22 - 24, indicate whether it is associated with
A only (A)
B only (B)
C both (A) and (B)
D neither (A) nor (B)

(A) Meiosis
(B) Mitosis
(C) Both
(D) Neither

22. nondisjunction
23. 47, XYY
24. 46, XY/45, X

DIRECTIONS for questions 25 - 31: For each of the questions below, ONE or MORE of the responses is correct. Select the best answer based on the following
A if 1, 2, and 3 are correct
B if only 1 and 2 are correct
C if only 2 and 3 are correct
D if only 1 is correct
E if only 3 is correct

25. A 35-year-old primigravida had an amniocentesis 3 weeks ago. The karyotype is reproduced in Figure 2-6. A description of the phenotype should state that the
    1. sex is male
    2. adult is usually tall
    3. adult is severely mentally handicapped
26. A family is suspected of carrying an X-linked recessive abnormality. One female member exhibits the trait. If this were an X-linked recessive, the possible explanations are that this is
    1. a function of the Lyon hypothesis
    2. a female who is homozygous
    3. an example of complete penetrance
27. An 18-year-old paraplegic seeks genetic counseling during the 21st week of her pregnancy. She is the only member of her family who has this condition, which is due to a meningomyelocele repaired at birth. There is no history of a neural tube defect (NTD) on the husband's side of the family. You should advise this patient
    1. to take folate
    2. there is a 2% risk of recurrence
    3. to have an amniocentesis for determination of amniotic fluid alpha-fetoprotein
28. A woman who has had three spontaneous abortions is found to have the karyotype

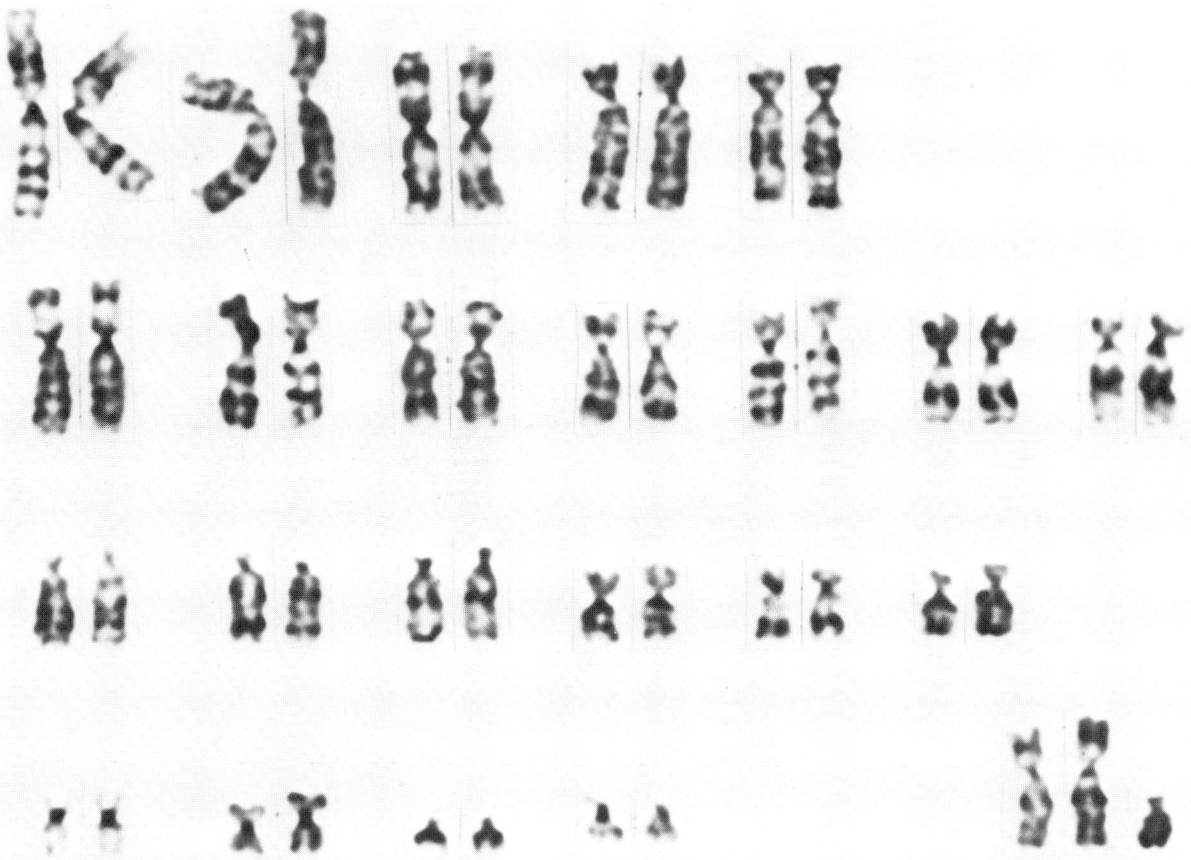

FIGURE 2-6.

shown in Figure 2-7. Rational options available to this couple include:
1. amniocentesis and selective abortion
2. ovum donation and embryo transplant
3. donor insemination

29. A chromosome break may result in
    1. a point mutation
    2. partial deletion
    3. a balanced translocation
30. When triploidy is associated with a partial mole, the
    1. likelihood of the subsequent development of a choriocarcinoma is increased over that seen after delivery of a complete mole
    2. fetal chromosomes are of paternal origin
    3. follow up should include monitoring of the β-Hcg
31. An oncogene may
    1. be the result of a point mutation
    2. alter normal cell-cell interactions controlling growth
    3. alter the cell's skeleton

ANSWERS

1. **A,** Pages 27, 40. Usually, if 50% of the protein produced by the gene pair is enough to give the usual phenotype, the condition is dominant. In this case, no generation is spared, the condition is equally represented between males and females, and all affected individuals have at least one affected parent. Male-to-male transmission rules out X-linked dominant inheritance.
2. **B,** Pages 28, 40. Since there is full penetrance, an autosomal dominant is unlikely. Both sexes are affected, making X-linked inheritance extremely unlikely. The parents are consanguineous and must be presumed carriers. Two of seven children are affected. With an autosomal recessive trait, one would expect 25% of the children to be affected on the basis of segregation.
3. **D,** Page 32. The karyotype is 47, XXX. Fifty percent of these women are fertile. While most of the offspring produced are

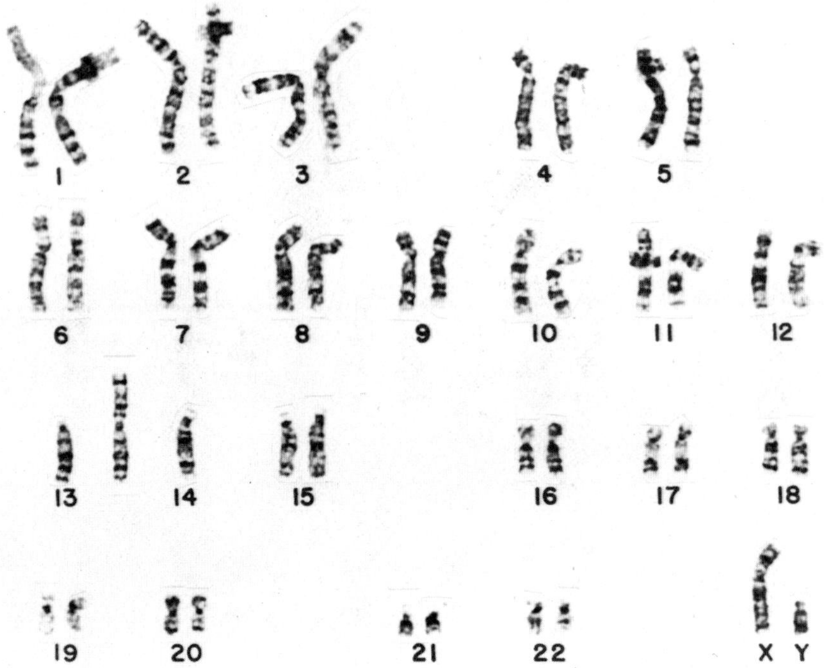

FIGURE 2-7.

normal, there is a slight increase of an offspring being produced with nondisjunctional events involving both the sex chromosomes and the autosomes.

4. **B,** Page 35. Of those abortuses with chromosome abnormalities, roughly 50% have autosomal trisomy. A trisomy of chromosome 16 has been noted in about one third of the cases, but since this has never been seen in living individuals, it must be considered universally lethal. In women who have produced a conception which is trisomic, the risk of a subsequent trisomic event is 1-2% being somewhat less for women under 35 and higher for women over 35.
5. **E,** Pages 23, 33, 34. In Robertsonian translocation (central fusion), two acrocentric chromosomes, such as 14 and 21, are involved. An isochromosome is the result of a transverse split rather than a longitudinal split of a metacentric chromosome during meiosis. The daughter chromosome has either two long or two short arms. With a reciprocal translocation, chromatin material is exchanged, but the chromosomal number does not change. When a chromosome breaks and turns on its axis, as is the case in this question, there is an inversion. In this example, the centromere was not involved, so the inversion is called paracentric. When the centromere is included, it is a pericentric inversion.
6. **C,** Pages 30, 33, 41. One would expect that 25% would be normal, 25% carriers, 25% unbalanced and affected, and 25% monosomic. If this involved the 21 chromosome, one would be dealing with Down syndrome. Since monosomy is lethal, the theoretical live-born risk is 33% normal, 33% carriers, and 33% Down syndrome.
7. **C,** Pages 30, 33, 41. The numbers in the above question, #6, do not turn out to be the case—the observed live-born risk of Down syndrome is 10%-15% if the mother has the translocation, and 1%-2% if the father is the carrier.
8. **E,** Pages 35, 41. It has been estimated that about 15% of ova penetrated by sperm fail to divide. Another 15% fail to implant, and 25% to 30% are aborted spontaneously at previllous stages. Of the roughly 40% of fertilized ova that survive the first missed menstrual period, as many as 25% are aborted spontaneously, so that only about 30% to 35% of all ova penetrated by sperm actually result in live-born infants. This information is being re-

fined as we gain more information with in vitro fertilization.

9. **E,** Pages 35-36, 38. Given these findings, one should predict that the karyotype is a polyploidy such as triploidy. The latter is associated with a partial hydatidiform mole. This patient should be followed as if she had a complete hydatidiform mole.
10. **B,** Pages 27-28. Each parent carries this autosomal dominant gene. It is highly unlikely that either is homozygous for the gene. The gene is not on the X or Y chromosome, but is on chromosome 17. The sex ratio for heterozygotes, therefore, is one male to one female. The gametes will be as pictured in Figure 2-8. Twenty-five percent will be normal (nn), 75% will be abnormal (NN or nN), 50% will have neurofibromatosis (nN), and 25% will be homozygous for this dominant gene and will have the lethal form (NN).
11. **C,** Page 28. Tay-Sachs disease is an autosomal recessive condition that is found most often in Jews of Eastern European origin. The carrier state can be detected by measuring serum hexosaminidase A. Death usually occurs by age 3 or 4. Although the carrier state can be determined during pregnancy, it is faster and cheaper to analyze blood for hexosaminidase A when the serum estrogens are at non pregnant levels.
12. **D,** Page 35. Figure 2-5 depicted a 47, XX +16 karyotype. A trisomy of chromosome 16 has been noted in about one third of trisomic abortus material. Since this has never been seen in living individuals, it must be considered universally lethal.
13. **A,** Pages 38, 40. The diagnosis of a chromosome abnormality in couples with chronic pregnancy wastage is important to rule out an abnormality incompatible with normal gestation, such as homologous translocations between identical members of the same group of chromosomes like 21-21. Roughly one in every 200 couples suffers from multiple abortions. Simpson discovered that the prevalence of chromosome abnormalities in women with chronic spontaneous abortion problems was about twice that of males (4.8% vs. 2.4%). It is important when counseling a couple to try to prevent either one from placing the blame on themselves or their partner. Although occasional sex chromosome abnormalities such as 47, XXX and 47, XYY, as well as a variety of mosaic representations, are seen among such couples, the majority demonstrate either balanced reciprocal translocations or Robertsonian fusion.
14. **B,** Pages 25, 27. Cystic fibrosis is the result of an abnormal gene, not a chromosomal abnormality. Identification of an affected individual or carrier may be accomplished by specifically identifying the mutant gene. The key to the localization of genetic information on the DNA molecule has been the discovery of a group of over 200 bacterial enzymes, restriction endonucleases, that recognize and cut specific nucleotide sequences in the double stranded DNA molecule. In the cases of cystic fibrosis, this has been achieved so that this determination should be offered to patients who are carriers. Although the "sweat test" was one of the first tests used to make the diagnosis in children, it could not be applied to amniotic fluid. There is usually not enough DNA from a chorionic villus biopsy to determine a nucleotide sequence by Southern Blot. Therefore, one has to use a cell culture or amplification of the DNA molecule (Polymerase chain reaction).

15-16. 15, **C;** 16, **B;** Pages 30, 41. Trisomy 13 and trisomy 15 are usually considered together. Trisomy 13 is known as Patau syndrome and is incompatible with extended life. Trisomy 18 is Edwards syndrome, also incompatible with extended life, while trisomy 21 is the more common and familiar Down syndrome. Nondisjunctional events resulting in a trisomy have been described in every autosome except 1 and 17.

17-18. 17, **A;** 18, **B;** Page 34. Wolf syndrome is due to the loss of a portion of the short arm of chromosome 4, and Cri-du-chat syndrome to the loss of the short arm of chromosome 5.

19-21. 19, **B;** 20, **C;** 21, **A;** Pages 34, 35, 41. Half of the abortuses with chromosomal abnor-

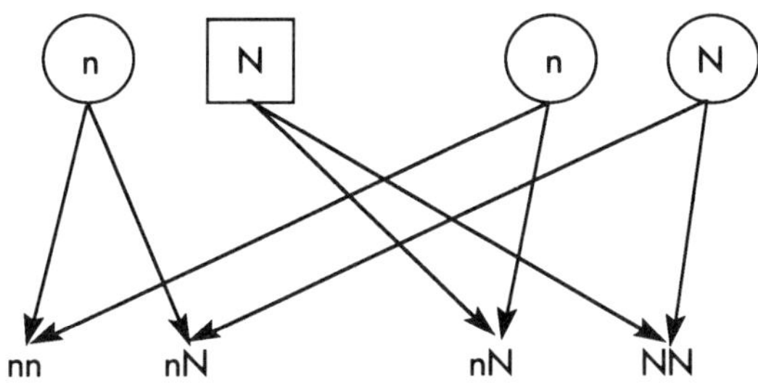

FIGURE 2-8.

malities have an autosomal trisomy; 20% have the karyotype 45,X; 14%-19% triploidy; 3%-6% tetraploidy; and chromosome rearrangements in 3%-4%.

22-24. 22, **C;** 23, **A;** 24, **B;** Pages 24, 30, 32. Nondisjunction is the faulty separation of chromosome pairs at anaphase in either meiosis or mitosis. Nondisjunction during spermatogenesis (meiosis) involving the Y chromosome can lead to the karyotype 47, XYY. Nondisjunctional events during mitosis in the early embryo will frequently produce individuals with cell populations containing different chromosome numbers.

25. **B** (1, 2), Page 32. The karyotype is that of 47, XXY, Klinefelter's syndrome. These men are characterized by tall stature and azoospermia. Although they may be mentally retarded, this is usually not severe. Gynecomastia is present in about one third of all cases.

26. **B** (1, 2), Pages 24, 28-29. Penetrance is the percentage of individuals in a population with the mutation who actually demonstrate the phenotypic change. In this case, the female either has the recessive gene on both chromosomes or the "normal" X is the one deactivated during "Lyonization." Usually the abnormal X is inactivated.

27. **C** (2, 3), Pages 29, 41. Although it has been suggested that neural tube defects might be prevented by administering folate supplements, these must be given preconceptually and during early gestation. The neural tube is formed by 4 weeks (postconception). This is a multifactorial disorder. The risk of recurrence in the United States is 11 times the population risk, which is approximately 2%. The sensitivity of amniotic fluid alpha-fetoprotein is better than maternal serum. Maternal serum alpha-fetoprotein is meant to be a screening test for a low risk population between 16 and 20 weeks of gestation. Amniocentesis is preferred for patients at risk, especially this late in pregnancy. Another possibility at 20 weeks in a similar clinical situation is an ultrasound evaluation, but this was not an option given in this question.

28. **B** (1, 2), Pages 37-38. The karyotype is of a Robertsonian fusion (translocation), 45, XY, t(13q14q). There is 33% theoretical chance that this woman would give birth to a trisomy 13 infant. The actual risk is listed as 10%. This is an abnormal maternal karyotype so that donor insemination will not help. Identifying an abnormal fetus and selective abortion or bypassing the abnormal mother are the only logical options listed.

29. **A** (1, 2, 3), Page 32. A chromosome break may simply heal, with or without a point mutation at the point of breakage. If a segment of the chromosome is lost during this healing process, partial deletion of chromatin material may take place. If two chromosomes break, they may exchange chromosome arms and give rise to a translocation.

30. **C** (2,3), Pages 38, 42. Choriocarcinoma has occurred after a partial mole, but it is much less likely than it is after a complete mole. Nevertheless, the patient should be followed as if she had a complete hydatidiform mole. This includes obtaining serial determinations of β-Hcg. See chapter 28 of Herbst, Mishell, Stenchever, and Drogemuller. In cases of triploidy where the nuclear material is of paternal origin, the placenta undergoes molar change.

31. **A** (1, 2, 3), Pages 24, 39, 42. Current theories suggest that perhaps the majority of human cancers arise from a genetic change in a single cell. Such genetic alterations may be of a variety of types but essentially involve either the somatic activation of cell oncogenes through point mutations, rearrangements or amplifications or the inactivation of tumor suppressor genes by point mutation or deletion in either germ or somatic cells. The tumor suppressor gene, may play a role in the pathogenesis of the cancer perhaps through the alteration of normal cell-cell interactions controlling growth. Oncogenes may also exert their effect through the alteration the cell's skeleton.

CHAPTER

3 Anatomy

DIRECTIONS for questions 1 - 15: Select the one best answer or completion.

1. On examination you find that a 40-year-old patient's uterus is anteflexed, firm, and approximately 9 cm long, 6 cm wide, and 4 cm thick, with an estimated weight of approximately 110 g. From this information *alone* you would be able to say that the patient was
   A. nulligravid
   B. multigravid
   C. 8 weeks pregnant
   D. afflicted with adenomyosis
   E. none of the above
2. A 63-year-old asymptomatic woman is found to have a 3 x 2 x 3 cm left adnexal mass that feels cystic. The most likely etiology is
   A. enlarged follicle cyst
   B. paraovarian cyst
   C. corpus luteum cyst
   D. hydrosalpinx
   E. ovarian neoplasm
3. At term, the pregnant uterus will increase in weight over the normal non-pregnant uterine weight approximately
   A. 2-3 times
   B. 4-5 times
   C. 10-20 times
   D. 30-50 times
   E. 100 times
4. A 24-year-old patient is seen for a routine exam and a 2 cm asymptomatic cystic structure is found submucosally at the junction of the lower and middle third of the vagina at approximately 10 o'clock. The most likely etiology is
   A. vaginal inclusion cyst
   B. clear cell adenocarcinoma
   C. Gartner's duct cyst
   D. Skene's duct cyst
   E. Bartholin's duct cyst
5. After a radical hysterectomy a patient complains of numbness over the medial aspect of her thigh. No muscle weakness is noted. This is most likely due to
   A. transection of the obturator nerve
   B. nonpermanent injury to the obturator nerve
   C. transection of the femoral nerve
   D. nonpermanent injury to the femoral nerve
   E. nonpermanent injury to the pudendal nerve
6. The correct sequence of the arterial blood supply to the uterus begins with the aorta and continues through the
   A. internal iliac, common iliac, uterine
   B. common iliac, hypogastric, uterine
   C. external iliac, internal iliac, uterine
   D. obturator, hypogastric, uterine
   E. common iliac, pudendal, uterine
7. A patient is most apt to have a trachelectomy performed if she
   A. is of Greek heritage
   B. has had a prior subtotal hysterectomy
   C. has a benign ovarian tumor
   D. has an unusual retroperitoneal pelvic mass
   E. has repeated episodes of dysfunctional uterine bleeding, unresponsive to D&C
8. A woman who has endometrial cancer can have metastases to the inguinal nodes, transported via which lymphatic chain?
   A. para aortic
   B. obturator
   C. round ligament
   D. lumbar
   E. iliac
9. A woman who has a vasovagal response during dilation of the cervix for a suction D & C done in the office is responding to stimulation of which of the following nerves?
   A. pudendal
   B. obturator
   C. sciatic
   D. femoral
   E. Frankenhauser's (paracervical) ganglion
10. The fallopian tube is anatomically divided into four segments. The longest segment is the

A. interstitial
B. isthmic
C. ampullary
D. infundibular

11. The major blood supply to each ovary arises from the
   A. common iliac artery
   B. internal iliac artery (hypogastric)
   C. obturator artery
   D. external iliac artery
   E. aorta.
12. A woman complains of sudden onset of pain beneath the umbilicus, which then moves to the right lower quadrant. She denies nausea, vomiting, or fever. Her last menstrual period was 7 weeks ago, and she has been sexually active without contraception. Assuming she has a right tubal pregnancy, how do you account for the initial subumbilical pain?
   A. the tube was located anatomically in the midline
   B. tubal pain is transmitted via L2, 3, 4
   C. tubal pain is transmitted via S2, 3, 4
   D. tubal pain is transmitted via T11-12
   E. tubal pain is transmitted via T 8-10
13. Cystocele and rectocele occur because of weakness of the
   A. uterosacral ligaments
   B. anal sphincter
   C. endopelvic fascia
   D. cardinal ligaments
   E. ischiocavernosus muscle
14. Urethral diverticula arise from
   A. mesonephric duct remnants
   B. an infection of the periurethral glands
   C. urethroceles
   D. straddle injury trauma to the urethra
   E. repetitive increase of intra-abdominal pressure
15. The inferior epigastric artery is a direct branch of the
   A. pudendal
   B. internal iliac
   C. external iliac
   D. inferior mesenteric
   E. internal mammary

DIRECTIONS for questions 16 - 30: For each numbered item, select the one heading most closely associated with it. Each lettered heading may be used once, more than once, or not at all.

16-18. Match the female genital structure with the homologous male structure.
   (A) prostate
   (B) penis
   (C) scrotum
   (D) penile urethra
   (E) cowper's gland

16. Labia majora
17. Skene's glands
18. Labia minora

19-21. Match the following with the labeled portions in Figure 3-1

19. zona basalis
20. myometrium
21. endometrium

22-24. Match the following structures with the labeled portions of Figure 3-2.

22. ovarian ligament
23. cervical portio
24. fimbria ovarica

25-27. Match the anastomotic connection with the following pelvic vessels.
   (A) superior gluteal artery
   (B) uterine artery
   (C) middle hemorrhoidal artery
   (D) inferior vesical artery
   (E) obturator artery

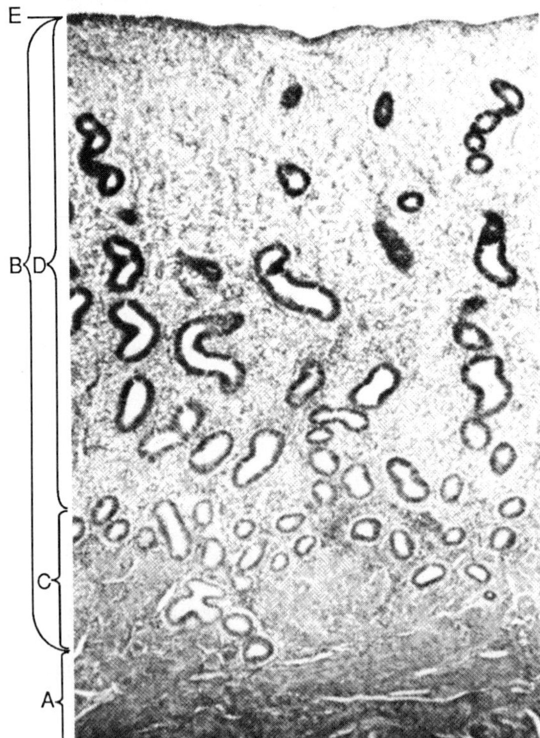

FIGURE 3-1.
A histologic view of the endometrium during the proliferative phase, demonstrating the strata in the endometrium.

(From Demopoulos RI: Normal endometrium. In Blaustein A, ed. Pathology of the female genital tract, 2nd ed., New York, Springer-Verlag, 1982, p. 216.)

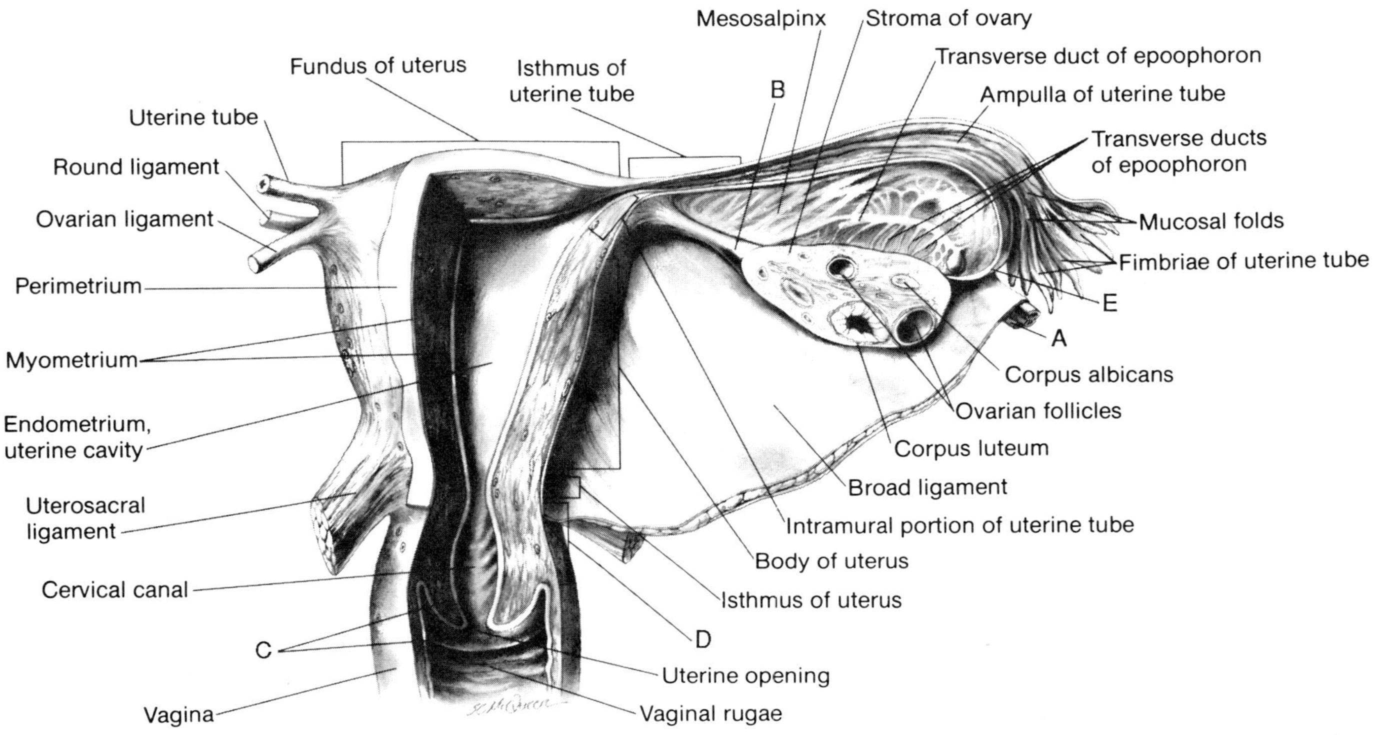

FIGURE 3-2.
A schematic drawing of a posterior view of the cervix, uterus, fallopian tube, and ovary.
(Redrawn from Clemente CD: Anatomy: A regional atlas of the human body, 3rd ed., Baltimore-Munich, Urban & Schwarzenberg, 1987)

25. Inferior mesenteric artery
26. Deep iliac circumflex artery
27. Medial femoral circumflex artery

28-30. Match the nodes with the labeled areas in Figure 3-3.

28. Internal iliac
29. Common iliac
30. Aortic

DIRECTIONS for questions 31 - 37: For each of the questions below, ONE or MORE of the responses is correct. Select the best answer based on the following

A if 1, 2, and 3 are correct
B if only 1 and 2 are correct
C if only 2 and 3 are correct
D if only 1 is correct
E if only 3 is correct

31. True statements about the normal cervix include:
    1. the cervical stroma is 60% connective tissue and 40% smooth muscle
    2. the endocervical lining is made up of many glands imbedded in the cervical stroma
    3. sperm may be stored in the lining folds of the endocervix for at least 48 hours
32. When a woman coughs or strains, the pelvic diaphragm prevents the abdominal contents from being extruded through the

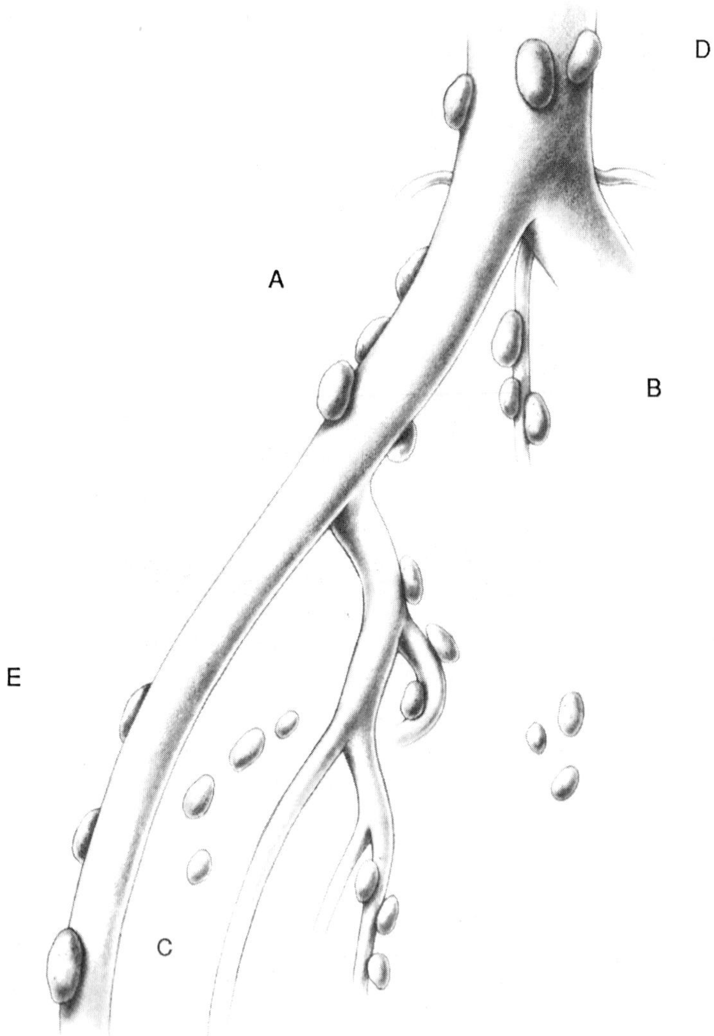

FIGURE 3-3.
Schematic view of the pelvic lymph nodes.
(From Plentl AA, Friedman EA: Lymphatic system of the female genitalia. Philadelphia, W.B. Saunders Co., 1971, p. 13.)

pelvic cavity. This pelvic diaphragm is made up of which muscles?
1. coccygeus
2. levator ani
3. deep transverse perineal

33. Patients with carcinoma of the cervix are likely to have metastases to the lymph nodes draining the cervix. These nodes include
    1. internal iliac
    2. visceral nodes of the parametria
    3. external iliac
34. After ligating the uterine arteries and removing the uterus from the abdominal cavity, the vaginal cuff was noted to bleed. Possible sources of this bleeding are
    1. pudendal artery
    2. inferior vesical artery
    3. middle hemorrhoidal artery
35. Following a rapid delivery, a large cervical tear is found to be bleeding. The vessels supplying blood to this site are
    1. descending branch of the uterine artery
    2. pudendal artery
    3. middle hemorrhoidal artery
36. Sympathetic nerve fibers to the pelvis
    1. are part of the autonomic nervous system
    2. generally cause vasoconstriction and muscle contraction
    3. originate from the cranial and sacral nerve roots
37. A woman has a uterus measuring 6 cm in length, 3 cm in width, and 1.5 cm in thickness, with a weight of 30 g. This is consistent with
    1. menopause
    2. amenorrhea
    3. adenomyosis

ANSWERS

1. **E,** Page 52. Although the size, shape, and consistency suggest a multigravid uterus, any of the listed possibilities could be true because of the great individual variation in anatomic size and configuration. It would not be possible to state that any one of the given reasons, or some other entity such as leiomyoma or a tumor was the reason for the upper limits of normal size and weight of this uterus.
2. **E,** Page 58. The size of the cystic structure would be normal in a menstruating female, but in a postmenopausal woman it is clearly abnormal, as no follicle or corpus luteum cysts should be present. Although the mass could be either a paraovarian cyst or a hydrosalpinx, these entities are very rare in postmenopausal women. Therefore, an ovarian neoplasm is the most likely finding. A malignant neoplasm is a definite concern. This finding in a postmenopausal patient usually warrants laparotomy after pre op evaluation.
3. **C,** Page 52. The normal non-pregnant uterus weighs 40-100 g. At term pregnancy, the uterus weighs 800-1000 g, which is a 10-20 fold increase. This increase is due to both hypertrophy and hyperplasia of muscle fibers, as well as an increase in decidua and the blood volume contained within the uterus. Postpartum, the uterus decreases in both size and weight, so that by 6-10 weeks postpartum it is back to a normal prepregnancy weight, though usually slightly larger than a nulligravid uterus.
4. **C,** Page 49. The anterior lateral position, size, lack of symptoms, and age of the patient make the most likely diagnosis a Gartner's duct cyst. Skene's ducts and glands are more anterior and distal in the vagina. Bartholin's gland is distal and posterior. Inclusion cysts generally are found in areas of prior trauma, such as childbirth tears or episiotomy. The patient's age and description of the cyst make clear cell adenocarcinoma unlikely. A Gartner's duct cyst is a dilation of a remnant of the embryonic mesonephros.
5. **B,** Page 67. The obturator nerve is motor to the adductor muscles of the thigh and sensory to the medial thigh. If it had been transected, motor weakness of the adductors would be present. Pressure injury, which involves the sensory fibers only or causes mild muscle weakness, will usually disappear in a few days or weeks. The femoral nerve is motor to the extensors of the leg and to the skin of the anterior thigh. The pudendal nerve is sensory to the perineum.
6. **B,** Pages 54, 59. The blood flows from the aorta to the common iliac to the hypogastric. The hypogastric (or internal iliac) has several branches that should be known by pelvic surgeons. They are superior gluteal, inferior gluteal, lateral sacral, uterine, internal pudendal, middle vesical, inferior vesical, iliolumbar, middle hemorrhoidal, and vaginal. The obturator and superior vesical arteries may also arise from the hypogastric artery. The hypogastric artery ends as the obliterated umbilical artery. Arterial blood that supplies the

uterus does not flow directly through the external iliac, obturator, or pudendal artery.

7. **B,** Page 49. The Greek word for neck is trachelos. The word cervix originates from the Latin word for neck. Therefore, the surgical removal of the cervix is called trachelectomy which is most apt to be performed in a woman whose cervix was left behind during a prior subtotal hysterectomy. Subtotal hysterectomies are done infrequently now and only if severe patient problems mandate rapid completion of surgery or if massive adhesions or other conditions prevent total removal of the uterus. These situations are very rare. Removal of a normal residual cervix is unnecessary.
8. **C,** Page 54. The inguinal nodes are not commonly involved with endometrial cancer, but the potential is present via the round ligament lymphatics. More commonly, the mode of spread is laterally through the lymphatics surrounding the iliac vessels and extending into the para aortic chain. Direct extension can also occur if the tumor penetrates the myometrium.
9. **E,** Pages 65-66. The nerve supply to the cervix is via a plexus of nerves in the uterosacral ligaments, known as the paracervical or Frankenhauser's ganglion. These then innervate the endocervix. The efferent pathway from Frankenhauser's ganglion is to the hypogastric plexus and enters the spinal cord at T11-12. The vasovagal response of bradycardia with nausea, sweating, and sometimes syncope is occasionally seen with cervical or intrauterine manipulation, as parasympathetic fibers run together with the sympathetics.
10. **C,** Pages 54-55. The whole fallopian tube is approximately 10-14 cm long. The ampullary portion is 4-6 cm long and is the segment where fertilization usually occurs. It has prominent folds, or plicae, which if disrupted by infection, inflammation, or trauma can result in blind pouches that can trap a fertilized ovum, leading to a tubal pregnancy. The other segments are shorter and have the following lengths: interstitial 1-2 cm, isthmic, 2-4 cm, infundibular, 1-2 cm.
11. **E,** Page 57. The major blood supply of each ovary arises from the aorta. In embryonic development, the gonads migrate caudally from their origin, bringing their blood supply, lymphatics, and nerves along with them. The right ovarian vein enters the inferior vena cava and the left ovarian vein enters the left renal vein. The lymphatics course cephalad in the infundibulopelvic chain and join the para aortic nodes at the level of the renal pedicle. Approximately 20% of early ovarian cancer will have microscopic spread to the para aortic nodes.
12. **D,** Pages 56, 66. Pain fibers in the tube are stimulated by tubal distention with referred pain in the dermatomes supplied by the T11-12 cord segment as the tube developed as a midabdominal structure. Therefore, initial midabdominal pain can be appreciated when tubal distention is occurring. When inflammation or rupture occurs, there is irritation of the overlying peritoneum and localization of the pain to the right lower quadrant. The same sequence may occur with appendicitis.
13. **C,** Page 70. Vaginal support is mainly from the endopelvic fascia surrounding it. The ischiocavernosus muscle is lateral and not involved in vaginal wall support. The ligaments support the uterus and apex of the vagina, but not the anterior and posterior walls.
14. **B,** Pages 46, 613. Chronic infection of the periurethral glands is felt to be the cause of urethral diverticula. The symptoms may be similar to a lower UTI, e.g. frequency, urgency, and dyspareunia. It may cause a small amount of urine leakage after voiding as the diverticulum empties as the subject stands.
15. **C,** Page 61, Table 3-1. The inferior epigastric is a branch of the exterior iliac. It runs in the rectus muscle and may be lacerated at the time of amniocentesis or insertion of a trocar during laparoscopy. Such a laceration can cause a rectus muscle hematoma.

16-18. 16, **C;** 17, **A;** 18, **D;** Pages 44-45, 74. The homologous anatomic structures in the male are the scrotum, prostate, and the penile urethra for the labia majora, Skene's glands, and labia minora, respectively. Embryologic development of genital structures is influenced by the presence of testosterone. The earlier excess androgen is present in embryonic development, the more likely it is that the configuration of the female genitalia will resemble the genitalia of a male. Knowledge of the homologous structures serves to remind us of this truism.

19-21. 19, **C;** 20, **A;** 21, **B;** Pages 52-53. The zona basalis, myometrium, and endometrium are as shown in Figure 3-1. The endometrium does not have a basement membrane separating it from the myometrium. Rather, the basal endometrium inserts itself in the interstices between the muscle fibers of the myometrium. This results in the gritty sensation and sound when curettage is performed. The visceral peritoneum envelops the uterus, so that the uterus is, in fact, a retroperitoneal structure. The endometrium varies during the menstrual cycle from 1 to 6 mm in thickness, with most of the change occurring in the zona functionalis.

22-24. 22, **B**; 23, **C**; 24, **E**; Figure 3-5 (from Herbst). Page 56. The ovary is suspended by three ligaments: the infundibulopelvic ligament, which attaches the ovary to the pelvic side wall and contains the ovarian arteries, nerves and lymphatics; the ovarian ligament, which attaches the ovary to the uterus; and the mesovarium, which is part of the broad ligament and contains anastomotic branches from the uterine artery. The cervical portio is that part of the cervix that extends freely into the vaginal canal and is covered by squamous epithelium. It may have varying amounts of columnar epithelium extending onto its surface. The fimbria ovarica is the long tubal fimbria that attaches the infundibulum of the fallopian tube to the ovary.

25-27. 25, **C**; 26, **A**; 27, **E**; Table 3-1 (from Herbst). Pages 59, 61. The high number of anastomoses in the pelvis allows many blood vessels to be sacrificed without ischemic compromise of the pelvic organs, particularly in younger women. For example, the inferior mesenteric artery can be ligated near the aorta without causing anoxic damage to the bowel, as anastomoses through the middle and inferior hemorrhoidal arteries maintain the blood supply. The deep iliac circumflex artery anastomoses with the superior gluteal and iliolumbar artey of the hypogastric and the medial femoral circumflex artery anastomoses with the inferior hemorrhoidal artery and the inferior gluteal artery of the hypogastric. Venous return has an even greater number of anastomotic channels.

28-30. 28, **C**; 29, **A**; 30, **D**; Figure 3-15 (from Herbst) and Pages 61-65. The lymphatics of the pelvis are important because metastatic spread of pelvic malignancies occur along their path. Therefore, they must be sampled in cases of pelvic malignancy to determine optimum treatment. The internal iliac nodes are found in the anatomic triangle made up of the external iliac artery, hypogastric artery, and pelvic sidewall. Deep femoral nodes are located in the femoral sheath and feed into the iliac and internal iliac chains. Common iliac nodes are located adjacent to the common iliac artery. Aortic nodes are adjacent to the aorta and require meticulous technique for safe sampling. Parauterine nodes are found immediately lateral to the uterus and are removed during radical hysterectomy.

31. **E** (3), Page 51. The cervical stroma is 15% smooth muscle and 85% connective tissue. The epithelium has only two cell types, secretory and ciliated. The epithelium is arranged in folds and crypts which are not true glands, although the crypts are frequently referred to as such. Sperm storage in the mucus-filled crypts is a well-known phenomenon. Near midcycle, the sperm may persist in these crypts for several days.

32. **B** (1, 2), Page 67. The pelvic diaphragm is made up of the coccygeus and levator ani muscles. The levator ani is divided into three parts: the pubococcygeus, the puborectalis, and iliococcygeus. The deep transverse perineal muscle with its fascia make up the urogenital diaphragm, and the psoas and iliacus both lie cephalad and lateral to the true pelvis. The pelvic diaphragm resembles a derby hat placed upside down in the bony pelvic cavity.

33. **A**, (All), Page 52. All of the listed nodes are part of the lymphatic drainage of the cervix. The obturator nodes also drain the cervix. The visceral nodes of the parametria should be removed during radical hysterectomy. If lymphadenectomy is performed, the obturator, external and internal iliac nodes are also removed as curative surgery for carcinoma of the cervix. Other possible drainage channels include nodes in the common iliacs, superior and inferior gluteal, sacral, rectal, lumbar, and aortic chains, as well as nodes on the posterior surface of the bladder.

34. **A**, (All), Page 48. Though the vaginal artery generally descends from the uterine artery, bleeding may still occur after the uterine artery has been ligated because of the highly developed collateral circulation. Collateral branches include the pudendal, middle hemorrhoidal, and inferior vesical arteries. The best method of

achieving hemostasis is to suture the vaginal cuff.

35. **A,** (All), Pages 51, 52. The descending branches of the uterine artery form the cervical artery. The pudendal artery feeds the vaginal artery, which anastomoses with the cervical artery. Middle hemorrhoidal arteries also anastomose with branches of the cervical artery.
36. **B** (1, 2), Pages 64, 65. The sympathetic and parasympathetic nerves make up the autonomic system. The parasympathetics originate in the cranial and sacral segments of the CNS and have ganglia near the visceral organs they serve. They generally cause vasodilation and muscle relaxation. The sympathetic fibers originate from the thoracic and lumbar portions of the spinal cord and cause constriction of the vessels and muscle contraction. Both enter the pelvis through rather ill-defined plexuses, namely the superior hypogastric.
37. **B** (1, 2), Pages 52, 58. A small uterus is consistent with the state of menopause or other causes of ovarian failure such as persistent hypothalamic amenorrhea. You would expect that such a woman would be amenorrheic. Adenomyosis generally increases the uterine size. The uterus of a normal menstruating woman would be larger in all dimensions and weigh approximately 50-80 g. The upper limits of normal size is approximately 110 g.

CHAPTER 4 Reproductive Endocrinology

DIRECTIONS for questions 1 - 20: Select the one best answer or completion.

1. Tanycytes are cells in the third ventricle thought to be important in the transfer of
   A. GnRH
   B. thyroxin
   C. cortisone
   D. FSH
   E. estrogens
2. The highest concentration of β-endorphin is found in the
   A. arcuate nucleus
   B. median eminence
   C. pituitary
   D. serum
   E. ovary
3. The reason gonadotrophin releasing hormone analogs can be used to inhibit FSH and LH is that
   A. the unoccupied receptors become refractory to binding
   B. the receptors are all bound and therefore can no longer respond
   C. a change in the ratio of the bound to the unbound receptors is needed to stimulate FSH and LH
   D. the analogs are not similar enough to GnRH and therefore do not cause stimulation
   E. the analogs do not bind the receptors but shield them from being bound by GnRH
4. Delta 5 (Δ^5) steroid compounds have
   A. a double bond between carbon atoms 5 and 6
   B. a double bond between carbon atoms 4 and 5
   C. five carbon atoms in the A ring
   D. five carbon atoms in the B ring
   E. a fifth benzene ring
5. Ovaries are unable to synthesize mineralocorticoids because they lack
   A. 3-beta-ol-dehydrogenase
   B. 17-hydroxylase
   C. 21-hydroxylase
   D. 11-hydroxylase
   E. 19-hydroxylase
6. The sex steroid present in the plasma in the greatest concentration during any part of the menstrual cycle is
   A. androstenedione
   B. testosterone
   C. estrone sulfate
   D. estradiol
   E. progesterone
7. FSH has the same beta subunit as
   A. LH
   B. ACTH
   C. TSH
   D. HCG
   E. none of the above
8. The hormone with the greatest affinity for steroid hormone binding globulin (SHBG) is
   A. progesterone
   B. estrogen
   C. testosterone
   D. dehydroepiandrosterone
   E. cortisol
9. If the preovulatory plasma concentration of estradiol is 250 picograms per ml and the metabolic clearance rate is 1350 liters per day, the daily production rate of estradiol is
   A. 0.19 mg
   B. 0.338 mg
   C. 5.4 mg
   D. 0.338 g
   E. 5.4 g
10. Compared to a female of normal weight, a grossly obese woman will have increased conversion of
    A. estradiol to estriol
    B. testosterone to progesterone
    C. progesterone to testosterone
    D. estradiol to androstenedione
    E. androstenedione to estrone
11. The reason that the concentration of protein hormones in the blood is expressed in international units or milli-international units per ml, rather than mg per dl is
    A. protein hormones metabolize so rapidly they cannot be measured by weight
    B. protein hormones are a combination of

different molecules that constantly change
C. protein hormones are hard to isolate in a pure form
D. protein hormones exist in such small amounts that milligram weights would be meaningless
E. the measurement of protein hormones was developed by arbitrary convention, which is difficult to change

12. Thromboxane differs from prostacyclin in that it
A. causes vasoconstriction
B. causes platelet aggregation
C. is **not** formed from arachidonic acid
D. is **not** an eicosanoid
E. has 20 carbons

13. The structure of the ovum that prevents its fertilization by sperm of another species is the
A. granulosa
B. theca interna
C. zona pellucida
D. vitelline membrane
E. theca externa

14. There is a direct correlation between the increase of serum estrogen during an ovulatory cycle and the
A. thickness of the theca externa
B. size of the dominant follicle
C. number of hilar cells in the ovary
D. number of follicles in the ovary
E. thickness of the ovarian cortex

15. An ovulatory sequence is characterized by the following order of steps, starting with increased FSH secretion:
A. follicular growth
increased estradiol production
the LH surge
ovulation
increased estradiol and progesterone production
B. increased estradiol and estrogen production
follicular growth
increased progesterone production
the LH surge
ovulation
C. follicular growth
increased progesterone production
the LH surge
ovulation
increased estradiol production
D. increased progesterone production
follicular growth
the LH surge
increased estradiol production
ovulation
E. the LH surge
follicular growth
increased estradiol production
increased progesterone production
ovulation

16. In serum obtained from a peripheral vessel the pulsatile nature of the secretion of LH is apparent, while the concentration of FSH is much less variable because
A. GnRH does not affect FSH secretion
B. FSH is not secreted in response to GnRH pulses, but only in response to the steady state of GnRH
C. FSH has a longer half-life than LH
D. inhibin decreases the amount of FSH secreted by the pulsatile GnRH
E. estrogen interferes with the measurement of FSH in immunoassays

17. The sensitivity of a laboratory test refers to
A. the ability to measure only one substance
B. the least amount of substance that can be measured
C. the ability to measure the exact amount
D. the variation between intraassays and interassays
E. none of the above

18. The sequence of events leading to menstruation is
A. Coiling of arteries
Vasoconstriction
Decrease in endometrial thickness
Vasodilation
Menses
B. Coiling of the arteries
Vasodilation
Vasoconstriction
Decreased endometrial thickness
Menses
C. Decrease in endometrial thickness
Coiling of arteries
Vasoconstriction
Vasodilation
Menses
D. Vasoconstriction
Coiling of the arteries
Decrease in endometrial thickness
Vasodilation
Menses
E. Vasoconstriction
Decrease in endometrial thickness
Coiling of arteries
Vasodilation
Menses

19. Ovulation in the human usually occurs
A. at the same time as the LH peak

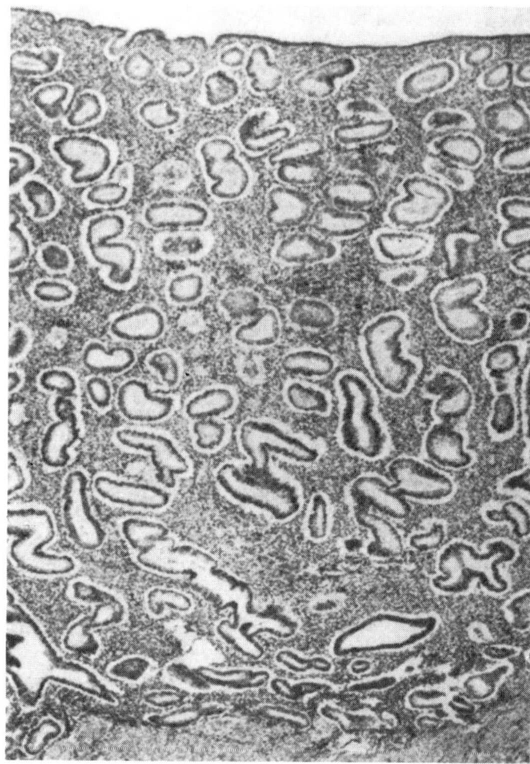

FIGURE 4-1.

(From Novak E, Novak ER, eds: Textbook of gynecology, 4th ed. Baltimore, Williams & Wilkins, 1952.)

B. within 24 hours before the LH peak
C. within 24 hours after the LH peak
D. at the same time as the estradiol peak
E. at the same time as the progesterone peak

20. The primary target of FSH activity is the
    A. adenohypophysis
    B. neurohypophysis
    C. ovarian theca
    D. ovarian hilum
    E. ovarian granulosa

DIRECTIONS for questions 21 - 29: For each numbered item, select the one heading most closely associated with it. Each lettered heading may be used once, more than once, or not at all.

21-23. Match the endometrium with the correct time of the cycle

(A) menstrual
(B) early follicular
(C) late follicular
(D) early luteal
(E) midluteal

21. Figure 4-1.
22. Figure 4-2.
23. Figure 4-3.

24-26. Match the times of the cycle with the appropriate serum level of hormone

(A) early follicular phase
(B) late follicular phase

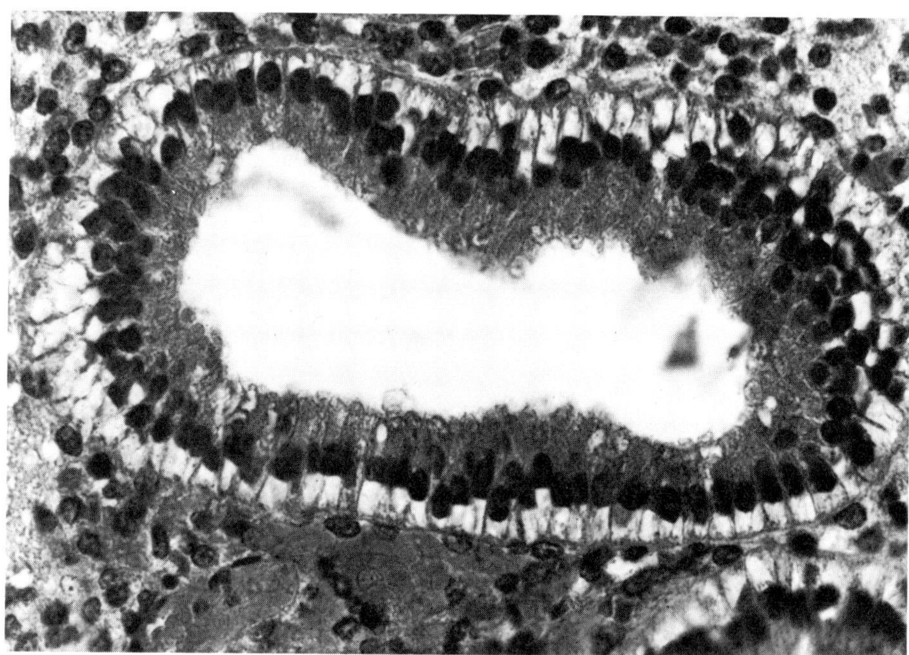

FIGURE 4-2.

(From March CM: The endometrium in the menstrual cycle. Reproduced with permission from Infertility, Contraception and Reproductive Endocrinology, 2nd ed., edited by Daniel R. Mishell, Jr., M.D., and Val Davajan, M.D. Copyright 1986 Medical Economics Books, Oradell, N.J. 07649.

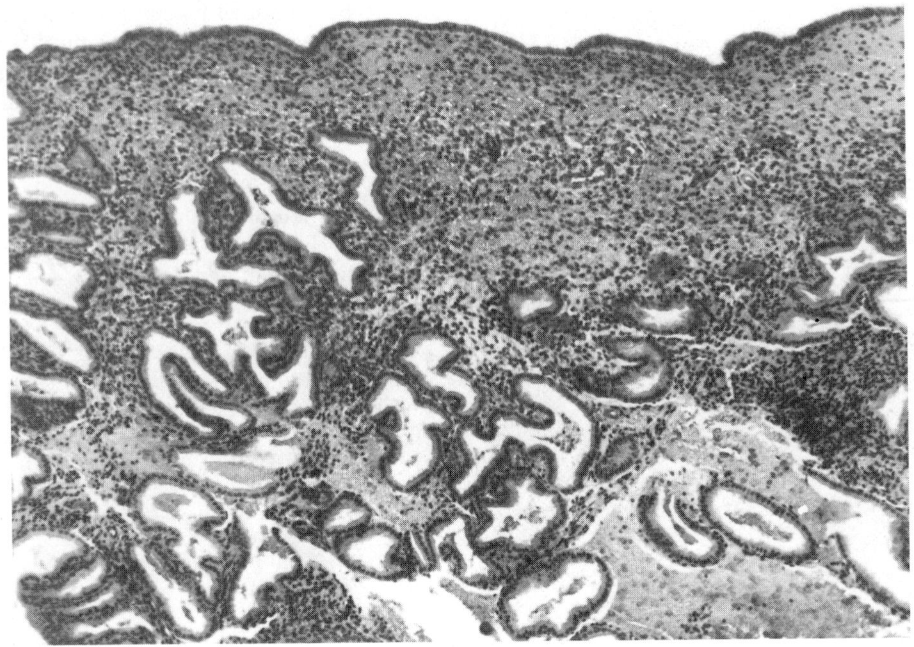

FIGURE 4-3.

(From March CM: The endometrium in the menstrual cycle. Reproduced with permission from Infertility, Contraception and Reproductive Endocrinology, 2nd ed., edited by Daniel R. Mishell, Jr., M.D., and Val Davajan, M.D. Copyright 1986 Medical Economics Books, Oradell, N.J. 07649. All rights reserved.)

(C) ovulation
(D) midluteal phase
(E) late luteal phase

24. Estrogen 100-150 picograms/ml, Progesterone 10-15 nanograms/ml
25. Estrogen >200 picograms/ml, Progesterone 1-2 nanograms/ml
26. Estrogen <50 picograms/ml, Progesterone <1 nanogram/ml

27-29. Match the listed substance with its action
(A) estrogen
(B) progestin
(C) glucocorticoids
(D) antiestrogens
(E) GnRH

27. inhibits synthesis of estrogen receptors
28. increases synthesis of estradiol dehydrogenase
29. binds estrogen receptors but initiates little transcription

DIRECTIONS for questions 30 - 35: For each of the questions below, ONE or MORE of the responses is correct. Select the best answer based on the following
A if 1, 2, and 3 are correct
B if only 1 and 2 are correct
C if only 2 and 3 are correct
D if only 1 is correct
E if only 3 is correct

30. Steroid hormone receptors
    1. are intracellular rather than on cell membranes
    2. enter the cell nucleus after binding with the steroid
    3. help determine a steroid's potency by their affinity for that steroid
31. The amplitude and frequency of GnRH secretion is known to be modulated by ovarian steroids and
    1. gonadotrophins
    2. catecholamines
    3. serotonin
32. Anovulation in a patient may be explained by
    1. an altered pulse frequency of GnRH
    2. a decreased concentration of dopamine in the central nervous system
    3. an increased secretion of GnRH
33. Progestins decrease the effect of estrogens by
    1. binding to the estrogen receptors
    2. inhibiting synthesis of estrogen receptors
    3. increasing synthesis of estrogen dehydrogenase
34. During menstruation,
    1. the entire functional layer of endometrium is shed

2. enzymes destroy part of the myometrial matrix supporting the endometrium
3. endometrial regeneration is already beginning

35. A 48-year-old woman asks you what her menstrual cycle will be like near menopause. You can accurately inform her that
    1. the mean age of menopause is approximately 51 years
    2. periods are apt to be irregular starting 3 years before actual cessation of flow
    3. the time between periods normally increases near menopause

ANSWERS

1. **A,** Pages 82-83. Tanycytes line the third ventricle and have microvilli which are postulated to absorb GnRH continuously and transport it into the portal system, thereby providing an alternative method for GnRH to reach the pituitary in contrast to the usual portal system transport.
2. **C,** Pages 87, 89. The reason for the high concentration of β-endorphins in the pituitary is unknown. The infusion of β-endorphins decreases LH by causing an inhibitory effect on GnRH neurons in the hypothalamus. This action is thought to contribute to anovulation in athletes who have high levels of β-endorphins.
3. **A,** Pages 89-90. GnRH analogs function in a fashion similar to native GnRH; that is, they bind some of the target cell membrane receptors and stimulate them maximally. The unoccupied receptors become refractory to further binding and the occupied ones are saturated and are not able to sustain the release of the second messenger, cyclic AMP, which maintains the activation of protein kinase. Protein kinase is needed to supply energy for the protein substrate that produces FSH and LH. The decreased FSH and LH results in anovulation.
4. **A,** Page 102; Figure 4-15 (from Herbst). Delta stands for a double bond between carbon atoms in the steroid molecule. When steroids are synthesized by the ovary, adrenal, or placenta, they follow specific pathways. Those with a double bond between carbon atoms 5 and 6 are called Δ^5 steroids. They have not yet been acted upon by the enzyme 4-5 isomerase, which changes the position of the double bond. This step is necessary to produce progesterone from pregnenolone and androsterone from dehydroepiandrosterone.
5. **C,** Page 103; Figure 4-16 (from Herbst). 21-hydroxylase is needed to hydroxylate carbon 21. This must be done before the steroids have a significant mineralocorticoid effect. 11-hydroxylase is needed to confer the glucocorticoid effect by hydroxylation of the carbon in position 11.
6. **E,** Table 4-4 (from Herbst). Estrogens are present in picogram levels. The concentration of estrone sulfate is greater than estradiol or estrone. However, it is conjugated and less potent than estradiol. Both androgens and progesterone are present in nanogram amounts. Although graphs often depict a higher curve for estrogen than for progesterone, the scales are different. Progesterone is present at levels of 4-19 ng/ml during the luteal phase. More important than concentration is the biological potency of a compound.
7. **E,** Pages 93-94. FSH, LH, TSH, and HCG have the same alpha subunit but different beta subunits. While also a pituitary hormone, ACTH has a different structure. Sensitive radioimmunoassay techniques utilize the beta subunit to identify the specific compound.
8. **D,** Page 103. Dehydroepiandrosterone, testosterone, and estrogen are bound to SHBG in order of decreasing affinity. Cortisone and progesterone are bound to cortisone binding globulin. Steroids are also bound to albumin and approximately 5% of steroids circulate as free hormone. SHBG is increased by estrogen, obesity, and increased T_4. It is decreased by androgens and hypothyroidism. Therefore, thyroid dysfunction may change the concentration of SHBG and may cause changes in the amount of free estrogen, which in turn may cause abnormal uterine bleeding.
9. **B,** Page 105. The production rate equals the metabolic clearance rate times the concentration; therefore, 1350 liters per day times 250 picograms per ml times 1000 ml per liter equals 337,500,000 picograms per day, or approximately 0.338 mg per day. Preovulatory estrogen levels are higher than at any other phase of the cycle. The dose of replacement estrogen should have a pharmacologic effect similar to approximately 0.3 mg per day of estradiol after systemic absorption.
10. **E,** Page 103. Androstenedione is converted to estrone in fatty tissue. In obese women, regardless of age, a greater percentage (up to 7%) of androstenedione is converted to estrone than occurs in women of normal weight. This conversion

can provide a constant pool of estrone, which inhibits ovulation and causes constant endometrial stimulation. This, in turn, can lead to the increased incidence of endometrial hyperplasia found in obese women.

11. **C,** Page 130. As most protein hormones are of high molecular weight and circulate attached to numerous other molecules, they are extremely difficult to isolate in pure form. Therefore, a reference standard is agreed upon and measurements are expressed in terms of that standard. If the standard is internationally agreed upon, the results will be expressed as international units or milli-international units.
12. **A,** Page 101. Both thromboxane and prostacyclin are formed from arachidonic acid and are eicosanoids having 20 carbons. Thromboxane has an oxane ring rather than a cyclopentane ring. Both cause platelet aggregation but thromboxane causes vasoconstriction while prostacyclin causes vasodilation. Both are inhibited by cortisol which decreases phospholipid hydrolysis and release and by type I (aspirin and indomethicin) nonsteroidal anti-inflammatory drugs (NSAID'S) which inhibit endoperoxide formation.
13. **C,** Page 108; Figure 4-24 (from Herbst). The zona pellucida is a mucopolysaccharide layer that allows only sperm of the same species to penetrate. When it is removed, as is done in a zona-free hamster egg penetration test, human sperm can penetrate the hamster egg. The sperm's ability, or inability, to penetrate the egg is used to determine fertilizing potential of the sperm. The theca interna and externa do not accompany the ovulated egg. The vitelline membrane blocks repeated penetration by sperm after one sperm has successfully entered the egg.
14. **B,** Page 111. The dominant follicle produces approximately 80% of the estrogen synthesized before ovulation. Its mean diameter is about 2 cm and its mean volume is approximately 3.8 ml. This increase in size, as monitored by ultrasound, is used in following women who are being stimulated for in vitro fertilization. Follicular size is a criterion used to indicate maximum potential for ovulation.
15. **A,** Pages 108, 111-112. Knowledge of the normal sequence of events in the menstrual cycle enables you to evaluate abnormalities and prescribe rational therapy. FSH stimulates the follicle, which in turn produces estradiol, which promotes the development of an LH-responsive dominant follicle and triggers the LH surge, resulting in ovulation. After ovulation the follicle develops into a corpus luteum, which produces both estrogen and progesterone. The progesterone causes secretion by an estrogen-stimulated endometrium preparing for the implantation of a fertilized ovum.
16. **C,** Pages 94, 116. GnRH does affect secretion and release of FSH, but because FSH has a half-life of approximately 4 hours, short bursts of its secretion are not apparent. LH has a half-life of 30 minutes so the episodic nature of its secretion is apparent. Although inhibin, a nonsteroidal hormone produced in the granulosa cells, does inhibit FSH, it is only manifest when the granulosa is large, and therefore it is not a constant inhibitor of FSH. Estrogen does not interfere with immunoassays used to measure FSH.
17. **B,** Page 132. The ability to measure only one substance is the specificity. The least amount of substance that can be measured is the sensitivity. The ability to measure the exact amount is accuracy. The variation between intraassays and interassays is the precision of a test.
18. **C,** Page 125. According to Markee's studies, first there is regression in the thickness of the endometrium with coiling of the spiral arteries and slowing of blood. This is followed by vasoconstriction, after which there is vasodilation, leading to escape of blood and menses. The initial decreased blood flow is thought to cause tissue ischemia, which releases lysosomal enzymes, which in turn break down the endometrium. This degraded tissue and blood from the coiled arteries of the functional layer of the endometrium make up the menstrual flow.
19. **C,** Page 111. In a normal cycle the rapid rise of estrogen from a growing follicle triggers a rise of LH at a time when the follicle is 18-25 mm in diameter and is ready to release an egg. The endometrium has been estrogen primed to respond to the progesterone, which will be produced by the post ovulatory corpus luteum. Ovulation usually occurs within 24 hours after the LH peak maintaining the exquisite timing needed to provide an egg at an optimum time for fertilization and subsequent implantation. The estradiol peak oc-

curs before ovulation and the progesterone peak after ovulation.

20. **E,** Pages 94-95. FSH receptors exist primarily on the granulosa cell membrane. When androgens or theca cells (which produce androgens) are added to FSH stimulated granulosa cells large amounts of estrogen are produced while only small amounts are produced without the androgen precursor. According to the 2 cell hypothesis of ovarian estrogen production, LH acts on theca cell receptors to stimulate production of androgens, which are transported to the granulosa cells. Granulosa cells, under the influence of FSH, aromatize androgens to estrogens. FSH and estrogen stimulate LH receptors on the granulosa cells, allowing LH to be bound and cause luteinization.

21-23. 21, **C**; 22, **D**; 23, **E**; Pages 121, 124. The endometrium undergoes specific, recognizable histologic changes during the menstrual cycle. These changes can be dated quite accurately to correlate with the days of the menstrual cycle. Endometrial biopsy and dating can be done to provide indirect evidence of ovulation. One should recognize that the cells lining the glands in Figure 4-1 are pseudostratified. In Figure 4-2 there is subnuclear vacuolization, and in Figure 4-3 the glands are tortuous, and the stroma vascular and edematous.

24-26. 24, **D**; 25, **C**; 26, **A**; Pages 116, 117. Estrogen rises throughout the follicular phase and peaks just before the LH surge. Progesterone is low until after ovulation when it rises along with the secondary rise in estrogen. Both estrogen and progesterone fall just before menses. The 17 hydroxyprogesterone level rises slightly before the LH surge and falls again just before menses.

27-29. 27, **B**; 28, *B;* 29, **D**; Page 107. Estrogens stimulate the synthesis of estrogen receptors and progesterone receptors in target tissues such as the endometrium. Progestins inhibit the synthesis of both estrogen and progesterone receptors. Progestins also increase the intracellular synthesis of estradiol dehydrogenase, which converts the more potent estradiol to the less potent estrone, further decreasing estrogenic activity in the target cell. Antiestrogens, such as clomiphene and tamoxifen, bind to estrogen receptors but do not initiate transcription and therefore decrease the usual effects of estrogen.

30. **A** (1, 2, 3), Page 105. Steroid hormone receptors are intracellular and bind a specific class of steroids after which the receptor steroid complex enters the cell nucleus. Estrogen receptors have the greatest affinity for estradiol, with less affinity for estrone and even less for estriol. Therefore, the affinity correlates with the observed potencies of these compounds. Once the hormone receptor complex is within the cell nucleus, messenger RNA is formed, which in turn enters the cytoplasm and translates its information to the ribosomes so that they will synthesize a new protein.

31. **B** (1, 2), Page 87. Steroids, gonadotrophins, and catecholamines modulate GnRH secretion. Estrogen and progesterone are transmitted to the anterior and medial basal hypothalamus via the systemic circulation, whereas the gonadotrophins (LH and FSH) are returned via the portal system. Catecholamines (dopamine and norepinephrine) and serotonin arrive via neural pathways. Serotonin has not been shown to regulate GnRH release directly, but it does stimulate the release of prolactin.

32. **A** (1, 2, 3), Page 87. Several experimental systems in both primates and humans have shown that high or frequent GnRH pulsations are inhibitory to FSH and LH release, as is too little GnRH. Dopamine appears to act in the median eminence to inhibit the release of GnRH. If too much dopamine is present, GnRH production drops, thereby decreasing FSH and LH. Without adequate FSH and LH, the usual sequence of follicle maturation, ovulation, and corpus luteum formation does not occur.

33. **C** (2, 3), Page 107. Progesterone inhibits synthesis of estrogen receptors and increases synthesis of estrogen dehydrogenase, which converts the more potent estradiol to the less potent estrone. As estrogen receptors are quite specific, progestin does not bind to them.

34. **E** (3 only), Pages 121, 127. As there is no basement membrane between the myometrium and endometrium, the basal endometrium is interdigitated between the muscle fibers of the myometrium. This produces the gritty sensation felt at the time of dilatation and curettage. During menses, many of the endometrial cells remain in both the functional and basal layers. Regeneration of cells begins even as

bleeding is continuing. Although enzymes may destroy endometrial cells, muscle cells are generally unaffected.

35. **A** (1, 2, 3), Page 121. The irregularity of periods that is common both at the beginning and the end of the menstrual years is more worrisome in the older woman, as the risk of endometrial carcinoma is much higher than in teenage years. A certain amount of irregularity is normal, with the normal pattern being a longer time between menses and a decreased flow averaging 4 1/2 days. The average age of menopause is 51.

PART TWO APPROACH TO THE PATIENT

CHAPTER 5 History and Examination of the Patient

DIRECTIONS for questions 1 - 4: Select the one best answer or completion.

1. Each of the following neoplasms can be screened during routine physical examination except
   A. carcinoma of the cervix
   B. carcinoma of the breast
   C. carcinoma of the ovary
   D. carcinoma of the endometrium
   E. carcinoma of the rectum
2. If the screening interval value is extended from two to three years, the increased risk of developing carcinoma of the cervix is approximately
   A. two-fold
   B. three-fold
   C. four-fold
   D. five-fold
   E. six-fold
3. The percentage of neoplastic bowel lesions that can be palpated on digital rectal examination is
   A. 30%
   B. 40%
   C. 50%
   D. 60%
   E. 70%
4. As the primary physician for *postmenopausal* women, gynecologists should obtain which of the following on an annual basis?
   A. mammography
   B. thyrotropin stimulating hormone (TSH)
   C. total cholesterol
   D. electrocardiogram
   E. PAP smear

DIRECTIONS for questions 5 - 8: For each numbered item, select the one heading most closely associated with it. Each lettered heading may be used once, more than once, or not at all.

5-8. Match the following diagnostic procedure with the *most* appropriate patient history listed below

(A) mammography
(B) colposcopy
(C) hysteroscopy
(D) endometrial sampling
(E) pelvic ultrasonography
(F) vaginoscopy

5. an 8-year-old girl with a 2 month history of vaginal bleeding
6. a 44-year-old nulligravid woman in clinic for an annual exam
7. a 44-year-old woman presenting with a problem of frequent "irregular periods"
8. a 21-year-old nulligravida with an unusually large cervical "erosion" (cockscomb-cervix)

DIRECTIONS For each numbered item 9 - 20, indicate whether it is associated with
A only (A)
B only (B)
C both (A) and (B)
D neither (A) nor (B)

9-11. Similarities and differences in pelvic relaxation

(A) cystocele
(B) rectocele
(C) both
(D) neither

9. represents a herniated peritoneal reflection
10. may present past the vaginal introitus
11. may be repaired vaginally

12-14. Bleeding manifestations

(A) of an **ovulatory** cycle
(B) of an **anovulatory** cycle
(C) both
(D) neither

12. consistent postcoital bleeding, regular menses
13. intermenstrual spotting any time during the cycle, regular menses

14. consistently regular, painful menses

15-17. Bimanual exam
(A) abdominal/vaginal
(B) abdominal/rectovaginal
(C) both
(D) neither

15. used to identify portio vaginalis
16. used to appreciate uterosacral ligament nodules
17. will identify a palpable postmenopausal ovary

18-20. Diagnosis
(A) *chlamydia*
(B) gonorrhea
(C) both
(D) neither

18. Papanicolaou smear likely to identify cellular changes
19. best identified by endocervical swab cultures
20. culture attempts should follow cytologic sampling for Papanicolaou smear

DIRECTIONS for questions 21 - 27: For each of the questions below, ONE or MORE of the responses is correct. Select the best answer based on the following
A if 1, 2, and 3 are correct
B if only 1 and 2 are correct
C if only 2 and 3 are correct
D if only 1 is correct
E if only 3 is correct

21. Reproductive (pregnancy) history of a patient includes previous
    1. molar pregnancy
    2. gestational diabetes
    3. paternity
22. Dermatologic findings of the vulvar and perineal skin of potential significance include
    1. hyperkeratosis
    2. pigmented nevus
    3. alopecia
23. Nonverbal clues given by patient behavior may be helpful in making the **clinical diagnosis** of
    1. endogenous depression
    2. anxiety neurosis
    3. hidden anger
24. Characteristics of the normal squamocolumnar junction (transformation zone) include
    1. areas of squamous metaplasia
    2. located at or near the portio vaginalis
    3. may shift in location in response to infectious or hormonal influences
25. Items in sexual history that usually relate to the presence of organic gynecologic pathology include
    1. anorgasmia
    2. dyspareunia
    3. postcoital bleeding
26. Papanicolaou testing should
    1. be performed yearly in all patients
    2. first be performed regularly with onset of coitus
    3. contain an adequate sampling of endocervical cells
27. Positive historical findings that help identify a 43-year-old patient at increased risk for endometrial neoplasia include
    1. chronic oligo-ovulation
    2. infertility
    3. use of a Lippes Loop IUD from age 30-35

ANSWERS

1. **D,** Page 154. Small endometrial tumors may not be appreciated by routine examination unless associated with a significant change in bleeding pattern. The others can be suspected by routine exam and diagnostic procedures such as pap smear and stool guaiac testing. Endometrial sampling is reserved for patients with abnormal menstrual histories, perimenopausal or postmenopausal bleeding, or it is advocated by some as a routine in postmenopausal estrogen users.
2. **C,** Page 154. Patients with later coital exposure who have had one sexual partner and who have had two successive negative annual smears may be considered low risk and should be screened by Papanicolaou testing every one to three years. Recently a study by Shy, et al showed that although no significant increase in cervical cancer was noted in women screened every two years compared with annually, the risk increased 3.9 times if the interval was three years and 12.3 times in women not screened for ten years.
3. **E,** Page 157. The value of the rectal examination should not be underestimated. This is the most efficient way to assess the uterosacral ligaments and to assess the size of the uterus in cases of retroflexion. By rectal examination it should be possible to palpate as many as 70% of bowel lesions with the rectal finger. Because bowel cancer is common in women particularly after the age of 35, this part of the examination should not be overlooked.
4. **A,** Page 158. Of the tests listed, the mammogram is mandatory on an annual basis as recommended by the American Cancer

Society and the American College of Obstetricians and Gynecologists. The other tests may be obtained when indicated but not as part of routine yearly screening. It is recommended that TSH be obtained every three years after the age of 60; a lipid profile including total cholesterol every three years after the age of 50; a PAP smear based on patient risk factors but not necessarily each year; and an electrocardiogram based on patients needs and symptomatology after one baseline exam at the age of 50. Guidelines for primary and preventive health care in postmenopausal women are still not well defined in all medical specialities, but with an aging population it will become incumbent on the gynecologist of the future to assume many roles in primary health care and preventive medicine.

5-8. 5, **E;** 6, **A;** 7, **D;** 8, **B;** Pages 158, 274, 281. A prepuberal girl with vaginal bleeding is at greatest risk for vaginal foreign body. A less likely source for this problem would be a functional ovarian neoplasm. A pelvic ultrasound might be helpful in ruling out both a neoplasm and possibly even the foreign body. Since ultrasound is noninvasive and more easily available, it represents a reasonable first step. If this is unrevealing, one would consider vaginoscopy under anesthesia to rule out a vaginal foreign body or a rare lower tract neoplasm. Mammography is indicated as a routine screening exam in gynecologic perimenopausal patients, particularly patients with any risk factors. Perimenopausal patients (over age 35) with a change in bleeding (menstrual) patterns should be screened by office sampling of the endometrium. Further assessment by dilation and curettage or hysteroscopy should be dictated by other pertinent history or physical exam features. An unusual configuration of the glandular cervical epithelium should alert the clinician to the possibility of material diethylstilbestrol (DES) exposure. If not done previously and found to be normal, this woman should have a colposcopic evaluation and careful palpation of the vaginal fornices.

9-11. 9, **D;** 10, **C;** 11, **C;** Pages 150-152. When performing a physical examination on patients with pelvic relaxation, a knowledge of potential herniations and loss of pelvic supporting structures is imperative. A cystocele and rectocele are usually apparent when present, but they are not always symptomatic. Both a cystocele and rectocele represent a protrusion of the wall of a hollow viscus. In the true sense they are not hernias. A enterocele is a herniated peritoneal surface and is often more subtle, necessitating a thorough working knowledge of this defect. This is especially important with regard to planning surgical procedures designed to correct disorders of pelvic support. All three can protrude through the vaginal introitus and all three can be repaired vaginally.

12-14. 12, **D;** 13, **C;** 14, **A;** Pages 144-145. Postcoital bleeding usually occurs as a result of some inflammatory or neoplastic disorder of the cervix and/or endometrium. It is not a reflection of an ovulatory or anovulatory endocrinologic milieu. Likewise, intermenstrual bleeding should be viewed as neoplastic or inflammatory until proven otherwise. Intermenstrual bleeding can also be associated with ovulation if it occurs near midcycle on a regular basis. This is due to the change in hormonal milieu at this time. Regular, painful menstruation is usually associated with ovulation, presumably because of the association of progesterone production with enhanced activity of prostaglandin on the smooth musculature of the uterus.

15-17. 15, **C;** 16, **B;** 17, **C;** Pages 155-156. The portio vaginalis is usually a visual landmark of the cervix and is seen by speculum examination, but it also can be palpated during either the abdominal/vaginal or abdominal/rectovaginal exams. Because the uterosacral ligaments insert onto the posterior cervicouterine junction and extend backwards to the hollow of the sacrum, they are best appreciated by the rectovaginal exam. An enlarged postmenopausal ovary is not necessarily better appreciated by either physical exam technique, depending on the anatomic relationships of the patient being examined. This finding suggests an ovarian neoplasm and needs further diagnostic assessment, regardless of how it is suspected.

18-20. 18, **D;** 19, **C;** 20, **C;** Page 155. Neither chlamydia or gonorrhea can be specifically identified by the cytologic techniques used in Papanicolaou screening. Koilocytosis which is seen on a Papanicolaou smear is suggestive of an infection by the human papilloma virus. Both *chlamydia* and gonorrhea are best identified by endocervical culture. Recent preliminary data suggest that cytologic screening for chlamydia may have promise, but this information is not yet generally accepted as a reliable, sensitive screen for this organism. (Kiviat NB, Peterson M, Kinney TE, Tam M, Stamm WE, Holmes KK. Cytologic manifestations of cervical and vaginal infections. II. Confirmation of Chlamydia trachomatis infection by direct immunofluorescence using monoclonal antibodies. JAMA 1985; 253 (7):997-1000.). Perform a Papanicolaou smear before obtaining endocervical cultures.

21. **A** (1, 2, and 3), Page 145. Any pregnancy in the patient's history should be recorded, including nonviable and preterm pregnancies as well as metabolic pregnancy complications and paternity. These events may help the clinician in predicting future reproductive outcomes and in offering a rationale for specific diagnostic or therapeutic measures such as ultrasonography, a-HCG testing, testing for carbohydrate intolerance, and identification of potential chromosomal problems.
22. **B** (1, 2), Page 149. Although skin findings such as hyperkeratosis and pigmented nevi may be normal variants, they warrant more careful follow-up. Usually a biopsy is necessary to make the diagnosis of intraepithelial neoplasia or atrophic dystrophy. Scattered cherry angiomata are not associated with more serious pathology when seen as an isolated incidental finding. Thinning of the pubic hair overlying the mons pubis may occur as women enter their later postmenopausal years.
23. **B** (1, 2), Page 144. Anger and seductiveness are not clinical diagnoses, but may be *part of* another pathological process. Depression and anxiety are diagnoses (DM III) and may be detected by nonverbal patient behavior.
24. **A** (1, 2, 3), Page 153. The transformation zone, by definition, is the functional zone between squamous epithelium of the ectocervix and the columnar epithelium of the endocervix It contains elements of both surfaces. This zone is dynamic and changes continually throughout the reproductive years in response to inflammation, trauma, pregnancy, and hormonal influences.
25. **C** (2, 3), Page 146. Whereas anorgasmia and vaginismus are usually related to psychological dysfunction, dyspareunia and postcoital bleeding are more likely to relate to potential nonsuppurative inflammation or neoplastic disorders. These historical findings warrant further assessment to rule out potential gynecologic pathology.
26. **C** (2, 3), Page 154. American College of Obstetricians and Gynecologists guidelines suggest that Papanicolaou testing begin at age 18 or when regular coital activity begins. In patients at higher risk—those with history of early coital activity and/or multiple partners or those with other risk factors such as prior herpes or condylomatous changes—this exam should occur **at least** annually. In patients with two successive negative smears and a single sexual partner, the interval between smears may safely be extended for up to 3 years. The Papanicolaou smear is inadequate and thus less diagnostic if it does not contain a sample of the endocervical canal.
27. **B** (1, 2), Pages 145, 896. Aspects of the gynecologic history that place the patient at risk are factors relating to her chronic anovulation which is also suggested by the infertility. Of course, more history is necessary, but as isolated fragments of information, oligo-ovulation and infertility should alert you about the potential for endometrial neoplasia.

CHAPTER 6

Significant Symptoms and Signs in Different Age Groups

DIRECTIONS for questions 1 - 20: For each numbered item, select the one heading most closely associated with it. Each lettered heading may be used once, more than once, or not at all.

1-3. Match the ovarian neoplasm with the description

(A) malignant teratoma
(B) serous cystadenocarcinoma
(C) cystic teratoma
(D) serous cystadenoma
(E) granulosa cell tumor

1. most common ovarian tumor in all age groups
2. most common neoplasm of adolescence
3. stromal cell tumor producing sex hormone

4-5. Match the adnexal mass with the description

(A) follicle cyst
(B) corpus luteum cyst
(C) cystic teratoma
(D) serous cystadenoma
(E) mucinous cystadenoma

4. accounts for the majority of adnexal masses during the reproductive years
5. most commonly mimics ectopic pregnancy

6-8. Assume ***EACH*** of the following pregnancies has progressed to approximately ***18*** weeks according to the patient's stated last normal menstrual period

(A) complete molar pregnancy
(B) twin pregnancy
(C) size/dates discrepancy
(D) polyhydramnios

6. quantitative HCG >210,000 mIUs
7. anomalous fetus
8. normal intrauterine pregnancy

9-11. Although any bleeding abnormality may occur with the conditions listed below, the classic association of each is

(A) menorrhagia
(B) metrorrhagia
(C) postmenopausal bleeding
(D) amenorrhea

9. endometrial carcinoma
10. uterine leiomyomata
11. carcinoma of the cervix

12-13. Match the condition with the symptom

(A) atrophic vaginitis
(B) endometrial carcinoma
(C) cervical carcinoma
(D) epithelial ovarian carcinoma
(E) urethral caruncle

12. most common cause for postmenopausal bleeding
13. least likely to be associated with post menopausal bleeding

14-17. Match the symptom with the inflammatory process

(A) right upper quadrant pain
(B) right lower quadrant pain
(C) left upper quadrant pain
(D) left lower quadrant pain
(E) bilateral lower quadrant pain

14. acute salpingitis
15. tubo-ovarian abscess
16. acute diverticulitis
17. acute mesenteric adenitis

18-20. Listed below are several conditions that can be associated with pain

(A) pelvic adhesions
(B) myofascial component
(C) major depressive disorder
(D) degenerating myoma
(E) ovarian torsion

18. responds to local anesthetic
19. associated with sexual abuse
20. is the most common finding in chronic pelvic pain patients

DIRECTIONS for questions 21 - 27: For each of the questions below, ONE or MORE of the responses is correct. Select the best answer based on the following

A if 1, 2, and 3 are correct
B if only 1 and 2 are correct
C if only 2 and 3 are correct
D if only 1 is correct
E if only 3 is correct

21. Characteristics of dysfunctional uterine bleeding include
    1. perimenopausal bleeding
    2. irregular menstrual interval
    3. nonsecretory endometrium
22. Pain in an individual is
    1. quantifiable
    2. unpleasant
    3. emotional

23. Most gynecologic processes that present with acute abdominal pain
    1. starts with periumbilical pain
    2. are associated with lower gastrointestinal symptoms
    3. are most often limited to the pelvic peritoneum (right or left lower quadrant)
24. Causes of ovarian enlargement between the ages of birth and menarche include
    1. follicle cysts
    2. dysgerminomas
    3. teratomas
25. Malignant adnexal neoplasms in adolescence include
    1. stromal cell tumors
    2. germ cell tumors
    3. epithelial cell tumors
26. In women over the age of 50, predictors of ovarian malignancy include
    1. cell type
    2. size
    3. menstrual status
27. The differential diagnosis of an adnexal mass in the postmenopausal patient should encompass
    1. endometriosis
    2. diverticular disease
    3. lymphoma

ANSWERS

1-3. 1, **D**; 2, **C**; 3, **E**; Pages 173-175; Tables 6.3 and 6.4. Bennington's cross-sectional study of a general gynecologic population by age group, revealed that the serous cystadenoma is the most common true neoplasm of the ovary in all age groups combined. The majority of patients with this tumor fell into the 20-44 year old age group. Of primary ovarian neoplasms seen in all age groups, the serous cystadenocarcinoma is most often bilateral. In adolescence a cystic teratoma is the most common, and is important clinically because of the possibility of torsion or rupture. True ovarian neoplasms that produce sex steroids are referred to as functioning tumors. An example is a granulosacell tumor which is associated with the production of estrogen. Functional enlargements on the other hand, refer to variations of ovarian follicular and/or ovulatory apparatus which in fact, are variants of normal reproductive anatomy.

4-5. 4, **A**; 5, **B**; Pages 172-173. In assessing patients with adnexal masses, it is important to differentiate between neoplasms and variations of normal functional ovarian anatomy. Cystic teratomas, serous and mucinous cystadenomas are true neoplasms of the ovary and occur less frequently than either of the functional cysts. During the reproductive years the majority of adnexal masses are follicle cysts. These may vary in size from 3 cm to 10 cm in diameter. They are often appreciated during the time of routine pelvic exam. They are unlikely to cause symptoms unless they become particularly large or rupture, releasing follicular fluid into the pelvic cavity. Even then, they will usually cause only transient symptoms. Often vaginal ultrasound is useful in assessing these cysts. One can follow their regression through one or two menstrual cycles. Characteristically they are unilocular and smooth without any evidence of internal excrescences. Corpus luteum cysts are also common during ovulatory years and usually do not enlarge significantly beyond 5 cm. They may be somewhat tender to palpation. On occasion, they bleed into the pelvic cavity and mimic an ectopic pregnancy. They persist past the time of anticipated menses. They may delay the expected period further suggesting ectopic pregnancy. Vaginal ultrasound, coupled with a negative HCG, is helpful in making this diagnosis ruling out an ectopic pregnancy. The intent of these questions is to create an appreciation for the clinical presence of functional cysts.

6-8. 6 **A**; 7, **D**; 8, **C**; Page 164. The unexplained enlarged uterus may create a diagnostic dilemma. This physical finding, when related to pregnancy, has a number of implications. Molar pregnancy is associated with massive proliferation of trophoblast and therefore generally associated with quantitative HCG levels of over 100,000 MIUs per ml. Although there may be a number of potentially serious causes for size/dates discrepancy, most often this is the result of poor menstrual history and thus associated with normal pregnancy. Although molar pregnancy may be associated with anomalous fetus (incomplete mole), and is somewhat more common in twin pregnancy, the finding of polyhydramnios should suggest this entity and diagnostic studies should be instituted to rule out the presence of the anomalous fetus in the case of polyhydramnios.

9-11. 9, **C**; 10, **A**; 11, **B**; Tables 6-1, Pages 164-165. The occurrence of endometrial carcinoma is greatest in the postmenopausal age group and thus usual bleeding manifestations of this tumor are not associated with true menstruation, but rather are manifested by irregular perimenopausal bleeding or more commonly postmenopausal bleeding. Menorrhagia is the occurrence of regular bleeding of a greater amount than usual for ten days or more and is most often associated with uterine myoma. Metrorrhagia is the occurrence of significant intermenstrual bleeding one or more times and is most commonly found with cervical carcinoma. Less commonly, it may present as post menopausal bleeding.

12-13. 12, **A**; 13, **D**; Table 6-2, Page 166. Although postmenopausal bleeding may be associated with a number of conditions, it must always be investigated because many causes are premalignant or malignant. The best way to rule out endometrial neoplasia is by outpatient endometrial sampling. This is possible in most patients. On occasion, technical difficulties require performance under anesthesia. The majority of women presenting with postmenopausal bleeding have atrophic vaginitis, as documented in a study by Dewhurst in which he analyzed 249 women. More than half of these patients presented with atrophic vaginitis. This should be compared to the approximately 15 or 20 percent of patients with postmenopausal bleeding who will have endometrial carcinoma. Unless the ovarian carcinoma is a granulosa cell tumor, and this is relatively uncommon, ovarian carcinoma is not associated with post menopausal bleeding. A urethral caruncle may be seen in post menopausal women and represents an eversion of the urethral epithelium. It is recognizable by sight, is benign, and needs no treatment.

14-17. 14, **E**; 15, **E**; 16, **D**; 17, **B**; Pages 167-168, Table 6-3. Abdominal and pelvic pain often occur together, and may be caused by a variety of gynecologic and non gynecologic entities. Pain of significant organic origin usually involves sudden onset, tenderness to palpation, mild to significant degrees of rebound tenderness, and an alteration in bowel sounds. Acute salpingitis and tubo-ovarian abscess are typically bilateral processes and thus elicit bilateral lower quadrant pain. Acute diverticulitis is most often manifest in the rectosigmoid thus presenting as acute left lower quadrant pain. Mesenteric adenitis often mimics appendicitis or right adnexal disease and thus presents as acute right lower quadrant pain. A clinician is frequently called upon to differentiate these and other entities based on the pain related history and physical findings.

18-20. 18, **B**; 19, **C**; 20, **A**; Pages 170-172. Handling patients with pain presents the clinician with a number of diagnostic problems. Acute pain is associated with more objective findings. Usually the differential diagnosis is more limited. With chronic pain, symptoms tend to be vague. These patients frequently have a significant psychologic component. Slocum has called attention to the presence of "trigger points" that are discernible by palpation along the myofascial junctions of the abdominal wall. These are often treated successfully by injections of a local anesthetic, such as 0.25% Bupivocaine, on one or several occasions. In analyzing the laparoscopic findings of 100 women who complained of constant pelvic pain in the same location for a minimum of six months, Kresch, et al reported that overall, 83% of the group with chronic pain had abnormal pelvic findings, whereas only 29% of a control group had abnormal findings. Of these findings, pelvic adhesions were the most common accounting for 38%. However, it should be mentioned that the role of adhesions in causing pain is still unclear. Clearly in a significant number of patients, who have otherwise unexplained chronic pelvic pain, major affective disorders may play a role. Of this group of patients suffering from past or current affective disorders, there is much greater likelihood of childhood or adult sexual abuse.

21. **A** (1, 2, 3), Page 164. Dysfunctional uterine bleeding implies irregular bleeding secondary to the lack of regular ovulation. This is most common shortly after menarche until regular ovulatory cycles are established as well as at the other end of the reproductive spectrum. Women in the perimenopausal period, who are undergoing early evidence of ovarian failure, have irregular periods. When the endometrium is sampled, it will most likely be proliferative.

22. **C** (2, 3), Page 167. Pain, as a subjective response, cannot be quantified by external standards and is usually described as unpleasant, making it an emotional experience. Pain is individualized through experience related to injury in early life. Although there are attempts to quantify pain

of both organic and emotional origin, assessment of this sensory experience is difficult.

23. **E** (3 only), Pages 167-168.

TABLE 6-1. Conditions That May Cause Signs and Symptoms of Acute Abdomen and Abdominal Quadrants in Which They Most Often Occur

Condition	Quadrant			
	Right Upper	Right Lower	Left Upper	Left Lower
Salpingitis	−	+	−	+
Tuboovarian abscess	±	+	±	+
Ectopic pregnancy	−	+	−	+
Torsive adnexa	−	+	−	+
Ruptered ovarian cyst	−	+	−	+
Acute appendicitis	−	+	−	−
Mesenteric lymphadenitis	−	+	−	−
Crohn's disease	−	+	−	−
Acute cholecystitis	+	±	−	−
Perforated peptic ulcer	+	±	+	±
Acute pancreatitis	+	−	+	−
Acute pyelitis	+	±	+	±
Renal calculus	+	+	+	+
Splenic infarct	−	−	+	−
Splenic rupture	−	−	+	−
Acute diverticulitis	−	−	−	+

+, More frequently; ±, may occur.

The common acute gynecologic entities listed in the table all share a common pattern; right or left lower quadrant pain. Some include bilateral pain depending on the pathologic process. Visceral pain from most gastrointestinal tract disorders is usually more specifically related to the part of the viscus involved. Urinary tract disease may present more diffuse pain depending on the part of the tract involved. Gastrointestinal symptoms and periumbilical pain are not characteristically associated with gynecological disorders.

24. **A** (1, 2, 3), Pages 176-177. Occasionally babies are born with adnexal cysts that present as abdominal masses. These are generally follicular cysts secondary to maternal hormone stimulation of the fetal ovaries. They generally regress within the first few months of life. Of the true ovarian tumors which present later in childhood, dysgerminomas and teratomas are the most common. Six to eight percent of these tumors are dysgerminomas and, while benign and malignant teratomas have been reported in childhood, they are quite rare before the age of ten.
25. **A** (1, 2, 3), Pages 176-177. Solid or cystic adnexal tumors, although rare in adolescence, are usually dysgerminomas or malignant teratomas. These are germ cell in origin. In a study by Diamond of tumors in women under the age of 21, all 6 malignant lesions were of germ cell origin. Likewise in a study by Norris and Jensen the 353 primary ovarian neoplasms found under the age of 20 years, germ cell tumors represented 28% of the cases. Of the remaining non germ cell tumors, 19% were of epithelial and 19% stromal in origin.
26. **B** (1, 2). Page 178. In a study by Rulin and Preston analyzing 150 adnexal tumors in women over the age of 50, 47 were malignant. Only one tumor of the 32 that were less than 5 cm proved to be malignant while 40 of 63 tumors larger than 10 cm were malignant. The majority of the larger tumors were of the epithelial cell type. There was no apparent association with menstrual status of these patients. Thus it would appear that size and cell type are reasonable predictors of malignancy in this age group.
27. **A** (1, 2, 3). Page 178. Adnexal masses occurring in postmenopausal women may be benign, but the chance of malignancy increases with age. Although endometriosis occurs primarily in women of the reproductive years, as many as 5% of cases appear postmenopausally. Masses from other organ systems are quite common in this age group including diverticulitis, accounting for painful left adnexal masses. Tumors such as lymphomas may present as rapidly growing, firm masses, which at times are accompanied by ascites.

CHAPTER 7 Counseling the Patient

DIRECTIONS for questions 1 - 8: Select the one best answer or completion.

1. A 68-year-old woman is concerned because her 70-year-old spouse, since undergoing prostatic surgery, is no longer capable of an erection. Initially you should
   A. recommend testosterone therapy for him
   B. recommend a penile prosthesis
   C. tell her that he should not be worried about this at his age
   D. refer both for sexual counseling
   E. discuss this with the spouse
2. A 21-year-old woman who has been married for 2 years, is referred by her family physician who was unable to obtain a pap smear. You find that you also are unable to insert a speculum; in fact, when you approach her, the levator muscles contract and she slides away from you on the examining table.
   From this information you can conclude that this woman
   A. has a phobic avoidance to the insertion of the speculum
   B. has an unhappy marriage
   C. has a vaginal septum or intact hymen
   D. will never respond adequately to sexual stimulation
   E. has never had intercourse
3. Acceptance of the inevitability of death proceeds in the following stages:
   A. Denial
   Anger
   Bargaining
   Depression
   Acceptance
   B. Denial
   Bargaining
   Anger
   Depression
   Acceptance
   C. Denial
   Depression
   Anger
   Bargaining
   Acceptance
   D. Anger
   Denial
   Bargaining
   Depression
   Acceptance
   E. Anger
   Denial
   Depression
   Bargaining
   Acceptance
4. The G-spot in a female
   A. is homologous to the seminal vesicle in a male
   B. is another name for the clitoris
   C. becomes exquisitely tender during sexual intercourse
   D. may be stimulated to the point of ejaculation of fluid during orgasm
   E. as the only source of orgasm indicates the individual has infantile sexuality, according to Freudian psychology

5-6. A 15-year-old states that she began her menses at age 11 and that during her 13th year she had a regular 26 to 30-day cycle. She has not had a period in the last 6 months, and she has never had intercourse. The medical history is unremarkable except that she feels that she is 20 pounds overweight.
Physical Examination
BP: 100/70 T: 97.8 P: 55
Ht: 5 ft 4 inches
Wt: 105 lbs
Breast: Tanner Stage IV
Abdomen: Unremarkable
Pelvic:
Escutcheon: Tanner Stage IV
Outlet: Unremarkable
Cervix: Unremarkable
Corpus: Normal size, smooth, firm
Adnexa: Unremarkable

5. Given the most likely diagnosis, you would expect all of the following **EXCEPT**:
   A. She abuses laxatives
   B. She has an increased likelihood of having a relative with the same problem
   C. She vomits frequently

D. She is an average student
E. She has had an adverse sexual experience

6. The therapy that will most likely be of benefit is
A. pergonal
B. insulin
C. psychoanalysis
D. cognitive behavioral therapy
E. high potency vitamins

7. Of the following gynecological procedures which is most likely to cause sexual dysfunction in a psychologically stable woman who is happily married?
A. total abdominal hysterectomy
B. total vaginal hysterectomy
C. anterior colporrhaphy
D. simple vulvectomy
E. retropubic urethropexy

8. Three years ago, after a lengthy illness, a 65 year-old woman's husband died. Since that time she has been depressed. This has manifested itself by chronic fatigue, irritability and anhedonia. The patient on one occasion said that she wanted to commit suicide and in the same breath said that she could not do that because it was against her religion.

In the above case, which of the following is not considered part of the normal grief reaction? The
A. length of the reaction
B. chronic fatigue
C. irritability
D. anhedonia
E. lack of decisiveness

DIRECTIONS: for questions 9 - 11: For each numbered item, select the one heading most closely associated with it. Each lettered heading may be used once, more than once, or not at all.

9-11. A large-boned 27-year-old is overweight. You recommend dieting. In addition, you would suggest (Table 7-1)
(A) Weight Watchers
(B) Medically supervised behavior modification
(C) Pharmacologic therapy
(D) Gastric restriction operation
(E) None of the above

9. if she is 5 feet 9 inches tall and weighs 255 pounds
10. if she is 5 feet 0 inches tall and weighs 275 pounds
11. if she is 5 feet 11 inches tall and weighs 238 pounds

TABLE 7-1. Height and Weight Table for Women*

Height		Weight (lbs)		
Feet	**Inches**	**Small Frame**	**Medium Frame**	**Large Frame**
4	10	102-111	109-121	118-131
4	11	103-113	111-123	120-134
5	0	104-115	113-126	122-137
5	1	106-118	115-129	125-140
5	2	108-121	118-132	128-143
5	3	111-124	121-135	131-147
5	4	114-127	124-138	134-151
5	5	117-130	127-141	137-155
5	6	120-133	130-144	140-159
5	7	123-136	133-147	143-163
5	8	126-139	136-150	146-167
5	9	129-142	139-153	149-170
5	10	132-145	142-156	152-173
5	11	135-148	145-159	155-176
6	0	138-151	148-162	158-179

*Weights at ages 25 to 29 based on lowest mortality. Weight in pounds according to frame (in indoor clothing weighing 3 pounds; shoes with 1-inch heels). (From 1983 Metropolitan Height & Weight Tables, Metropolitan Life Insurance Company, Health and Safety Division.)

DIRECTIONS: for questions 12 - 14: For each numbered item, indicate whether it is associated with
A only (A)
B only (B)
C both (A) and (B)
D neither (A) nor (B)

12-14. Phases of Female Human Sexual Response
(A) Excitement
(B) Orgasm
(C) Both
(D) Neither

12. can be affected by antihypertensive medication
13. response due to stimulation of the parasympathetic nervous system
14. development of the orgasmic platform

DIRECTIONS: for questions 15 - 21: For each of the questions below, ONE or MORE of the responses is correct. Select the best answer based on the following
A if 1, 2, and 3 are correct
B if only 1 and 2 are correct
C if only 2 and 3 are correct
D if only 1 is correct
E if only 3 is correct

15. A 25-year-old gravida 3, para 0, abortus 3 factory worker is seen 6 weeks postdeliv-

ery. Her last pregnancy ended at 20 weeks, and you feel that she has an incompetent cervix. Today she has multiple complaints, including tightness in the throat and chest, frequent sighing, and muscle weakness. You attribute this to a grief reaction. The patient continued to work during this last pregnancy despite your warning that this activity might lead to another pregnancy loss. Appropriate comments at this encounter include
   1. mentioning that she is still young and will have another chance
   2. acknowledging her feelings of grief
   3. referring her to a self-help group

16. A woman on oral contraception who is anorgasmic during coitus should
    1. use another form of contraception
    2. be allowed to masturbate during foreplay
    3. discuss this with her partner
17. Services included in a hospital-based hospice program are
    1. social work
    2. home care
    3. postdeath follow-up
18. The amounts of alcohol are approximately the same in:
    1. 12 ounces of beer
    2. a wine glass of wine
    3. 30 ml of whiskey
19. Childhood self-esteem is enhanced by
    1. praising
    2. setting limits
    3. intimidation

Questions 20 and 21

20. A 35-year-old stockbroker was to be married for the first time 6 months ago, but her fiance was killed in an auto accident on the way to the church. When she saw your partner a month ago, your partner decided that she was severely depressed and prescribed amitriptyline. She returns with a list of new symptoms which are listed below. These symptoms are frightening to her, but they do not prevent her from functioning as a normal human being. Those that are secondary to the medication and not her basic problem include:
    1. a dry mouth
    2. constipation
    3. hesitancy of urination
21. In addition to these symptoms, the woman is still depressed. You would now
    1. tell her to take a glass of wine at bedtime
    2. add another antidepressive medication
    3. offer her reassurance

ANSWERS

1. **E,** Page 197. The first step is to discuss this concern with both partners. The husband and his wife need to decide whether his lack of an erection is a problem. The husband may be concerned that he can no longer satisfy his wife. A physician can be useful in helping a couple sort out their needs and desire for sexual compatibility at this stage of life.
2. **A,** Pages 197-198. The question describes a woman who, according to Lamont's classification, has fourth-degree vaginismus, levator and perineal spasm, and retreat. This problem is generally due to a phobia to vaginal penetration based on a previous traumatic episode or a lack of appropriate knowledge about sex secondary to cultural or familial teaching that sex is evil, painful, or undesirable. Sexual dysfunction is not necessarily incompatible with a happy marriage. This couple could be very happy. The history did not suggest amenorrhea, so a septum or an intact hymen was ruled out. Treatment for this problem has a high success rate. Thus, one cannot assert that the woman will have an unhappy sex life. One cannot assert that she has never had intercourse. Traumatic intercourse, especially rape, could have been a precipitating factor.
3. **A,** Pages 205-206. The stages as suggested by Kubler-Ross are denial, anger, bargaining, depression, and acceptance. Unfortunately, many people die before all of these stages have been reconciled.
4. **D,** Pages 185, 193. The G-spot is an area on the anterior vaginal wall beneath the urethra believed to be homologous to the male prostate gland. During sexual arousal, it may be stimulated to the point of orgasm with ejaculation of fluid into the urethra. It was not mentioned by Freud, who felt that clitoral orgasm represented the hallmark of infantile sexuality.
5. **D,** Pages 188-189. These patients tend to be high achievers, usually A students. The occurrence of anorexia and bulimia is six times greater in first-degree relatives than in the general population. Vomiting and laxative abuse are common findings. The incidence of adverse sexual experience among anorectics may be underreported. These events occur in childhood or adolescence, and most usually involve a person known to the subject.
6. **D,** Page 189. A number of medications have been tried in the treatment of an-

orexia nervosa with varying success. These medications have included insulin, lithium, tricyclics, and phenothiazides as well as high potency vitamins. In many cases they have not been found to be better than a placebo. Psychoanalysis is a long-term approach and anorexia nervosa requires prompt intervention. More recently, however, cognitive behavior therapy has been used in the treatment of anorexia. This therapy is aimed at bringing to the attention of the individual the fact that her beliefs, assumptions, and style of thinking have brought about distorted body image, food aversion, phobias, and unreasonable fears of weight gain. In short the therapy is aimed at reshaping patients' thinking processes with respect to themselves and to their body images. Behavior modification and cognitive therapy have met with some success. Behavior modification is based on reward and punishment for a number of behaviors. Cognitive behavioral therapy is directed toward the specific thinking disorder rather than body image and food.

7. **D,** Page 194. Recently several lay publications have suggested a role for the cervix in sexual response, basing this theory on the fact that the cervix is related to a rich nerve supply. To date, no scientific data support this theory. Sexual gratification and orgasmic behavior seem definitely to be associated with nerve endings in the clitoris, mons pubis, labia, and possible pressure receptors in the pelvis. Loss or disruption of the clitoris seemed to be the single most important factor in the development of sexual dysfunction following surgery.
8. **A,** Page 200. Early symptoms of depression include chronic fatigue, anxiety and irritability, and anhedonia (loss of feelings of joy and pleasure), decreased interest in usual pursuits including sexual activity and personal appearance, and mental changes, including poor concentration and lack of decisiveness. The physician should determine whether the individual has suicidal thoughts and assess whether these thoughts are likely to be put into practice. If the patient seems to be seriously considering suicide, prompt referral to a mental health worker or facility should be made. The physician should be alert to patients who have suffered personal loss or grief but who are still deeply depressed after 6 to 18 months of grieving. While depression is normal in a grief situation, it should not last for a prolonged period.

9-11. 9, **B;** 10, **D;** 11, **A;** Pages 190-191, Table 7-2. All three patients have a large frame. Patient 9 is 50 lbs overweight and therefore moderately obese. Patient 10 is 100 lbs overweight and therefore severely obese. Patient 11 is 35 lbs overweight or mildly obese. Mild obesity can be successfully managed by diet and behavior modification under lay supervision. Most prescribe or sell foods low in fat in an attempt to achieve a diet containing about 20% fat. Moderate obesity is best managed under medical supervision. Good results have been obtained in the severely obese who have had a gastric restriction operation. Additional studies are needed to verify good long-term results.

12-14. 12, **B;** 13, **A;** 14, **D;** Page 192. The sympathetic portion of the autonomic nervous system influences the orgasmic phase. Medications, including the antihypertensive drugs reserpine and clonidine, may affect orgasmic response. Much of the response in the excitement phase is due to stimulation of the parasympathetic fibers of the autonomic nervous system. It is during the plateau stage that there is a marked degree of vasocongestion. This vasocongestion is prominent in the lower third of the vagina and is known as the orgasmic platform.

15. **C** (2, 3); Pages 201-202. In the immediate grief period, the bereaved often feels guilt. Although you should acknowledge her shock, guilt, and grief, you should not add to it. It is counterproductive to talk to her about working during her recent pregnancy. Self-help groups have a great deal to offer patients who suffer a pregnancy loss. If the local group is appropriate for the needs of a given patient, a referral should be made. One investigator has found that grieving couples prefer to receive support and help in dealing with the reality of the loss rather than focus on other life events, such as the next pregnancy.
16. **C** (2, 3); Pages 194, 197. Couples should be encouraged to communicate their sexual needs to each other so that appropriate stimulation is offered during the arousal period and during intercourse. If the patient is anorgasmic during intercourse but has experienced orgasms, her partner may aid in bringing about an orgasm during intercourse by allowing her to stimulate her

clitoral area or he may do so. Anorgasmia is not known to be secondary to oral contraceptive use. Furthermore, she would have to use a barrier method of contraception. As many as 10-15% of women have never experienced an orgasm through any form of sexual stimulation. The woman should not be made to feel abnormal. Sexuality is a question of pleasure or happiness, not of normalcy.

17. **A** (All); Page 207. Hospice organizations offer psychosocial support to patients and their families. The service includes post-death follow-up. Hospital-based hospice teams may include physicians, nurses, social workers, chaplains, and volunteers who may minister to any patient in any bed. Home care programs are often available.
18. **A** (All); Page 199. Alcoholic strength is often denoted by the percentage of alcohol present. Proof is twice the percentage volume of alcohol. A 12 ounce can of beer, a glass of wine, and 30 ml of either whiskey or a liqueur have the same quantity of alcohol.
19. **B** (1, 2); Page 186. Self-esteem begins to develop in early childhood and is the result of positive efforts. Touching, talking to the child in gentle ways, and praising the child's actions are reasonable steps in reinforcing the child's self-worth. Punishment should be limited to reinforcing the need for setting limits. Intimidation by verbal or physical means should be avoided.
20. **A** (All); Page 200. Most tricyclic drugs, including amitriptyline, have a parasympathomimetic effect. Dryness of the mouth, blurred vision, hesitancy of urination or dribbling, some menstrual disorders, and a decrease in sexual arousal are often complaints associated with their use.
21. **E** (3); Pages 200-201. Although patients may note a reduction in depressive symptoms after 1 or 2 weeks of drug use, real improvement may take as long as 1 month. It is unnecessary to add a second drug. A tricyclic may enhance the response to alcohol. This can increase the danger of a suicide attempt or overdosage. It would be best to reassure this patient and tell her it is too soon to expect improvement.

CHAPTER

8 Diagnostic Procedures

DIRECTIONS for questions 1 - 21: Select the one best answer or completion.

1. A 22-year-old, 5 feet 6 inch, 125 lb., gravida 0 says that her last normal menstrual period was 8 weeks ago. Two hours ago she had the acute onset of severe RLQ pain. Two days ago she noticed vaginal spotting.

   On examination, the BP is found to be 90/60 and the pulse 110. The abdomen appears distended. A pelvic examination is difficult to interpret because the patient is so tender that she does not allow a reasonable evaluation. Your next step would be a
   A. β-HCG
   B. hysteroscopy
   C. culdocentesis
   D. laparoscopic examination
   E. laparotomy
2. The optimal pressure in mm Hg for performing an adequate endometrial aspiration for an elective termination is
   A. 100-200
   B. 201-300
   C. 301-400
   D. 401-500
   E. 501-600
3. On examination a patient has moderately severe cervical stenosis. She is about to have an endometrial biopsy as part of an infertility investigation. The anesthesia of choice is a
   A. pudendal
   B. paracervical
   C. epidural
   D. spinal
   E. general
4. The complications associated with hysteroscopy when the distending media is 5% dextrose and water include all of the following **EXCEPT**
   A. uterine perforation
   B. bleeding
   C. pelvic infection
   D. circulatory overload
   E. cardiac arrest
5. The successful reversal of a previous sterilization procedure is most likely to follow a
   A. Pomeroy tubal ligation
   B. Irving tubal ligation
   C. laparoscopic tubal fulguration
   D. laparoscopic tubal application of Silastic bands
   E. laparoscopic tubal application of Hulka clips
6. All of the following are recognized procedures performed through a laparoscope **EXCEPT**
   A. evaluation of a 25 cm intra-abdominal mass
   B. laser ablation of an endometriotic implant
   C. ovarian biopsy for karyotype
   D. lysis of adhesions
   E. evacuation of a small ectopic pregnancy
7. Ultrasound is useful in all of the following **EXCEPT**
   A. determining when to give β-Hcg in ovulation induction
   B. assisting in the laparoscopic egg retrieval process
   C. assisting in the transvesical egg retrieval process
   D. documenting when ovulation has occurred
   E. preventing the hyperstimulation syndrome
8. An infertility patient has a history of a 28-day cycle. She has an endometrial biopsy performed as part of the investigation 6 days after her basal body chart temperature rises. The narrative of the report states that one strip of endometrium is day 19 and the other proliferative. You conclude that the patient has
   A. a luteal phase defect
   B. irregular shedding
   C. a normal ovulatory response
   D. an abnormal ovulatory response
   E. an uninterpretable result resulting from a lab error
9. The patient depicted in Figure 8-1 was referred for pelvic ultrasound because of increasing girth. The diagnosis is

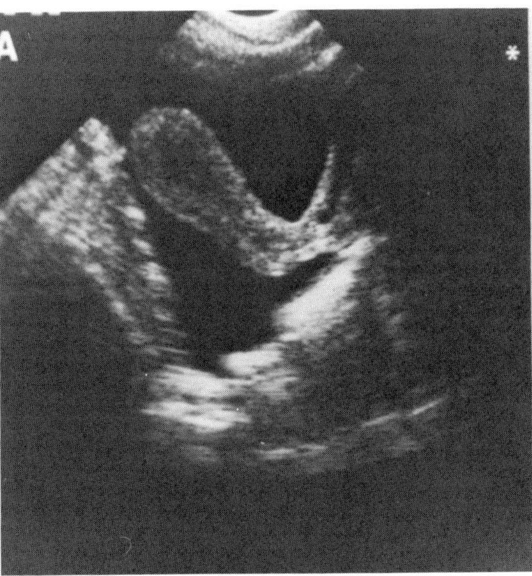

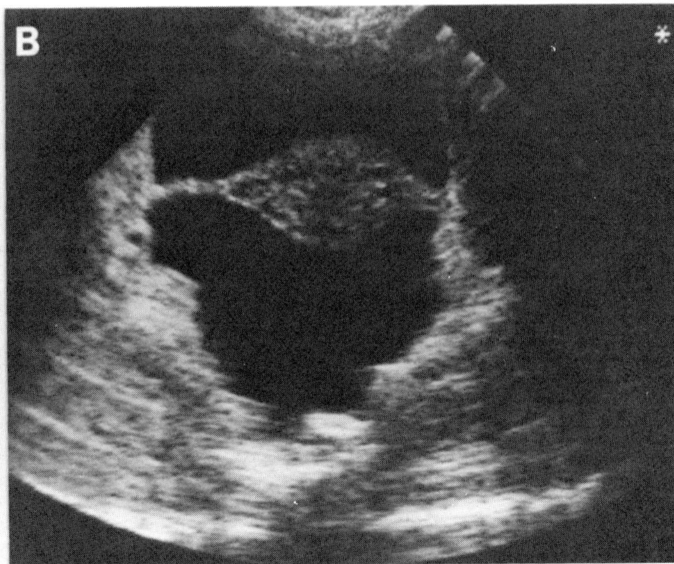

FIGURE 8-1.
(A) Longitudinal view of the pelvis. (B) Transverse view of the pelvis.

A. an early intrauterine pregnancy
B. a molar pregnancy
C. a ruptured tubal pregnancy
D. ascites
E. ovarian carcinoma

10. A 48-year-old woman who had an endometrial biopsy 6 months ago returns for a scheduled visit. The pathology report indicated proliferative endometrium. Since her biopsy, this patient has bled every 2 weeks for 8-12 days. She uses 10-15 pads a day, but states this is not a problem. You advise
A. a repeat visit in 6 months
B. an endometrial biopsy
C. endometrial cytological sampling
D. a dilation and curettage
E. a hysterectomy

11. A 35 year-old gravida 3, para 0-0-3-0 has been married to the same man for 15 years. The three losses were at 18, 22, and 25 weeks of gestation. While undergoing hysteroscopy the patient is found to have intrauterine septa. All other studies on both husband and wife are within normal limits. The next step in the care of this patient would be a
A. Tompkins metroplasty
B. Jones metroplasty
C. hysteroscopic metroplasty
D. verification by hysterosalpingography
E. MacDonald cerclage

12. All of the following are recognized indications for hysteroscopy **EXCEPT**
A. infertility
B. suspicion of uterine synechiae
C. repetitive abortions
D. abnormal vaginal bleeding
E. oligomenorrhea

13. The failure rate of laparoscopic tubal interruption procedures is around
A. <1/1000
B. 1/1000
C. 3/1000
D. 6/1000
E. >6/1000

14. Which of the following modalities utilizes beam attenuation that results from different densities in adjacent tissues?
A. ultrasonography
B. magnetic resonance imaging
C. computed tomography
D. scintillation scan
E. tomography

15. An endometrial biopsy is useful in the diagnosis of all of the following **EXCEPT**
A. pelvic tuberculosis
B. luteal phase defect
C. adenomatous endometrial hyperplasia
D. adenomyosis
E. abnormal uterine bleeding

16. Major complications attributed to laparoscopy include all of the following **EXCEPT**
A. cardiac arrhythmias
B. gas embolism

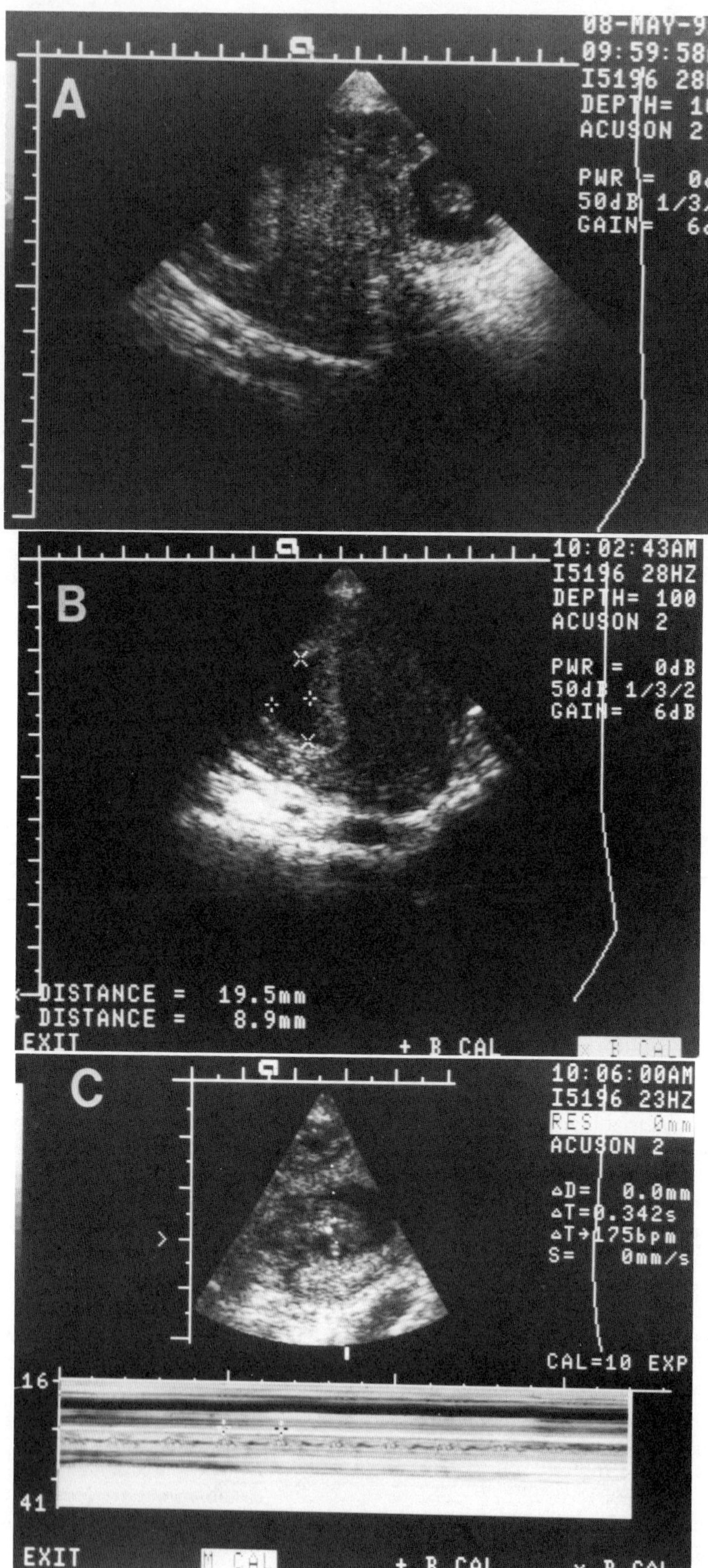

FIGURE 8-2.

Endovaginal scans. (A) Coronal View. (B) Enlargement of A taken slightly to the patient's right. (C) Enlargement of A taken to the patient's left.

C. laceration of the epigastric artery
D. intestinal perforation
E. hypocarbia

17. The patient is a 22-year-old gravida 0. Until 12 weeks ago she was taking a low dose oral contraceptive. Her last menstrual period was 9 weeks ago. For the last 6 weeks the patient has had intermittent spotting. An ultrasound done at another facility reported that the patient had an empty gestational sac. Quantitative β-Hcg determinations have been rising. The last β-Hcg, obtained 2 days ago, was 40,000 mIu/ml. The patient is referred to you for care.

    The endovaginal sonogram you ordered is depicted in Figure 8-2. Vital signs are normal and stable. Proper management includes

    A. a quantitative β-Hcg
    B. culdocentesis
    C. diagnostic laparoscopy
    D. pelviscopy
    E. laparotomy

18. Hysterosalpingography is useful in the diagnosis of all of the following **EXCEPT**

    A. an incompetent cervix
    B. intermenstrual spotting (metrorrhagia)
    C. peritubal adhesions
    D. acute endometritis
    E. a submucous myoma

19. Given the endovaginal ultrasound image depicted in Figure 8-3, one would conclude that the patient has

    A. a benign cystic teratoma
    B. a tubal ovarian complex
    C. a ruptured ectopic pregnancy
    D. an unruptured ectopic pregnancy
    E. no evidence of pathology

20. CS is a 41 year-old who is recovering from a saggiatal sinus thrombosis which occurred 2 months ago. This episode did not leave her with a neurological deficit. She has a blood dyscrasia, but her hematologists have not been able specifically to characterize the abnormality. Presently, the patient is on coumadin to prevent recurrence.

    CS had complained of extremely heavy flow. Her hemoglobin had been 8 gm/100 ml and the uterus was described as 10 week-sized, smooth, and regular. In the past she was placed on provera to diminish her menstrual flow, but she continued to have heavy periods.

    For the past month the patient has been on a parenteral gonadotropin releasing hormone agonist. Her flow has diminished to almost nothing.

    The long term management you would suggest is

    A. long term high dose provera
    B. long term releasing hormone agonist
    C. endometrial ablation
    D. bilateral hypogastric ligation
    E. hysterectomy

21. The use of high molecular weight dextran to expand the endometrial cavity during hysteroscopy is preferred because it

    A. is non-biodegradable
    B. is nonantigenic

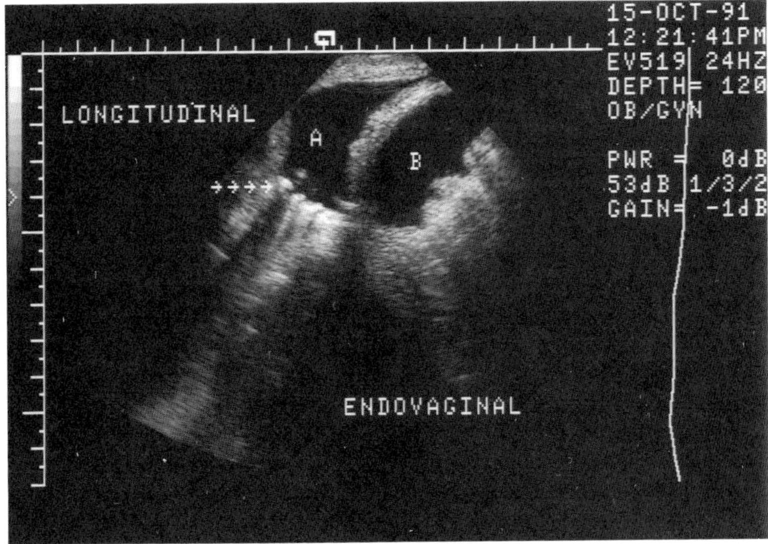

FIGURE 8-3.

C. is miscible with blood
D. is nonconductive
E. does not crystallize

DIRECTIONS for questions 22 - 30: For each numbered item, select the one heading most closely associated with it. Each lettered heading may be used once, more than once, or not at all.

22-23. A woman who has had severe PID is eventually found to have a ruptured tubal pregnancy with 300 ml of blood in the peritoneal cavity.

Match the culdocentesis results:

(A) 5 ml clotted blood, hematocrit 30%
(B) 5 ml unclotted blood, hematocrit 17%
(C) 5 ml unclotted blood, hematocrit 9%
(D) 5 ml serosanguineous fluid, hematocrit 7%
(E) no fluid after several attempts

22. extensive adhesions in the cul-de-sac
23. true positive

24-26. Pick the procedure that is the most definitive and cost effective in making the diagnosis:

(A) hysteroscopy with or without biopsy
(B) hysterosalpingogram
(C) dilation and curettage
(D) laparoscopy
(E) endovaginal ultrasound

24. a submucous myoma
25. peritubal adhesions
26. an unruptured tubal pregnancy at 6 weeks (menstrual dates)

27-30. Assume that your hospital is capable of supporting all the procedures listed below. Choose the appropriate initial procedure after a complete history and physical:

(A) hysteroscopy
(B) laparoscopy
(C) computed tomography
(D) pelvic ultrasound
(E) magnetic resonance imaging

27. A 28-year-old gravida 0 who is 5 feet 6 inches tall and weighs 134 pounds has been trying to get pregnant for 3 years. Her husband has a normal semen analysis. She ovulates and has good midcycle mucus.
28. A 30-year-old mentally retarded gravida 0 who is 5 feet 1 inches tall and weighs 190 pounds complains of pelvic pain. She is vague in her description of the pain and is impossible to examine.
29. A 25-year-old gravida 2, para 1 ab 1, had an induced abortion 1 year ago. Since then she has had amenorrhea and intermittent pelvic pain.
30. A 30-year-old gravida 6, para 6 who is 5 feet 6 inches tall and weighs 130 pounds has a 5 cm cervical lesion. This is histologically a squamous cell carcinoma.

DIRECTIONS For each numbered item 31 - 33, indicate whether it is associated with

A only (A)
B only (B)
C both (A) and (B)
D neither (A) nor (B)

(A) Sonogram labeled A in Figure 8-4
(B) Sonogram labeled B in Figure 8-4
(C) Both sonograms
(D) Neither sonogram

31. linear phased array
32. employs the piezoelectric effect
33. the transducer transmits 60% of the time and receives 40% of the time

DIRECTIONS for questions 34 - 44: For each of the questions below, ONE or MORE of the responses is correct. Select the best answer based on the following

A if 1, 2, and 3 are correct
B if only 1 and 2 are correct
C if only 2 and 3 are correct
D if only 1 is correct
E if only 3 is correct

34. M.S. is a 25-year-old gravida 0. She has been trying to conceive for 5 years. Her past history includes menses every 28-30 days and flow for 3 days with moderate dysmenorrhea the first 2 days. She had an acute pelvic infection at age 22 for which she had to be hospitalized. She has not had a clinical recurrence or reinfection. Her gall bladder was removed at age 20 for stones. She is allergic to shell fish. She smokes one pack of cigarettes a day and is a social drinker. Her physical examination, including a pelvic examination, is normal.

    This patient's investigation should include a(n)

    1. chromopertubation at laparoscopy
    2. pelvic ultrasound
    3. hysterosalpingogram

35. Complications following an endometrial biopsy include
    1. infection
    2. perforation
    3. hypotension
36. Hysterosalpingography is useful in the diagnosis of
    1. Asherman's syndrome (endometrial sclerosis)
    2. müllerian anomalies
    3. accessory ostia of the fallopian tubes
37. Procedures that can be performed through a hysteroscope include
    1. removal of a submucous myoma
    2. laser ablation of the endometrium

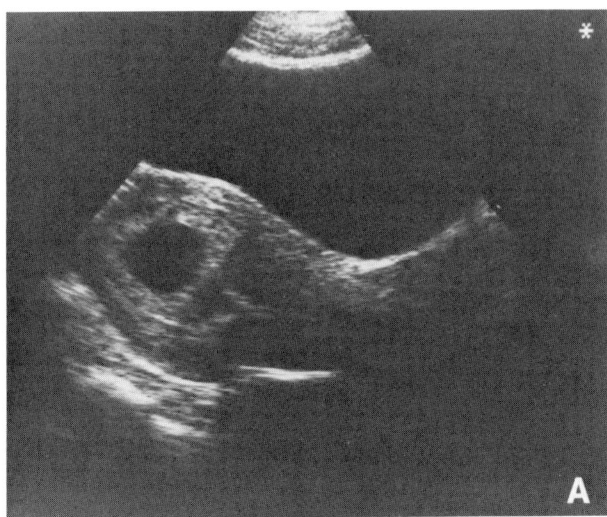

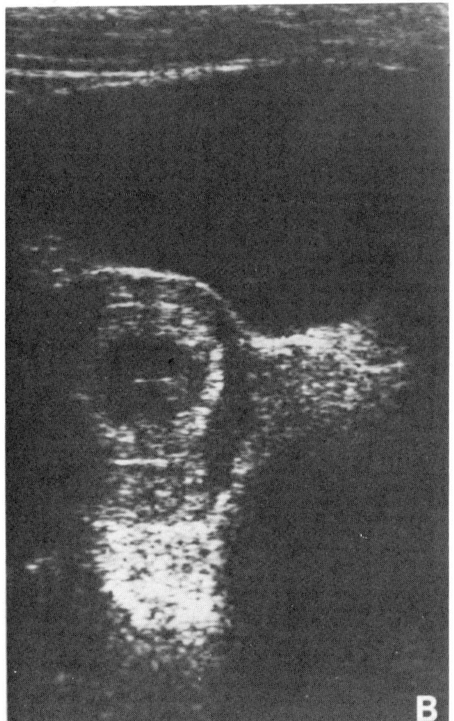

FIGURE 8-4.

3. cannulation of the ostia of the fallopian tubes

38. Figure 8-5 is a CT scan of a patient who on examination is felt to have a pelvic mass. One is able to say that
    1. there are metastases
    2. the patient is under 20 years of age
    3. the mass is thin walled
39. The patient pictured in Figure 8-6 is 25 years old and wishes to have children. You would recommend
    1. insertion of a Foley catheter
    2. premarin 7.5 mg per day
    3. transabdominal metroplasty
40. True statements about magnetic resonance imaging include:
    1. it does not penetrate air and bone
    2. it utilizes nonionizing radiation
    3. tomographic images are possible in coronal, sagittal, or transverse planes
41. A 1984 Consensus Conference issued a Statement of Caution in the use of diag-

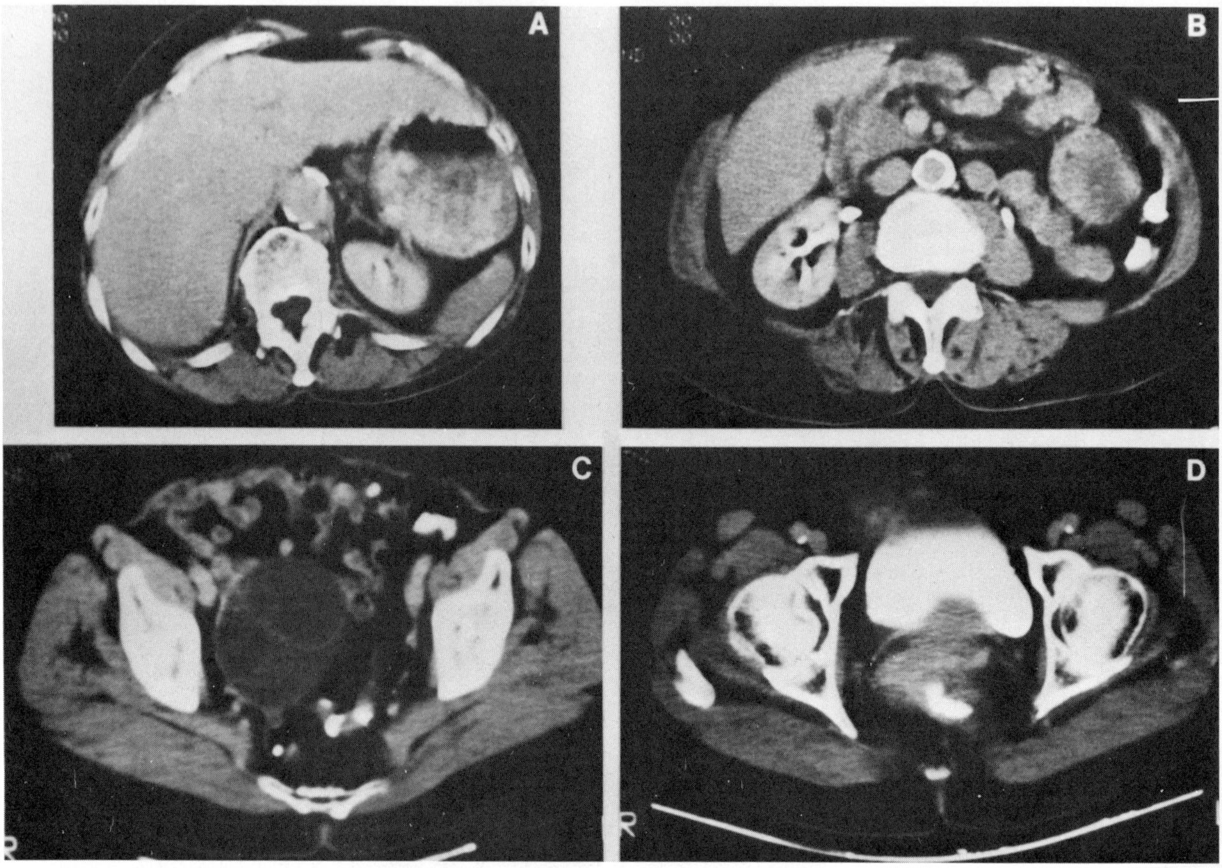

FIGURE 8-5.
(A) Computed tomography scan. (A), at the level of the liver; (B), below A; (C), above D; (D), at the level of the bladder.

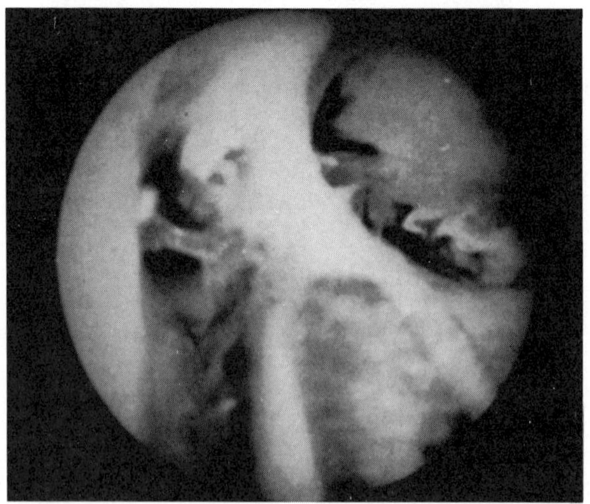

FIGURE 8-6.
Hysteroscopic view
(From Droegemueller W, Herbst AL, Mishell DR, Stenchever MA: Comprehensive Gynecology, St. Louis, 1987, The C. V. Mosby Co., p. 216.)

nostic ultrasound despite 20 years of clinical use with NO known adverse effects. The rationale was based on in vitro studies that demonstrated
1. changes in sister chromatid exchange frequency
2. an increase in the immune response
3. formation of new macromolecules

42. True statements about computed tomography include:
    1. the radiation dose to the midpelvis is 50% of the surface dose
    2. it is useful in confirming the diagnosis of ovarian thrombophlebitis
    3. the radiation dose is similar to a barium enema
43. Endometrial cytological sampling
    1. should be placed in Bouin's
    2. has a false negative rate of 5% to 15%
    3. can not be performed in women over 70 years of age
44. A 40 year-old gravida 0 who is diabetic is felt on pelvic examination to have 18 week-sized myomata. Before performing a total abdominal hysterectomy, one should obtain
    1. a pelvic ultrasound
    2. an endometrial biopsy
    3. a random blood glucose

ANSWERS

1. **C,** Pages 225-227. This patient is acutely ill. There is not time to get a β-Hcg. Besides, a positive test won't differentiate an intrauterine from an extrauterine pregnancy. An ultrasound was not a choice. If it had been, one would have to consider how long it would take to perform this examination. Is the ultrasound unit in the immediate area? Is endovaginal scanning possible or does the patient need to have a full bladder before adequate visualization can be accomplished? There are few contraindications to hysteroscopy. Active bleeding is a relative contraindication. This patient had noted vaginal spotting. Pregnancy is a contraindication to hysteroscopy and this patient's last period was 8 weeks ago. Although invasive, a culdocentesis is likely to be helpful and it is inexpensive. A laparoscopy would be unnecessary, even contraindicated in the presence of a massive hematoperitoneum and this patient's signs and symptoms suggest that possibility. A laparoscopy might be indicated if the culdocentesis were negative. A laparotomy is not in order until there is more evidence that the patient has a surgical abdomen.
2. **E,** Page 229. To denude the endometrium completely, the optimum pressure for aspiration is 500 to 600 mm Hg.
3. **B,** Page 228. An endometrial biopsy is usually performed without any anesthesia. In the presence of cervical stenosis, a paracervical will block transmission from fibers in the cervical ganglion. Occasionally, the endocervical application of viscous lidocaine 2-4% may decrease discomfort. Twenty percent benzocaine gel applied topically to the cervical os on a cotton-tipped applicator may also serve as an effective anesthetic.
4. **E,** Page 240. Complications of hysteroscopy include uterine perforation, pelvic infection, and bleeding. The potential complications of the distending media include circulatory overload with 5% dextrose and water. Anaphylaxis is a complication associated with the use of dextran. The potential of gas embolism exists with the use of carbon dioxide as the distending media. Cardiac arrests have been reported with uterine insufflation with CO_2 when unmonitored amounts of gas were used.
5. **E,** Page 242. The spring-loaded clip causes necrosis of less than 1 cm of the tube and is the easiest sterilization procedure to reverse successfully.
6. **A,** Page 243. An absolute contraindication to laparoscopy is a large intraperitoneal or pelvic mass. Laser ablation of an endometriotic implant, ovarian biopsy, lysis of adhesions, and evacuation of a small ectopic pregnancy are recognized therapeutic laparoscopic procedures.
7. **B,** Pages 214-217. When a dominant follicle has reached a size of 18 to 20 mm, one can give β-Hcg to induce ovulation. Since the ovary is visible at laparoscopy, ultrasound would offer little or nothing to egg retrieval via the laparoscope. On the other hand, eggs have been successfully retrieved using a percutaneous transvesical, transurethral transvesical, or transvaginal approach under direct ultrasonic guidance. If the dominant mature follicle, seen a day or two prior, disappears, it is good presumptive evidence that ovulation has occurred. In most cases, the hyperstimulation syndrome can be avoided in patients undergoing ovulation induction if β-Hcg is withheld when multiple follicles have reached a critical size, i.e., 16 mm or greater.

8. **C,** Page 228. The endometrium of the isthmus may be out of phase and give a false impression of lack of progesterone production. In this case one of the strips in all probability came from the isthmus. The description is that of a normal ovulatory response. If there is a luteal phase defect, the endometrium should be more than 48 hours less than the 20 days expected given this patient's menstrual history. It should be noted, however, when doing an endometrial biopsy as a part of an infertility investigation, one should perform the biopsy later in the cycle in order to be in a position to make the diagnosis of a luteal phase defect. Irregular shedding should be diagnosed on the fifth or sixth day of bleeding.
9. **D,** Pages 215-217. Water, urine, and ascitic fluid are all extremely echolucent. Blood is usually more complex. In the longitudinal view there is no evidence of a gestational sac, blood, or tissue inside of the uterus. The ovaries are not seen in the transverse view shown in Figure 8-1. There is no mass in the pelvis. This is a woman with ascites due to cirrhosis.
10. **D,** Pages 231-232, 237. The diagnostic accuracy of endometrial biopsy in diagnosing malignancy is 90% to 98% when compared to subsequent findings at dilation and curettage or at hysterectomy. The gold standard is dilation and curettage. Therefore, if abnormal perimenopausal bleeding recurs following an endometrial biopsy, a dilation and curettage should be performed to rule out carcinoma. In the future, hysteroscopy may replace many diagnostic D&C procedures. No matter how meticulous the surgeon is, he or she may miss a focal lesion, particularly pedunculated structures. Dilation and curettage is a blind hit-or-miss procedure.
11. **C,** Pages 238, 239. A cerclage is indicated if the recurrent abortions are the result of an incompetent cervix. Both the Tompkins and Jones procedures are done abdominally. Transabdominal metroplasty involves a uterine incision, necessitating that future pregnancies be delivered by cesarean. Hysteroscopy is superior to hysterosalpingography in discovering intrauterine disease. In comparative studies, the use of hysteroscopy revealed synechiae, polyps, or myomas in 40% of patients with normal hysterosalpingograms. Hysteroscopic metroplasty of intrauterine septa has been very successful and is safer with fewer complications than laparotomy. However, concurrent laparoscopy is advocated by most investigators to evaluate the rest of the pelvis.
12. **E,** Pages 235, 237. Indications for hysteroscopy include recurrent abnormal bleeding, repetitive abortion, uterine synechiae, abnormal hysterosalpingograms, and infertility. A patient with oligomenorrhea probably has an ovulatory problem that would not be diagnosed by hysteroscopy. Furthermore, the procedure should not be done if there is any chance of an existing intrauterine pregnancy.
13. **C,** Page 241. The failure rate of laparoscopic tubal sterilization is approximately 1 in 250 to 1 in 500 cases.
14. **C,** Pages 214, 218, 227. Sonography utilizes sound waves that are reflected from interfaces back to the transducer. A CT scan identifies gross distortions in local anatomy by using the difference in x-ray beam attenuation that results from different densities in adjacent tissues. Magnetic resonance imaging uses radiofrequency radiation and a varying magnetic field. Prior to a scintillation scan, a radioisotope is injected. The liquid or crystal radiation detector "records" the x or gamma rays emitted from the subject. To perform tomography, objects out of the plane of interest are blurred during an x-ray study by simultaneously moving the x-ray tube and the recording plate.
15. **D,** Pages 227, 230. There are endometrial changes with pelvic tuberculosis and adenomatous endometrial hyperplasia. A timed biopsy is one of the principal methods used to establish a luteal phase defect. In this era of cost containment endometrial biopsy, not a dilation and curettage in the hospital under general anesthesia, is the preferred first step in the evaluation of abnormal uterine bleeding. Adenomyosis is a disease of the myometrium, not the endometrium. The diagnosis cannot be made by endometrial biopsy; it is a clinical diagnosis confirmed only on microscopic evaluation of the myometrium. Several reports in the past five years have documented the advantage of magnetic resonance imaging in diagnosing and evaluating adenomyosis.
16. **E,** Pages 246, 250. The major complications of laparoscopy are laceration of vessels, intestinal injuries, and complications of the pneumoperitoneum, which include pneumothorax, diminished venous return,

gas embolism, and cardiac arrhythmias. The most frequent complication of laparoscopy is **hypercarbia**, not hypocarbia, associated with hypoventilation.

17. **D,** Pages 215, 225, 240. Figure 8-2A shows a uterus and a left adnexal mass which is compatible with a tubal pregnancy. The fluid within the uterine cavity has been measured in Figure 8-2B, while cardiac activity is demonstrated by M mode in Figure 8-2C. The latter is an endovaginal view of the left adnexal mass seen in Figure 8-2A. With an endovaginal ultrasound, intrauterine pregnancies may be visualized as early as 4 weeks after the last menstrual period with an β-Hcg titer of approximately 1,000 mIu. A pregnancy should be routinely visualized by 5 postmenstrual weeks, at which time the gestational sac is 4 mm in diameter. Since an ectopic pregnancy has been established, a quantitative β-Hcg, diagnostic laparoscopy, and a culdocentesis are unnecessary. The latter would be negative since the scan suggests that the pregnancy is unruptured. If there were fluid in the cul-de-sac, on ultrasound one would expect to see an echolucent area behind the uterus. The question is whether to treat by laparotomy or pelviscopy. This is a small gestation and could easily be removed through a laparoscope.
18. **D,** Pages 232, 235. Although the anatomical changes in the diameter of the internal os in the nonpregnant state may have little predictive value for future competency in pregnancy, hysterosalpingography measurements are used by some to make the presumptive diagnosis. Metrorrhagia might be secondary to endometrial polyps or submucous myoma, both of which can be seen on hysterosalpingogram. Heavy acute abnormal uterine bleeding and acute pelvic infection are contraindications to the procedure. Hysterosalpingography discovers only 50% of peritubal disease diagnosed by direct visualization via the laparoscope.
19. **E,** Page 214. In figure 8-3 Labels A and B are within a cystic structure. Note that the contour of these structures is wavy. Using real time one would note movement. The arrows point to an echodense line beneath which there is shadowing. This represents gas within bowel (labels A and B). Hence, there is no pathology. A disadvantage of ultrasound is its poor penetration of bone and air. Thus the symphysis pubis and air-filled bowel loops often inhibit visualization.
20. **C,** Page 240. This patient has previously failed on provera. Besides, the use of provera in a patient who has recently had a thrombotic episode should be questioned. Use of a releasing hormone agonist is extremely expensive. Its long term use has not been approved. This patient is at risk for any operative procedure, particularly a major procedure such as a hypogastric ligation or hysterectomy. There is no reason to suspect that a hypogastric ligation would be of any benefit to this patient. The incidence of thrombotic problems following hysterectomy are well known. Laser ablation of the endometrial lining is a viable option. The laser photovaporizes the epithelium. This procedure is performed in women with severe dysfunctional uterine bleeding, who are not candidates for hysterectomy. The procedure usually takes one hour and is most effective in producing amenorrhea in women over 40. Electrocoagulation with a resectoscope or a rollerball may also be used for endometrial ablation. Although these procedures are generally safe and effective, long-term follow-up and information about endometrial carcinoma in unablated foci has not been determined. Endometrial ablation, by either electrocautery or laser, produces amenorrhea in approximately half of patients, with substantially decreased bleeding in another 40%.
21. **D,** Page 237. High molecular weight dextran is biodegradable, nontoxic, nonconductive, and immiscible with blood. It is antigenic, sometimes causing anaphylaxis. It also rapidly crystallizes; thus, endoscopic instruments must be cleaned shortly after the procedure.

22-23. 22, **E;** 23, **B;** Page 225. It is conceivable that in this patient with a history of severe PID the cul-de-sac was obliterated. Thus, no fluid was obtained which was probably the case in question 22. The diagnosis of a hemoperitoneum is made when 5 ml of unclotted blood with a hematocrit of 15% is withdrawn, the case in question 23.

24-26. 24, **A,** Page 238; 25, **D,** Page 232; 26, **E,** Page 216. Hysteroscopy is superior to hysterosalpingography in discovering and diagnosing intrauterine pathology. Likewise, the laparoscope is better than hysterosalpingography in discovering and diagnosing peritubal pathology. Comparative studies have documented that hysterosalpingography discovers only 50% of the peritubal disease diagnosed by direct visualization via the laparoscope. The only listed options to be considered in answering the question about the unruptured tubal pregnancy are laparoscopy and endopelvic ultrasound. At 6 weeks it is possible that an unruptured ectopic would be missed at the time of laparoscopy. In addition although the question indicates that the patient has this diagnosis, you would be approaching the patient not knowing that this was the problem. The differential would be an intrauterine pregnancy and this diagnosis should be ruled out before an operation, such as laparoscopy, is undertaken. This is probably the most cost effective method of handling this patient although studies substantiating this point have not yet been reported. With an endovaginal probe, intrauterine pregnancies may be visualized as early as 4 weeks after the last menstrual period with an β-Hcg titer of approximately 1,000 mIu. A pregnancy should be routinely be visualized by 5 postmenstrual weeks. In the case of an ectopic pregnancy, the gestational sac, fetal pole, and fetal heart beat can be visualized outside the uterus by 6 weeks.

27. **B,** Page 240. In this hypothetical infertility patient, the male factor and cervical factor would appear to be normal. The patient is said to ovulate. As yet the tubal factor has not been evaluated. This could be done with a hysterosalpingogram or by laparoscopy. Authorities differ in approach. Another option that was not given is an endometrial biopsy to evaluate the luteal phase.
28. **D,** Page 214. The patient is a poor historian. She will not permit a pelvic examination. The least expensive, least invasive procedure possible should be attempted first. This young patient may or may not have pathology. She is difficult or impossible to examine. Although the patient may not allow an endovaginal scan, she probably will cooperate for an abdominal pelvic evaluation. An ultrasound may demonstrate pathology. If there is pathology, a specific diagnosis may only be possible if a more invasive procedure is utilized. If no pathology is found, the best course to follow is observation, providing the history given above is complete and accurate. Another consideration is an examination under anesthesia with laparoscopy if the ultrasound is negative and symptoms continue.
29. **A,** Pages 236-237. It is likely that this patient developed intrauterine synechiae (Asherman's syndrome) following the therapeutic abortion. The intermittent pain that she has could be dysmenorrhea secondary to cervical stenosis, also a possible-consequence of the induced abortion.
30. **C,** Page 218. This is a patient with cervical carcinoma. Often a CT scan will help in the initial evaluation of a pelvic neoplasm, particularly staging. It is more accurate in diagnosing retroperitoneal metastases than intraperitoneal ones. The CT is useful in detecting obstructed ureters and enlarged pelvic and paraaortic nodes that are suspicious for involvement of tumor. MRI also has been used to evaluate local spread but there is only limited experience.

31-33. 31, **B;** 32, **C;** 33, **D;** Pages 214-216. (Ziskin, MC: Basic physics of ultrasound. In Fleischer, AC, Romero, R, Manning, FA, Jeanty, P, and James AE (eds.): The principles and practice of ultrasonography in obstetrics and gynecology, ed. 4, New York, 1991, Appleton & Lange, p. 7.) The picture obtained with a sector scan format is pie-shaped as seen in Figure 8-4 (A). Although the transducer is held stationary, incorporated within the transducer is an oscillating acoustic mirror for beam steering. The format of a linear array is rectangular which is demonstrated in Figure 8-4 (B). The transducer of the sector scan is usually small, and thus it is easier to use to look at nonpregnant pelvic structures. Most endovaginal probes employ sector technology. Because the transducer is closer to the pelvic organs than when a transabdominal approach is used, the resolution is often superior. In Figure 8-4 (A) the bladder is full. An endovaginal scan is performed with an empty bladder and the sound encounters the cervix, not the anterior abdominal wall first. The piezoelectric effect is the generation of an electric voltage when a crystal is compressed. Ultrasound transducers are made up of piezoelectric crystals. When the crystals receive an electric charge, they vibrate and emit acoustic pulses. Acoustic echoes return from the tissues being scanned and cause the piezoelectric crystals to vibrate again and release an electric charge. The electric charges from the various crystals are then integrated by a computer in the machine to display a two-dimensional image. The transducer emits sound only

0.01% of the time. Most of the time it is receiving, **NOT** sending, sound pulses.

34. **D** (1 only), Page 235. A pelvic sonogram is not indicated in the investigation of an infertility patient if the physical examination is normal. The problem is this patient's previous infection and her allergy to fish. People who are allergic to shellfish often are allergic to iodine, which is found in the dye used for hysterosalpingography. The incidence of allergic reactions and the severity of these reactions, if they occur, are much less with the newer non-ionic contrast media. [Katayama, H., et al., *Adverse reactions to ionic and nonionic contrast media. A report from the Japanese Committee on the Safety of Contrast Media.* Radiology, 1990. **175**(3): p. 621-8.] Acute pelvic infection serious enough to require hospitalization develops in 0.3% to 3.1% of patients who have a hysterosalpingogram. This incidence of pelvic infection is directly related to the population studied, being more common in women with dilated tubes. For this reason, it would be wise to look at the tubes directly. If they are grossly distorted, the diagnosis has been made. If they appear relatively normal, chromopertubation at laparoscopy can be carried out. Prophylactic antibiotics would be appropriate.
35. **A** (1, 2, 3), Page 229. The major complication related to an endometrial biopsy is uterine perforation, which occurs in 1 or 2 cases per 1000. Infection and postoperative bleeding are rare. Some women develop a severe vasovagal reflex.
36. **A** (1, 2, 3), Pages 232-235. Asherman's syndrome (endometrial sclerosis) can be identified by slowly injecting a water-soluble medium under fluoroscopic control. Hysterosalpingography is a safe and rapid means of investigating abnormalities of the müllerian ducts. Tubal anomalies, including diverticula and accessory ostia, can be diagnosed by hysterosalpingography.
37. **A** (1, 2, 3), Pages 236-237. Procedures performed under hysteroscopic guidance include location and removal of intact or fragmented IUDs, resection of submucous myomas, lysis of synechiae, incision of uterine septa, removal of endometrial polyps, laser ablation of the endometrium, and placement of silicone plugs into the tubes for sterilization.
38. **E** (3 only), Pages 218, 221-222. The scan depicted in Figure 8-5 D is that of a bladder filled with contrast medium, indented by a uterus that appears normal in this view. In Figure 8-5 A there is a scan of a normal liver. None of the scans suggests lymph node involvement. The patient is probably older than 20, since her aorta is calcified (Figure 8-5 B). Figure 8-5 C shows a thin-walled pelvic mass, probably benign, probably ovarian.
39. **B** (1, 2,), Page 239. Figure 8-6 is a hysteroscopic view of uterine synechiae which can be cut with a pair of microscissors. Then a large Foley catheter is placed in the cavity as a splint. For the next two months the patient should receive 7.5 mg of conjugated estrogen per day. This procedure and postoperative therapy avoids a transabdominal metroplasty.
40. **C** (2, 3), Pages 222-223, 248. Magnetic resonance imaging utilizes nonionizing radiation. Because it can penetrate both bone and air, it allows identification of soft tissue pathology inaccessible to other imaging techniques. It has the capacity to differentiate between normal and malignant tissue. Images are tomographic and may be visualized in coronal, sagittal, or transverse planes.
41. **D** (1 only), Page 214. The National Institutes of Health has recently reviewed the potential harmful effects of ultrasound studied in laboratory experiments. They discovered reduction in immune response, changes in sister chromatid exchange frequency, cell death, changes in function of cell membranes, and degradation of macromolecules. Greater attention has been directed toward the safety of ultrasonic equipment. The 1981 AIUM/NEMA *Safety Standard for Diagnostic Ultrasound Equipment* (J. Ultrasound Med., 2:S1-S49, April, 1983) was revised in late 1986. The current recommendation for clinical obstetrical ultrasound equipment is an intensity of energy waves of less than 100 mW/cm_2 of tissue being exposed.
42. **A** (1, 2, 3), Pages 218, 221-222. The radiation dose of computed tomography to the midpelvis is approximately 50% of the 2 to 10 rad surface dose. This radiation exposure is similar to that of a barium enema. This modality is more accurate in diagnosing retroperitoneal metastases than intraperitoneal ones. A CT scan is able to identify a node when it reaches a diameter of 1.5 to 2 cm, and it is an excellent technique for confirming the diagnosis of ovarian vein thrombophlebitis.

43. **B** (1, 2), Page 230. To preserve cytonuclear detail, the cellular material from endometrial cytological sampling should be placed in Bouin's solution rather than in formalin. The false negative rate is between 5% and 15% when compared to material from dilation and curettage or hysterectomy. This is identical to the false negative rate of cytological screening associated with invasive carcinoma of the cervix. Although endometrial cytological sampling can be difficult in older women, age is not the limiting factor. Sampling success is determined by the status of the endocervical and endometrial canal. Women in this age group who are not on estrogen replacement therapy often have a pinpoint os.
44. **E** (3 only), Pages 217, 231-232. It is unnecessary and expensive to verify the obvious [Johnson, H.A., *Diminishing returns on the road to diagnostic certainty.* JAMA, 1991. **265**(17): p. 2229-31.] Therefore, ultrasound is not indicated. One can only condemn the practice of substituting a pelvic ultrasound for a pelvic examination. Routine preoperative endometrial biopsy in asymptomatic women undergoing hysterectomy has not been shown to be necessary. Since this patient is a diabetic, the degree to which this is controlled must be ascertained.

PART THREE GENERAL GYNECOLOGY

CHAPTER 9 Congenital Abnormalities

DIRECTIONS for questions 1 - 6: Select the one best answer or completion.

1. A 25 year old female treated by another physician for congenital adrenal hyperplasia (CAH) presents for a premarital examination. This patient
   A. is likely to be infertile
   B. is likely to be grossly overweight
   C. will transmit the syndrome to all her offsprings
   D. will require cortisol replacement therapy
   E. is likely to have uterine anomalies
2. Laparoscopy is useful during the surgical management of patients with
   A. Rokitansky-Küster-Hauser syndrome
   B. hematocolpos
   C. uterine septum
   D. longitudinal vaginal septum
   E. congenital adrenal hyperplasia
3. If an infant is born with ambiguous genitalia, the physician should
   A. assign the sex as male and change it later if needed
   B. assign the sex as female and change it later if needed
   C. delay gender role assignment until an investigation is complete
   D. assign male sex with no subsequent change
   E. assign female sex with no subsequent change
4. A newborn is seen in the nursery with an enlarged clitoris, hypertension and fusion of the labia. An older sister was diagnosed as having congenital adrenal hyperplasia. The most likely enzyme deficiency is
   A. 5-α-reductase
   B. 21 hydroxylase
   C. 11 hydroxylase
   D. 20,22 desmolase
   E. 3-β-ol dehydrogenase
5. A supernumerary ovary is
   A. the presence of a third ovary separated from the normally situated ovaries
   B. the presence of one large ovary in the midline
   C. the presence of two ovaries, one normal size and the other much larger, both situated on one side
   D. The presence of an ovary in a male with two testes
   E. the presence of excess ovarian tissue near a normally placed ovary and connected to it.
6. In patients with the Rokitansky-Küster-Hauser syndrome, vaginal reconstruction should be performed
   A. when the patient is well motivated
   B. as soon as the condition is diagnosed
   C. in childhood
   D. only after marriage
   E. after coital attempts have been unsuccessful

DIRECTIONS: For each of the questions below, ONE or MORE of the responses is correct. Select the best answer based on the following

A if 1, 2, and 3 are correct
B if only 1 and 2 are correct
C if only 2 and 3 are correct
D if only 1 is correct
E if only 3 is correct

7. Enlargement of the clitoris is often the result of
   1. a müllerian duct defect
   2. an estrogen deficiency
   3. androgen stimulation
8. True statements concerning congenital adrenal hyperplasia (CAH) include
   1. CAH is an autosomal recessive disorder
   2. the most common form is a deficiency of 21 hydroxylase

3. the gene for this enzyme is coded on chromosome 6

9. A newborn is found to have the findings seen in Figure 9-1. Explanations for this finding include
   1. in utero exposure to 19 nor-progestins
   2. congenital adrenal hyperplasia
   3. the child is a true hermaphrodite
10. Guidelines for treatment of children losing salt due to congenital adrenal hyperplasia include
    1. serial measurements of 17 hydroxy-progesterone
    2. frequent determination of blood electrolytes
    3. maintenance of growth chart
11. Obstructive lesions of the vagina in a 15-year-old girl may result in
    1. amenorrhea
    2. hematocolpos
    3. abdominal pain
12. A significant number of patients with the Rokitansky-Küster-Hauser syndrome often have
    1. primary amenorrhea
    2. urinary tract malformation
    3. ovarian failure
13. A short blind vagina is a clinical finding in patients with
    1. Rokitansky-Küster-Hauser syndrome
    2. androgen insensitivity
    3. congenital adrenal hyperplasia
14. A 16-year-old girl with primary amenorrhea is seen in the clinic. On examination, she is found to have a short blind vagina and no uterus. Proper initial management of a patient with vaginal agenesis includes
    1. vaginoplasty
    2. karyotype
    3. intravenous pyelogram (IVP)
15. In cases of vaginal agenesis, vaginal reconstruction can be achieved by
    1. creating a coital pouch (Williams vulvovaginoplasty)

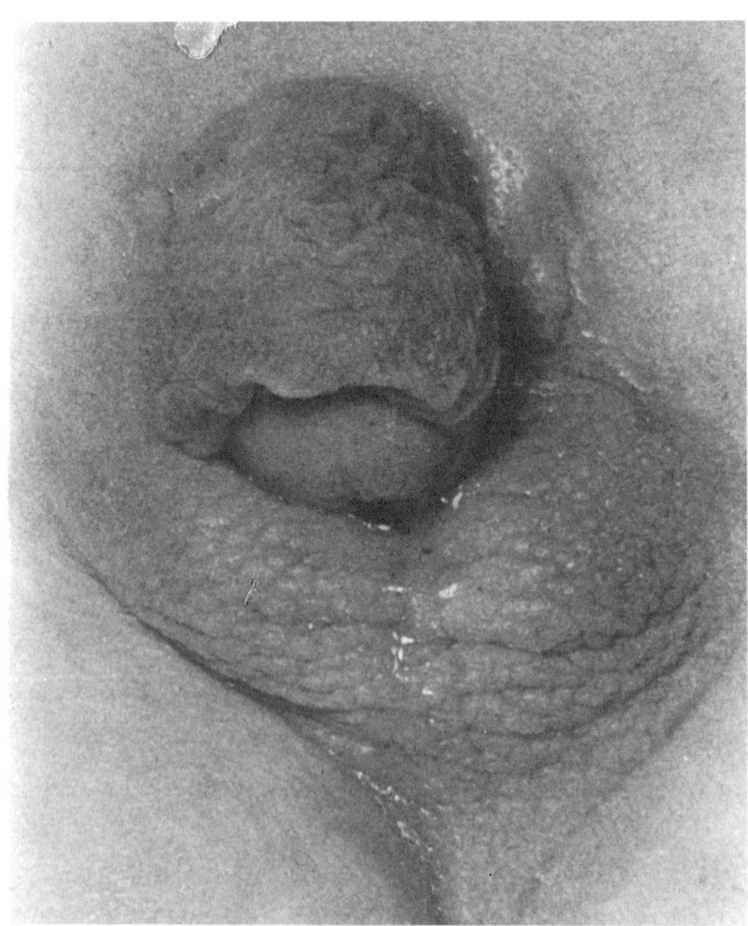

FIGURE 9-1.

2. McIndoe-Reed reconstruction
3. graduated dilatation (Frank's method)

16. True statements concerning transverse vaginal septum include
    1. having menstrual periods excludes the possibility of a transverse vaginal septum
    2. lower vaginal septa are more likely to be complete
    3. upper vaginal septa are more likely to be incomplete
17. Failure of lateral fusion of the müllerian duct may result in
    1. uterus didelphys
    2. a longitudinal vaginal septum
    3. transverse vaginal septum
18. Pregnancy in a rudimentary uterine horn is associated with
    1. fetal death
    2. missed abortion
    3. uterine rupture
19. A non-communicating rudimentary uterine horn
    1. needs to be removed as soon as the diagnosis is made
    2. is often associated with dysmenorrhea
    3. increases the risk of ectopic pregnancy if not removed
20. Anomalies that should be corrected surgically include
    1. a uterus didelphys
    2. an imperforate hymen
    3. a rudimentary uterine horn
21. A septate uterus can be unified by
    1. hysteroscopic division of the septum
    2. a Strassman procedure
    3. a Tompkins procedure
22. Findings helpful in determining whether a child with ambiguous genitalia is a male or female include palpation of
    1. the gonads in the labia or inguinal canal
    2. a uterus on rectal examination
    3. small breast buds
23. A 15 year-old presents with complaints of abdominal pain, a palpable abdominal mass and primary amenorrhea. Diagnoses that should lead the list of considerations include
    1. congenital adrenal hyperplasia
    2. imperforate hymen
    3. transverse vaginal septum
24. Considering the differential diagnosis you generated for question 23, diagnostic tests apt to be helpful in the work-up of the patient described in question 23 include
    1. ultrasound
    2. laparoscopy
    3. an intravenous pyelogram (IVP)
25. Conditions that tend to be diagnosed prior to puberty or adolescence include
    1. congenital adrenal hyperplasia
    2. uterus didelphys
    3. rudimentary uterine horn
26. A patient with five repetitive first trimester abortions underwent a hysterosalpingogram that showed a uterine septum. Proper additional diagnostic studies include
    1. genetic studies on both partners
    2. laparoscopy
    3. endometrial biopsy
27. Absence of the uterus is found in women with
    1. androgen insensitivity syndrome
    2. Rokitansky-Küster-Hauser syndrome
    3. a hematocolpos
28. Impairment of sexual activity is expected in patients with
    1. vaginal agenesis
    2. a transverse vaginal septum
    3. an arcuate uterus
29. A longitudinal vaginal septum is commonly associated with
    1. recurrent vaginal infections
    2. irregular menses
    3. uterus didelphys
30. If untreated, an imperforate hymen may cause
    1. endometriosis
    2. urinary obstruction
    3. abdominal pain

ANSWERS

1. **D,** Pages 257-258. Patients with congenital adrenal hyperplasia have accelerated growth during childhood, but the epiphyseal plates close prematurely, reducing final adult height. When adequately replaced with cortisol, the growth pattern is expected to be normal. As with all autosomal recessive disorders, when both parents are affected, all children are expected to inherit the syndrome. Infertility is not a predominant feature of the disorder, since ovarian function is expected to be normal in patients who are adequately treated. However, some studies have shown that these patients suffer from relative infertility. These patients are not typically obese. Depending upon the defect, there may be masculinization of the external genitalia.
2. **C,** Pages 258-259, 266. Hysteroscopic division of a uterine septum is the preferred method of surgical management. It is monitored by laparoscopy to ensure that

the incision does not extend through the myometrium. Laparoscopy is not indicated for patients with Rokitansky-Küster-Hauser syndrome, in whom the diagnosis is made clinically, and supported by a pelvic sonogram. Similarly, it has no role in the care of patients with hematocolpos or with a longitudinal vaginal septum.

3. **C,** Pages 256-257. An infant born with ambiguous genitalia presents a neonatal emergency. The majority of the virilized females have congenital adrenal hyperplasia (CAH). Some are salt losers, and unless treated with cortisol, they may die of an Addisonian crisis. In order to avoid future change in gender assignment, it is recommended that the decision regarding the newborn's sex be deferred until the investigation is complete.
4. **B,** Page 257. The newborn described has ambiguous genitalia. Most female infants with ambiguous genitalia suffer from congenital adrenal hyperplasia (CAH). In addition, this child has an older sister with CAH, which is an autosomal recessive disorder. Congenital adrenal hyperplasia is not associated with a 5-α-reductase deficiency. The remaining three enzymes listed as options are essential steps in the production of cortisol. Deficiency of 20,22 desmolase, which converts cholesterol to pregnenolone, is usually incompatible with life. Since the child has an older sister, this enzyme is not likely to be affected. The most commonly affected enzyme in patients with CAH is 21 hydroxylase. The second most common is 11 hydroxylase, accounting for about 5% of all patients; it is associated with hypertension.
5. **A,** Pages 255, 268. A supernumerary ovary is defined as the presence of a third ovary separated from the normally situated ovaries, while an accessory ovary is defined as the presence of excess ovarian tissue near a normally placed ovary and connected to it.
6. **A,** Pages 258-259. Patients with vaginal agenesis require vaginal reconstruction. Graduated dilation is probably the preferred method, and should be delayed until the patient is motivated and therefore cooperative. It should be performed after puberty, when the adolescent girl is contemplating sexual activity or marriage. Since sexual activity may commence prior to marriage, marriage should not be a precondition for vaginal reconstruction.
7. **E** (3 only), Pages 256-257. Clitoral enlargement often is the result of excessive androgen stimulation. Estrogen deficiency states or müllerian duct defects do not cause clitoral enlargement. The genital tubercle, from which the clitoris develops, is very sensitive to androgenic stimulation in utero. With age, the sensitivity diminishes, but even late in adult life, prolonged exposure to androgens causes clitoral enlargement.
8. **A** (1, 2, 3), Pages 257-258, 269. Congenital adrenal hyperplasia (CAH) is an autosomal recessive disorder caused by an enzyme deficiency in the pathway of cortisol production. As a result, cortisol levels are low leading to increased ACTH production. Accumulation of cortisol precursors occur. These are converted to androgens that virilize the female infant. In 90-95% of patients with CAH, the deficient enzyme is 21 hydroxylase, the gene for which is coded on chromosome 6.
9. **A** (1, 2, 3), Page 256. An infant with ambiguous genitalia may be a virilized female, an under virilized male or a true hermaphrodite. Female infants may be virilized in utero when exposed to androgens ingested by the mouth (i.e. 19 nor-progestins in oral contraceptive pills, Provera, etc.), or androgens produced by the infants (congenital adrenal hyperplasia, etc.).
10. **A** (1, 2, 3), Pages 257-258. 17 hydroxyprogesterone is the best indicator of adequate cortisol replacement. A less sensitive method is determination of the growth pattern. Too much cortisol replacement retards growth whereas too little accelerates growth. In addition, in patients who are salt losers like this patient, frequent determinations of electrolytes are necessary to monitor replacement therapy.
11. **A** (1, 2, 3), Pages 258, 259, 261, 263. Obstructive lesions of the vagina can cause accumulation of fluid or blood behind the obstructive membrane. Initially, the accumulation is in the vagina, forming a mucocolpos in a child, or hematocolpos in a postmenarcheal girl. As the fluid accumulates, it backs up into the uterus, causing a hematometra and retrograde menstruation through the tubes. The latter results in abdominal pain and the development of endometriosis. The obstruction prevents egress of blood from the vagina, and pri-

mary amenorrhea is one of the diagnostic features of obstructive lesions of the vagina.

12. **B** (1, 2), Pages 258-259. Patients with Rokitansky-Küster-Hauser syndrome suffer from vaginal agenesis and, in most cases, absence of the uterus. They often present with primary amenorrhea. In over 50% of the patients, urinary tract malformation coexists. An intravenous pyelogram (IVP) is indicated for all patients who are diagnosed as having vaginal agenesis. Ovarian development is normal in these patients, and secondary sexual development is expected to be normal. Patients with Rokitansky-Küster-Hauser syndrome usually have a normal (46, XX) karyotype.
13. **B** (1, 2), Page 259. A short blind vagina indicates either vaginal absence, or a transverse septum which shortens the vagina and prevents one from seeing the cervix. Patients with congenital adrenal hyperplasia may have a narrow introitus, but the vagina is of normal length and the cervix is visible.
14. **C** (2, 3), Pages 258-261. A patient with vaginal agenesis will probably desire a functional vagina. This can be accomplished by gradual dilatation or vaginoplasty. This procedure should be considered when the patient is contemplating intercourse (See answer to question 9-6). An IVP should be requested at this visit to rule out the presence of an urinary tract anomaly. A karyotype should also be ordered to identify those in whom the vagina did not develop because of müllerian inhibiting factor produced by a testis (androgen insensitivity syndrome).
15. **A** (1, 2, 3), Pages 259-262. There is a potential space filled with loose areolar tissue between the bladder and the rectum, which can be developed to reconstruct a vagina. This can be achieved by graduated dilation (Frank's method). In this method, graduated dilators are pressed against the location in which the vagina should be present, and with time a vagina is created. It requires a well-motivated patient and is successful in about 60% of patients. Alternatively, this space can be created surgically and lined with a split thickness skin graft or amnion graft (McIndoe-Reed). If such a space cannot be created, a coital pouch is created from the labia minor and perineal skin (Williams vulvovaginoplasty).
16. **C** (2, 3), Page 261. Transverse vaginal septa may be complete, obstructing the vagina, or incomplete, allowing menstrual flow to egress through a central opening. Vaginal septa located in the upper vagina are often incomplete, while those in the lower vagina are often complete.
17. **B** (1, 2), Pages 262-263. The uterus and vagina are formed from paired müllerian ducts that fuse in the midline. When fusion fails to occur in the distal portion, the patient has a longitudinal vaginal septum. When fusion fails to occur in the proximal portion, a bicornuate uterus is found. Complete failure of lateral (longitudinal) fusion results in genital tract duplication: a longitudinal vaginal septum and uterus didelphys. A transverse vaginal septum is an example of failure of vertical fusion between the müllerian tubercle and the sinovaginal bulb.
18. **A** (1, 2, 3), Pages 263-264. Pregnancy in a rudimentary uterine horn is often associated with a missed abortion or fetal death. The blood supply to a rudimentary horn is often compromised and insufficient to support a pregnancy. On occasion, when the blood supply is adequate, as the fetus grows, rupture of the horn occurs.
19. **A** (1, 2, 3), Pages 263-264. The cavity of a rudimentary uterine horn is lined with endometrium. When the effluent sheds, it escapes through the tube into the peritoneal cavity, causing abdominal pain. Such retrograde menstruation is considered by some to cause endometriosis. These women often complain of dysmenorrhea. Pregnancy in a noncommunicating uterine horn is considered to be an ectopic gestation. Pregnancy in a rudimentary horn often results in missed abortion, fetal death and uterine rupture. When rupture occurs, it often causes a massive intraperitoneal hemorrhage. Unless the bleeding is controlled, it may lead to maternal death. It is therefore recommended that a noncommunicating rudimentary uterine horn be removed as soon as the diagnosis is made.
20. **C** (2,3), Pages 258-263. A rudimentary uterine horn exposes the patient to the risks of ectopic gestation, uterine rupture, endometriosis and infertility. It needs to be removed as soon as the diagnosis is made. An imperforate hymen leads to a hematocolpos, and should be incised. A uterus didelphys requires no surgical treatment.

21. **A** (1, 2, 3), Page 266. A uterine septum should be removed if the patient is having repetitive fetal losses. It is assumed that the septum provides an unfavorable area for implantation and leads to abortion. There are many techniques for the removal of a uterine septum, including the Strassman procedure, in which a coronal incision is made through the fundus and the septum is excised. The Tompkins procedure is another choice. With this operation a sagittal incision is made through the fundus and the septum is excised. In both these methods, a laparotomy is performed and the full thickness of the myometrium is incised. The preferred method uses an operative hysteroscope, which is inserted through the cervical os. The procedure is monitored by laparoscopy. The advantages of this procedure are: 1) it does not require a laparotomy, 2) risk of pelvic adhesions are reduced, and 3) the risk of future uterine rupture is less.
22. **B** (1, 2), Page 256. Certain physical findings may support an initial impression of the true sex of a newborn with ambiguous genitalia. When gonads are palpable in the labia or the inguinal canal, the infant is likely to be a male. Palpation of a uterus on rectal examination suggests that the newborn is a female. The presence or absence of breast tissue is a reflection of maternal hormones that crossed the placenta and not infant gonadal sex.
23. **C** (2, 3), Pages 258-259. The triad of primary amenorrhea, abdominal pain and a palpable mass is suggestive of vaginal obstruction. The diagnoses to be considered in this particular instance are an imperforate hymen or a complete vaginal septum.
24. **D** (1 only), Page 259. The patient presented has an obstructed vagina trapping menstrual blood. A sonogram may show the level of obstruction and provide useful information prior to surgical correction. GU abnormalities are not associated with either an imperforate hymen or a transverse vaginal septum. Laparoscopy would not be helpful.
25. **D** (1 only), Pages 256-257, 263-264. Genital anomalies of the upper genital tract are often not diagnosed until later in life when they interfere with menstruation or with fertility. The diagnosis of a uterus didelphys or a rudimentary uterine horn is rarely made in childhood. Congenital adrenal hyperplasia, with its increased androgen production, is often diagnosed at birth in the virilized female. The male infant, even if not virilized at birth, may be diagnosed if he is a salt loser or when he virilizes during childhood.
26. **D** (1 only), Page 264. The patient has had five repetitive first trimester abortions and, during her work-up, is found to have a septate uterus. Division of the septum, which represents an unfavorable site for implantation, is indicated. A complete work-up of both parents is indicated to exclude other causes for fetal wastage. It is recommended that a karyotype of both parents be done to identify chromosome abnormalities. Endometrial biopsy and laparoscopy, though important steps in the evaluation of the infertile couple, are not required. The patient has no difficulty in conception, but suffers from recurrent abortions.
27. **B** (1,2), Pages 258-259. Absence of the uterus is caused by a failure of the müllerian ducts to form properly, as in patients with Rokitansky-Küster-Hauser syndrome. Patients with testicular tissue (androgen insensitivity) produce müllerian-inhibiting factor, which causes regression of the müllerian ducts. These individuals are born without a uterus. Patients with a hematocolpos have a normal uterus.
28. **B** (1, 2), Pages 258-259, 261-262. Sexual activity is impaired in patients with vaginal anomalies which make the vagina either too short or too narrow. Patients with vaginal agenesis often have difficulties during intercourse. Most of them have only a short vagina that requires vaginal reconstruction. A transverse septum, particularly if situated in the lower vagina, prevents adequate penetration. An arcuate uterus has no effect on sexual activity.
29. **E** (3 only), Pages 263-264. A longitudinal vaginal septum is an example of failure of lateral fusion and is associated with uterus didelphys. The presence of a septum may interfere with sexual function and the patient may complain of dyspareunia. Vaginal infections and irregular menses are unrelated to the presence of a longitudinal vaginal septum.
30. **A** (1, 2, 3), Page 258. Patients with imperforated hymen accumulate blood behind the obstructive membrane. As the blood

accumulates, the pressure within the vagina increases, and urethral obstruction may occur causing urinary retention. As the blood flows from the uterus through the tubes into the peritoneal cavity, abdominal pain is a frequent symptom. As a result, endometriosis may develop.

CHAPTER

10 Pediatric Gynecology

DIRECTIONS for questions 1 - 9: Select the one best answer or completion.

1. The most common ovarian neoplasm in premenarchal females is a(n)
   A. dysgerminoma
   B. mature teratoma
   C. immature teratoma
   D. serous cystadenoma
   E. thecoma
2. A neonate is found to have an ovarian mass. The most likely diagnosis is
   A. a mature teratoma
   B. an immature teratoma
   C. a dysgerminoma
   D. a serous cystadenoma
   E. a functional luteal cyst
3. A complete gynecologic examination of a pediatric patient includes all of the following **EXCEPT**
   A. history
   B. visualization of the cervix
   C. cultures of the vagina
   D. bimanual rectal-vagina examination
   E. bimanual rectal-abdominal examination
4. A 4-year-old child is seen with symptoms of dysuria and bloody discharge. Inspection of the external genitalia reveals a small hemorrhagic mass with a central aperture situated in the midline above the anterior aspect of the vaginal opening as depicted in Figure 10-1. The most likely diagnosis is
   A. an endometrial polyp
   B. sarcoma botryoides
   C. a urethral prolapse
   D. a vaginal polyp
   E. a sacro-coccygeal tumor
5. The ovarian tumor that most commonly causes pseudoprecocious puberty is a
   A. thecoma
   B. granulosa cell
   C. luteoma
   D. Sertoli-Leydig cell tumor
   E. teratoma
6. In a child, a neutral pH obtained from vagina fluid is the result of
   A. a higher than usual vaginal sodium content
   B. the predominance of anaerobic bacteria
   C. a lack of glycogen in the epithelial cells
   D. poor perineal hygiene
   E. contamination of the vagina with urine
7. The classic symptom of a pinworm infection is
   A. vulvar pain
   B. nocturnal vulvar itching
   C. dysuria
   D. vaginal bleeding
   E. fever
8. The single most important factor in the treatment of childhood vulvovaginitis is
   A. the application of topical estrogen
   B. the application of topical corticosteroids
   C. the application of topical antibiotics
   D. oral broad-spectrum antibiotics
   E. improvement in local perineal hygiene
9. The most common foreign body found in the vaginas of small children is
   A. a piece of toilet paper
   B. a toy
   C. a hair pin
   D. a crayon
   E. sand

DIRECTIONS: For each numbered item 10 - 16, indicate whether it is associated with
A only (A)
B only (B)
C both (A) and (B)
D neither (A) nor (B)

10-13. Match the appropriate diagnostic method with the problem
(A) vaginoscopy
(B) rectal examination
(C) both
(D) neither

10. Suspicion of foreign body
11. Pelvic pain
12. Recurrent vulvovaginitis
13. Abnormal bleeding

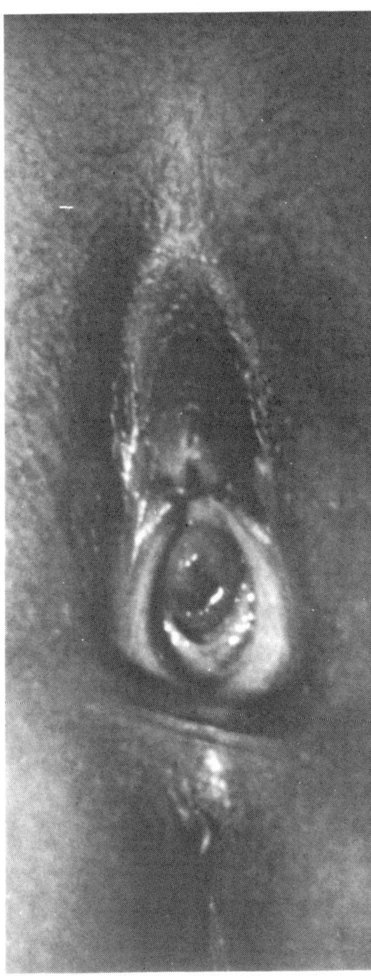

FIGURE 10-1.

14-16. Match the statement with the type of precocious puberty

(A) complete precocious puberty
(B) incomplete precocious puberty
(C) both
(D) neither

14. ovulation
15. uterine bleeding
16. related to central nervous system disease

DIRECTIONS for questions 17 - 31: For each of the questions below, ONE or MORE of the responses is correct. Select the best answer based on the following

A if 1, 2, and 3 are correct
B if only 1 and 2 are correct
C if only 2 and 3 are correct
D if only 1 is correct
E if only 3 is correct

17. A patient with true precocious puberty characteristically has
    1. a premature menopause
    2. normal intellectual development
    3. a uterus of normal size
18. In performing a pelvic examination on a normal 9 year-old, one would expect to
    1. be unable to palpate the ovaries
    2. palpate a uterus whose length approximates 6.5 cm
    3. visualize a extremely, pale pink vaginal epithelium
19. Characteristics of the physiological vaginal discharge encountered in a perimenarchal girl include
    1. association with an increase in estrogen level
    2. microscopic evidence of sheets of epithelial cells
    3. complaints of vulvar irritation
20. A 5-year-old presents to the office with a history of a small amount of bloody vaginal discharge that occurred three days ago. The discharge subsided and now she is free of symptoms. General physical examination and inspection of the external genitalia are normal. Proper management includes performing a
    1. wet prep for *Trichomonas vaginalis*
    2. urinalysis and urine culture
    3. vaginal endoscopic examination under anesthesia
21. Comparing a gynecological exam of a prepubertal child with that of an adult, the child's exam will
    1. take longer
    2. emphasize medical rather than surgical therapy
    3. focus on preventative health care measures
22. Causes of precocious puberty include
    1. McCune-Albright syndrome
    2. hypothyroidism
    3. granulosa cell tumor
23. A child is found to have pinworms. Other family members who should be treated include
    1. pregnant mother
    2. 5 year-old brother
    3. father
24. A 9 year-old girl is brought to the emergency department following a straddle injury on a bicycle bar. A large, non expanding vulvar hematoma is noted. One should
    1. obtain an I.V.P
    2. incise and drain the hematoma
    3. prescribe an ice pack and observe the child

25. Drugs used to treat true precocious puberty which slow advancement of bone age include
    1. GnRH agonist
    2. danazol (Danocrine)
    3. depo-provera (medroxyprogesterone acetate)
26. In a premenarchal child with vulvovaginitis, the identification of organisms in the vagina indicative of sexual molestation include
    1. *Neisseria gonorrhoeae*
    2. *Chlamydia trachomatis*
    3. *Trichomonas vaginalis*
27. Examination of a 3 year-old reveals labial adhesions. The child is able to void without difficulty. One should initially recommend
    1. topical estrogen
    2. surgical separation
    3. a work-up for sexual abuse
28. Figure 10-2 is photograph of a 7 year-old girl. It would be appropriate to tell this patients family that
    1. without proper treatment hirsutism is likely to occur
    2. this child should have a laparoscopic examination
    3. without proper treatment this child will likely be under 5 feet tall
29. A child is more susceptible than an adult to vulvovaginitis because children
    1. often maintain poor perineal hygiene
    2. have a vaginal mucosa that lacks the protective effects of estrogen
    3. have a vagina with neutral pH
30. A 7 year-old girl presents with accelerated growth and breast enlargement. Appropriate initial studies include
    1. a x-ray for bone age
    2. an abdominal ultrasound
    3. a FSH level
31. Bacterial infections causing a bloody vaginal discharge in a preadolescent female encompass
    1. *Shigella boydii*
    2. Group A β-hemolytic streptococcus
    3. *Escherichia coli*

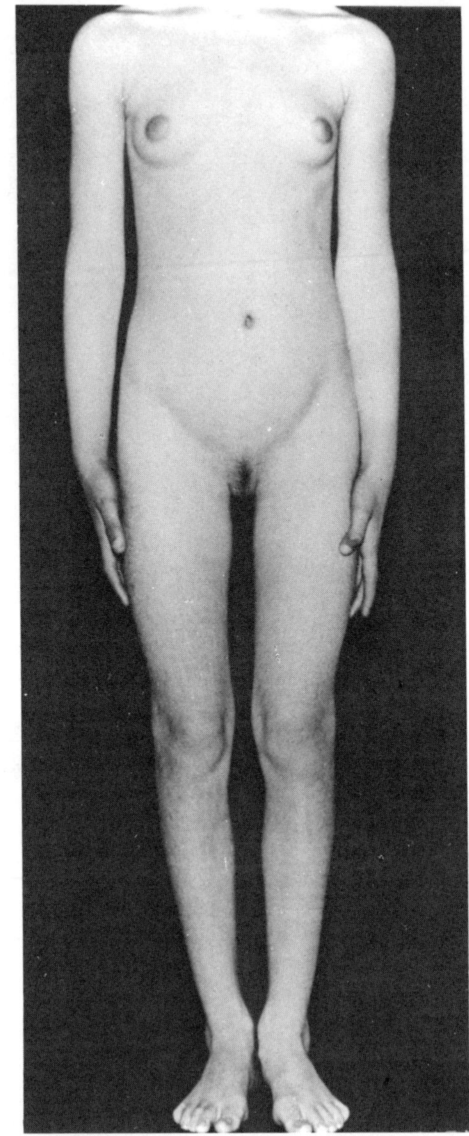

FIGURE 10-2.

ANSWERS

1. **B,** Page 281. Approximately 3 out of every 4 ovarian neoplasms in a premenarchal female are a benign cystic teratoma. In one series, the dysgerminoma was the most common malignant neoplasm, but the benign teratoma was the most common tumor overall.
2. **E,** Page 281. Functional luteal cysts of the ovary are not uncommon in neonates because of maternal levels of gonadotrophins. These cysts regress spontaneously and therefore, do not require operative intervention.
3. **D,** Page 272. The successful gynecologic examination of a child requires a slow pace on the part of both the physician and staff with ample time taken to be gentle and patient. All instruments should be of a size appropriate for the individual. In an infant it may be ill advised to attempt to visualize the cervix unless the child is sedated or anesthetized. A bimanual rectal-vaginal examination is not recommended.

Instead, a rectal examination should be performed if the patient has vaginal bleeding or abdominal or pelvic pain. It is even sometimes best to defer the pelvic examination to a second visit in order to allay the child's anxiety. It should be noted, however, that in the area of pediatric gynecology, clinical errors tend to be those of omission rather than commission.

4. **C**, Page 278. Careful physical examination will aid in making this differential diagnosis. A series from the Chelsea Hospital for Women showed that the four leading causes of vaginal bleeding in girls under ten years of age were: genital tumors, precocious puberty, vulvar lesions and urethral prolapse.
5. **B**, Page 287. Granulosa cell tumors account for 60% of the cases of pseudoprecocious puberty. Incomplete or pseudoprecocious puberty is premature female sexual maturation and uterine bleeding without associated ovulation. Granulosa cell tumors are usually quite large when associated with pseudoprecocious puberty and approximately 80% can be palpated abdominally. Thecomas and luteomas are much smaller and usually cannot be palpated abdominally. Overall, only 5% of granulosa cell tumors and 1% of thecomas occur prior to puberty.
6. **C**, Pages 273, 276. The thin vaginal epithelium of a prepubertal child has a neutral pH, thus providing a better medium for bacterial growth than a woman of reproductive age. This higher pH is due to a paucity of lactobacillus that produce acid from the glycogen in the vaginal epithelium of a woman of reproductive age.
7. **B**, Page 277. The classic symptom of a pinworm infestation is nocturnal, perianal and vulvar itching. At night, the pin-sized adult worms migrate from the rectum to the skin of the vulva to deposit eggs. They may be discovered by using a flashlight or by dabbing the vulvar skin with clear cellophane adhesive tape and then examining the tape under the microscope.
8. **E**, Page 278. The foundation of treating childhood vulvovaginitis is the improvement of local perineal hygiene. Approximately one in four cases is cured by improved local hygiene alone. Most cases respond to a combination of topical estrogen cream and oral antibiotics given for ten to 14 days. The estrogen cream is to be applied to the vulvar area at night. The cream should not be used longer than three to four weeks because of systemic absorption.
9. **A**, Page 278. Symptoms related to a vaginal foreign body constitute 4% of all pediatric gynecologic outpatient visits. Neither the mother nor the child typically remembers inserting a foreign body, most often pieces of toilet paper. Large objects may be removed by bayonet forceps, and small objects such as sand may be washed out by irrigation.

10-13. 10, **C**; 11, **B**; 12, **A**; 13, **C**; Pages 273-274. Both vaginoscopy and bimanual rectal-abdominal examination provide important information in evaluating various problems in the young child. Depending on the symptoms, different evaluation techniques must be utilized. Recurrent vulvovaginitis, persistent bleeding, suspicion of a foreign body or neoplasm, and congenital anomalies are indications for vaginoscopy. Introduction of any instrument into the vagina of a young child takes patience and time. The prepubertal vagina is narrower, thinner, and lacking in the distensibility of the vagina of a woman in her reproductive years. There are many narrow-diameter endoscopes that will suffice, including the Kelly air cystoscope, contact hysteroscopes, pediatric cystoscopes, small diameter laparoscopes, plastic vaginoscopes, and special virginal speculums. A nasal speculum or otoscope is usually too short. The physician can divert the child's attention from the endoscope in the vagina by simultaneously gently compressing oneof the patient's buttocks. Sometimes, it is possible to divert the attention of the child by having her blow-up a latex glove like a balloon. The last step in the pelvic examination is a rectal examination. This most distressing aspect of the examination may sometimes be omitted, depending on the child's symptoms. Common reasons to perform a rectal examination include genital tract bleeding, pelvic pain, and suspicion of a foreign body or pelvic mass. The child should be warned that the rectal examination will feel similar to the pressure of a bowel movement.

14-16. 14, **A**; 15, **C**; 16, **A**; Pages 282-283. The syndrome of precocious puberty is subdivided into complete (true) or incomplete (pseudo) and isosexual and heterosexual disorders. These definitions are only of clinical value after the eventual diagnosis has been established. The pathophysiology of precocious puberty is divided into two distinct categories: a normal physiologic process occurring at an abnormal time, or an abnormal physiologic process that is independent of an integrated hypothalamic pituitary-ovarian axis. Complete or true precocious puberty involves premature maturation of the hypothalamic pituitary-ovarian axis and includes normal menses, ovulation, and the possibility of pregnancy. Incomplete or pseudoprecocious puberty involves premature female sexual maturation and uterine bleeding but without associated ovulation. In the latter syndrome, secretion of estrogens is independent of hypothalamic-pituitary control. Obviously, depending on when the patient is first seen in relationship to the natural history of her disease, it may be necessary to observe patients at regular intervals for 2 to 3 years to distinguish one syndrome from another. Follow-up is sometimes necessary to rule out subtle, slow-growing lesions of the adrenal gland, brain or ovary.

17. **C** (2, 3), Pages 285-286. The cause of premature maturation of the hypothalamic-pituitary-ovarian axis is unknown. Idiopathic (constitutional) development accounts for 70% of cases of complete (true) precocious puberty. Emotional problems in these young girls arise from the fact that they are put under extremesocial pressures. The child may be exposed to sexual exploitation and ridiculed by her peers. The child needs extensive sex education and help in anticipating such difficulties. Most of these patients are shy and withdrawn from their peers. These individuals do not necessarily have a premature menopause. Menopause and intellectual development are normal. Genital development is also normal.
18. **D** (1 only), Pages 273-274. Normal findings in a prepubertal child differ from that of an adult. These findings include a vaginal wall that appears redder and thinner. The cervix appears as a transverse ridge that is redder than the vagina. Neither uterine corpus nor ovaries should be palpable. In addition, the vagina is narrower, thinner and lacking in the distensibility of the vagina of a woman of reproductive age.
19. **B** (1, 2), Pages 277-278. In the six to 12 months prior to menarche, a grayish-white, nonirritating discharge may be seen. This leukorrhea contains sheets of vaginal epithelial cells and is due to an increase in circulating estrogen levels. The mother and child should be reassured that this is a normal physiologic process that will diminish with time.
20. **C** (2, 3), Page 278. Both urinary and vaginal etiologies for this type of complaint must be followed up on the first episode. Therefore, vaginal inspection and evaluation of the urinary tract should be done initially in cases of bloody discharge. Persistent vaginal bleeding is an extremely rare symptom in a preadolescent female. The differential diagnosis of vaginal bleeding includes neoplasia, precocious puberty, urethral prolapse, trauma, sexual assault, vulvar vaginitis, and possible exposure to exogenous estrogens either from oral preparations or skin creams. The differential diagnosis of a bloody vaginal discharge includes the consideration of two bacterial infections of the vagina: shigella and group A β-hemolytic streptococcus which usually occurs 7 to 10 days following a sore throat and upper respiratory tract infection. Because of the serious sequelae of some of these diseases it is mandatory to adequately visualize the entire lower reproductive tract. Generally, endoscopy for vaginal bleeding is performed under general anesthesia. Trichomoniasis is a sexually transmitted disease and would not be anticipated in this child unless there was some suggestion or evidence of child molestation.
21. **B** (1, 2), Pages 271-272. The outpatient visit for a child should be structured differently from a visit by a woman of reproductive age. More time is needed to gain the child's confidence. That child's relationship with physicians will be affected if her initial encounter is a negative one. In addition, a child's visit to a gynecologist usually focuses on a perceived problem rather than on preventive medicine, such as occurs with the usual appointment with the pediatrician. Typically, children's gynecologic problems are treated by medical rather than surgical means. The physician and the nursing staff should be prepared to approach a child's visit with these important considerations in mind.
22. **A** (1, 2, 3), Pages 282, 286-287. Precocious puberty is the appearance of any signs of secondary sexual maturation at an age more than three (3) standard deviations below the mean. It is found in patients with the McCune-Albright syndrome, hypothyroidism, and estrogen-producing ovarian neoplasms such as granulosa cell tumors.

23. **C** (2, 3), Pages 277-278. Vermox is the treatment of choice for pinworms and is given as one chewable tablet for each **non pregnant** family member over the age of two years. Approximately 20% of female children who are infected with pinworms then develop vulvovaginitis.
24. **E** (3 only), Pages 279-281. The usual causes of genital trauma during childhood are accidental falls, the majority of which involve straddle injuries. If a sharp object is involved, a laceration with potential deep damage may occur. In most cases, the hematoma will stop growing when the pressure from the expanding hematoma exceeds venous pressure. If an artery has been traumatized, bleeding may continue until the artery is surgically ligated. The treatment of a non-expanding vulvar hematoma is the use of an ice pack. Only rarely is surgical evacuation and ligation of bleeding vessels necessary. Extensive lacerations require general anesthesia for diagnosis and management. Children with vulvar trauma should have a booster injection of tetanus toxoid if the last immunization was more than five years prior to the event.
25. **D** (1 only), Page 289. The present drug of choice for the treatment of true precocious puberty is one of the potent agonists or analogues of gonadotrophin-releasing hormone. The agonists bind to the pituitary's GnRH receptors and remain attached for a prolonged period, rendering the pituitary incapable of response to endogenous GnRH. Such a mechanism is called **down regulation**. Danazol and medroxyprogesterone acetate suppress menstruation and inhibit further breast development, but have no effect on growth rate.
26. **A** (1, 2, 3), Page 276. Vulvovaginitis is the most common gynecologic problem in the premenarchal patient. Approximately 80% to 90% of visits of children to gynecologists involve introital irritation and discharge. When cultures of the vagina are taken, it must be remembered that the normal vagina is colonized by an average of nine different species of bacteria. There are specific pathogens, however, that indicate sexual molestation. These include *Neisseria gonorrhoeae*, *Chlamydia trachomatis*, and *Trichomonas vaginalis*.
27. **D** (1 only), Pages 278-279. Adhesive vulvitis is a self-limiting consequence of chronic vulvitis. Denuded epithelium agglutinates. This occurs most commonly in young girls between two and six years of age. Most infants are asymptomatic; early stages of the process reveals posterior agglutination. In more advanced cases, fusion over both the urethral and vaginal orifices may occur. No treatment is necessary unless the child has difficulty voiding. Topical estrogen cream will result in spontaneous separation within two to four weeks. Most mothers prefer treatment of the condition. Forceful separation should not be done. Labial agglutination may be associated with sexual abuse, but agglutination alone is so common that suspicion of child abuse is unwarranted.
28. **E** (3 only), Page 282. Precocious puberty is arbitrarily defined as the appearance of any signs of secondary sexual maturation at an age more than 3.0 standard deviations below the mean. The principal concerns of parents of these children are the social stigma and the diminished height caused by premature closure of epiphyseal growth centers. Without therapy, approximately 50% of patients will be under five feet tall. Early in the course of this disease, the girls are taller and heavier than their chronologic peers who have not yet experienced their growth spurt. Precocious puberty is five to six times more frequent than pseudoprecocious puberty. Thus, it is unlikely that this child has an estrogen producing ovarian tumor. Besides, prior to laparoscopy one would most likely perform an imaging procedure such as a pelvic ultrasound. If the secondary sex characteristics are discordant with the genetic and phenotypic sex, then the condition is termed "heterosexual precocious puberty." Figure 10-2 does not raise a suspicion of heterosexual precocious puberty.
29. **A** (1, 2, 3), Page 276. There are both physiologic and behavioral reasons why a child is more susceptible to vulvar and vaginal infections than a reproductive age woman. In addition to lacking estrogen's protective effect, the vagina at this age lacks glycogen, lactobaccilli and an adequate level of antibodies to fight infection. The thin vaginal epithelium of a prepubertal child has a neutral pH, thus providing a better medium for bacterial growth than a woman of reproductive age. This higher pH is due to a paucity of lactobacillus that produce acid from the glycogen in the vaginal epithelium of a woman of reproductive age. In addition, many children wipe their anus from posterior to anterior,

thereby inoculating the vulvar skin with intestinal flora.

30. **A** (1, 2, 3), Pages 287-288. The initial evaluation of patients with possible precocious puberty places an emphasis on the exclusion of neoplasms of the central nervous system, ovaries or adrenal glands. Hand-wrist films are typically repeated at six-month intervals to evaluate the rate of skeletal maturation and the necessity for active treatment. Advancement of bone age of more than 95% of the norm for the child's chronological age documents a peripheral estrogen effect. Ultrasound or computer axial tomography of the abdomen should be performed to discover enlargement of the ovaries, uterus, or adrenal grands. In addition, serum levels of FSH, LH, prolactin, TSH, estradiol, testosterone, or dehydroepiandrosterone sulfate all may be of value in establishing the differential diagnosis.
31. **B** (1, 2), Page 278. Persistent vaginal bleeding is an extremely rare symptom in a preadolescent female. The differential diagnosis should include the possibility of two bacterial infections of the vagina: *Shigella boydii* and Group A β-hemolytic streptococcus, which usually occur seven to ten days following a sore throat and upper respiratory tract infection.

CHAPTER 11

Contraception, Sterilization, and Pregnancy Termination

DIRECTIONS for questions 1 - 11: Select the one best answer or completion.

1. The major undesirable effect of Depo-Medroxyprogesterone Acetate (DMPA) when used as a contraceptive is
   A. hot flashes because of lower FSH levels
   B. a disruption of the menstrual cycle
   C. an increase in body weight
   D. an increase in facial hair
   E. a lowering of total cholesterol
2. The major mechanism of action of Depo-Medroxyprogesterone Acetate (DMPA) is the
   A. inhibition of the mid cycle gonadotropin surge
   B. production of an unfavorable endometrial environment
   C. alteration of tubal motility
   D. alteration of cervical mucous
   E. development of long standing amenorrhea
3. When compared to methods in which coitus related activities are not needed such as oral contraceptives and intrauterine device, methods used at the time of coitus such as diaphragm, condom and spermicides have a much lower
   A. method effectiveness
   B. use effectiveness
   C. continuation rate
   D. complication rate
4. A contraindication to use of contraceptive sponges containing Nonoxynol-9 is prior
   A. contraceptive failure using this technique
   B. herpes genitalis
   C. cervical dysplasia
   D. history of toxic shock syndrome
   E. Chlamydial cervicitis
5. Evidence exists to suggest that the use of latex condoms prevents the transmission of
   A. herpes virus
   B. HIV virus
   C. *Chlamydia trachomatis*
   D. Human Papilloma Virus
   E. all of the above
6. The rationale for developing the multiphasic combination oral contraceptives is to
   A. lower the total dose of steroid administered
   B. increase the contraceptive effectiveness
   C. decrease the incidence of breakthrough bleeding
   D. decrease the incidence of fluid retention
   E. decrease the incidence of weight gain
7. All oral contraceptive formulations now in the United States consist of varying amounts of one of the following 19-nortestosterone progestins **EXCEPT**
   A. Norethindrone
   B. Norethindrone Acetate
   C. Ethynodiol Diacetate
   D. Gestodene
   E. Norgestrel
8. Ovulation inhibition, by combination contraceptive steroids occurs primarily by
   A. direct FSH suppression
   B. direct LH suppression
   C. alteration of ovarian responsiveness to gonadotropin stimulation
   D. interfering with release of gonadotropin-releasing hormone (GNRH)
   E. inhibition of endogenous estradiol production by the ovary
9. All of the following are considered non contraceptive benefits of oral contraceptives **EXCEPT** a
   A. decrease in endometrial proliferation
   B. reduction in the incidence of benign breast disease
   C. reduction in the occurrence of functional ovarian cysts
   D. reduction in ovarian cancer
   E. reduction in the incidence of cholelithiasis
10. The active progestin contained in Norplant is:
   A. Gestodene
   B. Depo-Medroxyprogesterone Acetate (DMPA)

C. Norethindrone Acetate
D. Levonorgestrel
E. Norethindrone Enanthate (NET-EN)

11. Risk factors associated with development of pelvic inflammatory disease among IUD users include all of the following **EXCEPT**
A. use of the IUD four months or less
B. nulliparity
C. women less than age 25
D. use of copper bearing devices
E. previous history of pelvic inflammatory disease

DIRECTIONS For each numbered item 12 - 20, indicate whether it is associated with
A only (A)
B only (B)
C both (A) and (B)
D neither (A) nor (B)

12-14. Evaluation of contraceptive methods
(A) Method Effectiveness
(B) Use Effectiveness
(C) Both
(D) Neither

12. highest for oral contraceptives
13. used in the calculation of the Pearl Index
14. pregnancy after tubal sterilization is an example of

15-17. Physiologic effect
(A) Ethyinyl Estradiol
(B) 19-Norgestagens
(C) Both
(D) Neither

15. increase in globulin factor precursors of angiotensinogen responsible for blood pressure elevations
16. increase in factors VII and X associated with hypercoagulability
17. component in oral contraceptives responsible for increased incidence of breast cancer in users

18-20. Estrogens
(A) Ethinyl Estradiol
(B) Mestranol
(C) Both
(D) Neither

18. synthetic estrogen found in United States manufactured oral contraceptives
19. binds to estrogen cytosol receptors
20. enzymatic conversion necessary to render biologically active in humans

DIRECTIONS for questions 21 - 29: For each of the questions below, ONE or MORE of the responses is correct. Select the best answer based on the following
A if 1, 2, and 3 are correct
B if only 1 and 2 are correct
C if only 2 and 3 are correct
D if only 1 is correct
E if only 3 is correct

21. The major mechanism(s) of action of Norplant include
1. increase in mean estradiol levels
2. inhibition of ovulation
3. inhibition of sperm penetration

22. Side effects of Norplant include
1. breast atrophy
2. lower mean hemoglobin levels in long-term users
3. irregular uterine bleeding

23. Effective postcoital contraception can be achieved by use of
1. Ethinyl Estradiol
2. Diethylstilbestrol
3. Danazol

24. The main mechanism(s) of action of the intrauterine contraceptive device is the
1. alteration in tubal motility
2. alteration in cervical mucous
3. localized sterile inflammatory reaction it causes within the uterine cavity

25. The majority of women discontinuing the use of intrauterine devices for contraception do so because of
1. excess uterine cramping during menstruation
2. fear of pelvic infection
3. the development of abnormal uterine bleeding

26. Complications related to pregnancy and IUD wearers include
1. an increase in congenital anomalies
2. an increase in septic abortion
3. an increase in spontaneous abortion

27. True statements regarding the performance of elective abortion in the United States include
1. most pregnancy terminations occur with gestations of greater than 12 weeks menstrual age
2. complication rates are similar for first and second trimester pregnancy terminations
3. twenty five percent of abortions are obtained by married women

28. In comparing methods of second trimester legal abortion, which of the following are true?
1. dilatation and evacuation (D&E) is substantially safer than the use of prostaglandins between 13 and 16 weeks
2. dilatation and evacuation (D&E) is substantially safer than installation of hypertonic saline between 13 and 16 weeks

3. The use of osmotic dilators such as Laminaria in second trimester abortions reduces the risk of uterine trauma and cervical injury

29. Demographic figures most commonly associated with the use of sterilization in the United States include a(n)
   1. female over 30 years of age
   2. couple married over ten years
   3. upper middle class socioeconomic status

ANSWERS

1. **B,** Pages 328-330. Depo-Medroxyprogesterone Acetate (DMPA) has mechanisms of action similar to oral combination contraceptives. This includes suppression of midcycle LH and maintenance of FSH in the follicular phase range. A major side effect of DMPA is the complete disruption of the menstrual cycle. As the duration of therapy increases, the incidence of frequent bleeding steadily declines. By the end of two years 70% of women are amenorrheic. Levels of triglycerides and HDL cholesterol, but not total cholesterol, are significantly lower in long term users. DMPA is extremely effective with failure rates ranging in the 0-1.2 per 100 woman year range. It has little effect on facial hair.
2. **A,** Page 329. MPA acts by inhibiting the mid cycle gonadotropin surge. Mean estradiol levels remain fairly constant at about 40 mg/ml for up to five years of treatment. These estradiol levels are higher than menopausal levels. Although the endometrium becomes atrophic as a result of the high progestin level this is not the major mechanism of action. Likewise, cervical mucous changes as a result of decreased estrogen production but it is not the primary mechanism of action. The influence on tubal motility is assumed to be similar to that of oral contraceptives. As a result of endometrial atrophy, patients become amenorrheic after long-term treatment. This is an effect secondary to the high progestin-induced changes.
3. **B,** Pages 297-299 including Table 11-2. Although the actual effectiveness of a contraceptive method is difficult to ascertain, method effectiveness and use effectiveness have been used to differentiate whether conception occurred while the contraceptive was being used correctly or incorrectly. In general, methods used at the time of coitus such as diaphragm, condom and spermicides have a much greater method effectiveness than use effectiveness. The overall value of a contraceptive method as used by a couple is determined by a calculation of the actual effectiveness as well as the continuation rate. Continuation rates for the so-called barrier methods are the lowest for diaphragm, condom and spermicide and the highest for an IUD, which necessitates a visit to a health care facility to discontinue use. Complication rates for the so-called barrier rates are also quite low.
4. **D,** Page 300. The most popular spermicide is a contraceptive sponge containing nonoxynol-9. In large clinical trials the one year failure rate for the sponge is slightly, but significantly, higher to that with the diaphragm or about 15%. A study by McIntire and Higgins indicated that the increased risk of pregnancy occurred only in women who had a previous sponge failure, but this does not constitute a contraindication. The incidence of the Toxic Shock Syndrome appears to be slightly increased in users of the sponge, but it is still a rare entity. However, if the patient previously had the Toxic Shock Syndrome, she should be advised against the use of the contraceptive sponge. Other gynecologic infectious disease entities do not constitute contraindication to use of the sponge and in fact, the active ingredient, nonoxynol-9 is an effective agent in inhibiting pathogenic bacterial and/or viral growth.
5. **E,** Page 301. Several epidemiologic studies have shown that spermicides reduce the frequency of clinical infection with sexually transmitted diseases both bacterial and viral. Specifically, transmission of the Herpes virus, the Human Papilloma virus, and the HIV virus as well as Chlamydia Trachomatis and Neisseria Gonorrhea are inhibited by condom use.
6. **A,** Page 304. Biphasic and triphasic formulations are generally referred to as multiphasic. The rationale for this type of formulation is that a lower total dose of steroid is administered without increasing the incidence of breakthrough bleeding. Other side effects of oral contraceptives appear to be unchanged.
7. **D,** Page 304. Of the progestins listed in the question, Gestodene is currently available only in Europe. Two other progestins are also used in Europe—Desogestrel and Norgestimate, which have greater progestational activity but are less andro-

genic than the currently used progestins. These have been marketed for a number of years in Europe and currently. Clinical testing with these formulations in the United States is underway or has been completed.

8. **D,** Page 308. Contraceptive steroids prevent ovulation mainly by interfering with the release of gonadotropin-releasing hormone (GNRH) from the hypothalamus. In animal studies, as well as a few human studies, this inhibitory action of contraception steroids has been overcome by the administration of GNRH. In addition, some studies suggest that despite a GNRH administration, there is residual suppression of LH and FSH suggesting a direct pituitary effect as well. This effect is thought to be less important than the effect on GNRH secretion by the hypothalamus.
9. **E,** Pages 326-327. As a result of the antiestrogenic action of progestins contained in oral contraceptives, a number of non contraceptive benefits exist. These include endometrial atrophy, inhibition of the synthesis of estrogen and receptors in breast tissue exerting an antiestrogenic action on the breast and decreasing benign breast disease. There is significant decrease in symptomatic functional ovarian cysts because of gonadotropin inhibition. There is a decreased incidence in the development of future ovarian cancer secondary to incessant ovulation. The likelihood of cholelithiasis increases slightly in oral contraceptive users.
10. **D,** Pages 331-332. Subdermal implants made of Silastic capsules of Levonogestrel have been developed and are now currently available in the United States. Clinical trials of this long-acting, effective reversible method of contraception were initiated in 1975 and currently it has been studied in more than one half million subjects in forty-five countries. The other progestins mentioned above are contained in other contraception delivery systems both in the United States and Europe (Gestodene). Norethindrone Enanthate (NET-EN) is another form of a long-acting injectable progestational agent.
11. **D,** Page 347. Detailed analyses are available from CDC data published in 1988 outlining risk factors for the occurrence of pelvic inflammatory disease among IUD users. In a group of married or cohabitating women who had only one sexual partner and who had an IUD inserted more than four months earlier, the relative risk for developing PID compared to no method was 1.0. Other populations at high risk for PID include those with a prior history of PID, nulliparous women under the age of 25, and a woman with multiple sexual partners. No increased risk for PID has been shown in other groups for currently available devices including copper bearing devices.

12-14. 12, **C;** 13, **D;** 14, **A.** Pages 297-299. The term method effectiveness and use effectiveness have been used to differentiate whether conception occurred while a contraceptive was used properly or improperly. Failure rates in both categories are lowest for oral contraceptives. The overall value of a method as used by a couple (correctly or incorrectly) is determined by the calculation of actual effectiveness as well as continuation rate. These rates can be estimated by either actuarial or non actuarial methods such as the Pearl Index. The Pearl Index is the number of events divided by total woman months of contraceptives used. This figure is then multiplied by 1,200. An example of method failure would be tubal sterilization, provided that the procedure had been done properly and provided that the patient was not pregnant at the time of the sterilization procedure.

15-17. 15, **A;** 16, **A;** 17, **D.** Pages 310-312, 318, including Tables 11-5 and 11-6. Synthetic estrogens have been associated with increase in globulins for which one, angiotensinogen, may cause increase angiotensin II resulting in hypertension while other globulins such as factor VII and factor X may be associated with development of hypercoagulable states. This may lead to development of thrombosis in susceptible oral contraceptive users. No long term study documents an increase in breast cancer rates in oral contraceptive users since the progestin component of the pill counteracts the stimulatory action of estrogen on target tissues.

18-20. 18, **C;** 19, **A;** 20, **B.** Pages 304-306. Both the above synthetic estrogens are present in oral contraceptives, although compounds containing mestranol require conversion to ethinyl estradiol to become biologically active. This is because human estrogen cytosol receptors do not bind to mestranol. Therefore, human endometrial response and the effect on liver corticosteroids-binding globulin differs with these two estrogens. When mestranol is used, they depend on the rate of conversion to ethinyl estradiol.

21. **C** (2 and 3). Page 333. Analyzing daily ultrasonographic scans of the ovaries of Norplant users with regular cycles and elevated luteal phase progesterone levels, it has been noted that about a third of these cycles have ovarian change consistent with an anovulatory pattern. Since only about half of the cycles of Norplant users have a fairly regular menstrual pattern, probably less than 20% of cycles are ovulatory. A number of these are progesterone deficient. Thus, inhibition of ovulation is mechanism of action of this method of contraception. Cervical mucous remains scanty and viscid and normal sperm penetration does not take place as demonstrated in both in vivo and in vitro studies.
22. **E** (3 only). Pages 334-335. The major side effect of Norplant use is irregular uterine bleeding. Bleeding episodes tend to be more prolonged and irregular during the first year of use although the mean number of days of bleeding decline steadily with time. Mean total blood loss in Norplant users is about 25 ml/month, which is slightly less than the average. Several studies have shown that the mean hemoglobin concentration in the first three years of Norplant use tends to rise slightly. Although mastalgia is a complication of Norplant use, no evidence exists to show that there is breast atrophy.
23. **A** (1, 2, and 3). Pages 335-337. Various preparations have been used effectively as a postcoital contraceptive or what is often referred to as the "morning after pill." The most commonly used estrogen compounds include DES, Ethinyl Estradiol, and conjugated estrogens. The overall mean effectiveness of the estrogen compounds is greater than 99%. Danazol has also been administered in two separate doses of 400-600 mgs separated by 12 hours. Effectiveness of this is slightly less at about 98%.
24. **E** (3 only). Page 338. The IUDs main mechanism of contraception action in the human is spermicidal. It is produced by a local sterile inflammatory reaction caused by the presence of the foreign body in the uterus. Moyer and Mishell found a nearly 1,000% increase in the number of leukocytes in washings of the human endometrial cavity eighteen weeks after the insertion of an IUD compared with the washings obtained before insertion. Tissue breakdown products of these leukocytes are toxic to all cells including sperm and the blastocyst.
25. **E** (3 only). Pages 341-342. Increased cramping is noted by IUD users, but usually decreases significantly by the third cycle. Nearly all the medical reasons accounting for IUD removal involve one or more types of abnormal bleeding. These are heavy or prolonged menses or intermenstrual bleeding. The amount of blood loss during each menstrual cycle is significantly greater in IUD users. The mean blood loss per cycle more than doubles increasing from approximately 35 ml to 80 ml. The exact mechanism causing an increased mean blood loss is not completely understood although histologic studies of endometrium obtained by biopsy and hysterectomy demonstrate both vascular erosions as well as increased vascular permeability. Mefenamic acid ingested in a dosage of 500 mgs 3 times per day during menstruation has been shown to reduce mean blood loss significantly in the IUD users.
26. **E** (3 only). Pages 343-345. All reported series of pregnancies with any type of IUD in situ include an increase in incidence of spontaneousabortion. This rate is approximately three times that which would be expected without IUD use. There is no increase in the rate of congenital anomalies and since removal of the Dalkon Shield from the market, there is no conclusive evidence of an increased incidence of sepsis with currently available designs.
27. **E** (3 only). Page 350. Since 1980, the number of legal abortions performed has been relatively stable. In 1988 there were an estimated 1.6 million elective abortions performed in the United States. Approximately one fourth of these were obtained by married women. Ninety percent of abortions are performed within the first 12 weeks of pregnancy. After 10 weeks of menstrual age, abortion complication rates increase progressively with gestational age.
28. **A** (1, 2, and 3). Page 351. Dilatation of the cervix for second trimester abortions can

be facilitated by osmotic dilators. This will decrease the risk of uterine trauma such as perforation and cervical injury. Early studies suggest that D&E was substantially safer than induction of labor by any method for abortions between 13 and 16 weeks from the last menstrual period.

29. **B** (1 and 2). Page 348. In the United States in 1988 sterilization of one member of a couple was the most widely used method of preventing pregnancy. The popularity of sterilization is greatest if 1) the wife is over 30 years old; and 2) the couple has been married more than ten years. No information suggests that couples of more advantaged socioeconomic status choose this method.

CHAPTER 12 Rape, Incest, and Abuse

DIRECTIONS for questions 1 - 20: Select the one best answer or completion.

1. A young woman was seen 2 weeks ago in the emergency room after a rape that occurred in her apartment. She was not injured physically. She now complains of difficulty sleeping, fear of being alone in her apartment, and withdrawal from her usual personal contacts. This behavior is
   A. paranoid and delusional
   B. part of the rape-trauma syndrome
   C. a manifestation of preexisting psychoses
   D. an unusual response in the absence of physical injury
   E. rapidly resolved by moving from her apartment
2. You see a 22-year-old woman who has come alone to the emergency room after an alleged rape. Examination reveals no physical injury, and although there is evidence of recent coital exposure, she is calm, well-organized, and answers all questions regarding the incident. She states she is fine and wants to return to her apartment after all the information and appropriate tests are obtained. The most appropriate action at this time is
   A. discharge her to return to the health care facility in 2 weeks
   B. give her an appointment to see a qualified social worker in the next week
   C. have her see a qualified social worker before she leaves
   D. refer her to a local minister for counseling if she needs it
   E. ask her to call a friend to take her home
3. You see an apparently healthy 28-year-old woman, who gives a history of recent loss of interest in men and demonstrates increasing anxiety as you question her about her feelings. She states she has become fearful and has had a loss of self-esteem. She has numerous minor physical complaints that include pelvic pain, but there are no objective findings. Of the following, the most likely etiologic factor is
   A. recent loss of a loved family member
   B. low grade pelvic inflammatory disease
   C. drug reaction
   D. AIDS-related complex
   E. a recent history of sexual assault
4. A 14-year-old is referred to you from a youth center. Her school grades have suddenly dropped, and she has run away from home and becomes involved in prostitution. She appears intelligent and healthy. Of the following, the most plausible explanation for her behavior is
   A. the excitement of street life
   B. nymphomania
   C. psychoses
   D. incest
   E. disenchantment with school
5. A victim of a sexual assault sustained no injuries, did not acquire any sexually transmitted disease (STD), and did not become pregnant. She feels very guilty, however, and has lost self-esteem and confidence. Of the following, which is the most appropriate action?
   A. assure her that over time all will be well
   B. reevaluate her for sexually transmitted diseases and the normalcy of her pelvis to assure her that everything is all right
   C. provide professional counseling that attaches no blame to her
   D. point out that rape happens to a lot of women and they usually do well
   E. tell her that most women who are raped are asking for it and she should feel guilty
6. A victim of an alleged rape is examined. The incident occurred approximately 8 hours ago. She states vaginal penetration occurred. She is calm, has no injury, and has no motile sperm in her cervical mucus on examination. You should record
   A. that no recent intercourse took place
   B. that no rape occurred
   C. that the assailant probably wore a condom or had a vasectomy

D. that sperm "die" in 4 to 6 hours
E. the findings as you discovered them

7. Studies of individuals who have had long-term incestuous relationships in childhood have found that
A. only a small percent (less than 10%) of them have abnormal psychosocial sexual development
B. anxiety and psychosomatic complaints tend to get worse with time
C. incestuous relationships with siblings is more damaging than with parents
D. the closer the family member, the more damaging the incestuous relationship
E. most incestuous relationships continue for years

8. Which of the following history or physical findings would constitute sufficient evidence for you to make a diagnosis of rape on the patient's record when seeing her in the emergency room?
A. a vaginal laceration
B. a patient's statement that she was sexually assaulted
C. non motile sperm in the vagina
D. motile sperm in the cervical mucus
E. none of the above

9. When seeing an injured female in the office or emergency department, one should remember that many such patients are there as a result of domestic violence. What percentage of injured women seen in emergency departments are victims of battering?
A. <1%
B. 5%
C. 10%
D. 25%
E. >40%

10. When you discover a case of marital, family, or elderly abuse, what is the most appropriate action?
A. notify the police
B. have a stern talk with the abuser
C. involve community social resources
D. ignore the incident, as it will probably be resolved by the participants
E. refer to a psychiatrist

11. The most accurate method of ruling out an individual as the perpetrator of rape is by
A. a lie detector test
B. the individual's sworn statement
C. finding no evidence of trauma to the alleged victim
D. finding no sperm or acid phosphatase in the alleged victim's vagina
E. DNA typing of specimens from the alleged victim

12. Sperm will survive for the longest time in which anatomic site?
A. rectum
B. vulva
C. pharynx
D. vagina
E. endocervix

13. Forensic evidence in a case of possible rape should be
A. submitted to the general hospital lab
B. given to the emergency room nurse
C. left in the emergency room "out" basket for routine collection
D. sent to the county police lab
E. handled according by a specific protocol that insures security

14. The risk of pregnancy from a single random, unprotected coital exposure is approximately
A. 1 in 5
B. 1 in 15
C. 1 in 30
D. 1 in 60
E. 1 in 100

15. The legal definition of rape varies from state to state, but it must include
A. force or threat of force
B. lack of mutual consent
C. penile penetration
D. presence of semen
E. none of the above

16. How long does the reorganization phase of the rape/trauma syndrome usually last?
A. a few hours
B. a few days
C. a few weeks
D. a few months
E. many months

17. Cases of forcible rape resulting in injury requiring surgery and/or hospitalization occur in what percentage of victims?
A. 1%
B. 5%
C. 20%
D. 40%
E. >50%

18. What is the recommended prophylactic treatment for sexually transmitted diseases following an alleged rape?
A. benzathine penicillin
B. ampicillin
C. ampicillin and probenicid
D. ceftriaxone, followed by doxycycline
E. gentamicin and clindamycin

19. Prophylaxis against an unwanted pregnancy after rape is best achieved by

A. performing a D&C
B. inserting a Progestasert IUD
C. using diethylstilbesterol (DES), 25 mg b.i.d. for 5 days
D. using ethinyl estradiol, 2.5 mg b.i.d. for 5 days
E. using *dl*-norgestrel 0.5 mg (Ovral), 2 tabs every 12 hours for 2 doses

20. The most likely abuser of an elderly woman living with her family is a(n)
A. adult son or daughter
B. husband
C. sibling
D. social case worker
E. stranger who enters the home

DIRECTIONS for questions 21 - 23: For each numbered item, select the one heading most closely associated with it. Each lettered heading may be used once, more than once, or not at all.

21-23. You see a suspected rape victim who is worried about several sexually transmitted diseases. Match the disease with the appropriate test at the time of the initial examination.
(A) culture on living cells
(B) obtain serology
(C) culture in agar
(D) examine a saline preparation
(E) none of the above

21. *chlamydia*
22. syphilis
23. hepatitis

DIRECTIONS for questions 24 - 29: For each of the questions below, ONE or MORE of the responses is correct. Select the best answer based on the following
A if 1, 2, and 3 are correct
B if only 1 and 2 are correct
C if only 2 and 3 are correct
D if only 1 is correct
E if only 3 is correct

24. The described phases of the rape trauma syndrome are divided into acute (short-term) and reorganization (long-term). Manifestations of the acute phase include
1. physical symptoms
2. loss of emotional control
3. lifestyle changes.

25. You have been asked to give an inservice talk on sexual assault to the emergency department nursing staff. Correct statements that you might include are
1. perpetrators of rape are commonly known to the victim
2. the very young, the handicapped, and the very old are especially at risk for sexual assault
3. more than half of all rapes are reported

26. During an examination for alleged rape, no sperm are found on a vaginal wet mount. Further appropriate diagnostic tests include
1. sampling the cervical mucus for sperm
2. determining the acid phosphatase concentration of the vaginal contents
3. ABO typing of vaginal secretions

27. Initial evaluation of a sexual assault victim who is seen in the emergency room should include
1. specific tests for common sexually transmitted diseases
2. examination for the possibility for existing pregnancy
3. collection of evidence for medical-legal purposes

28. You suspect marital abuse upon seeing a woman with bizarre injuries. If that is true, sympathetic questioning may reveal that abuse is occurring. What else might be revealed?
1. the woman is afraid that she will not be able to support herself if she leaves the marriage
2. the abuse has been repetitive over a long period of time
3. more than one member of the family is regularly abused

29. An 82-year-old woman, apparently healthy, is seen with multiple circular sores on both her lower legs, which do not correspond to any physiologic pattern. You discover that she lives with her daughter and son-in-law and has recently become unable to control her urine. She seems confused and somewhat frightened in the strange emergency room surroundings. The differential diagnosis includes
1. diabetic ulcers
2. bed sores
3. domestic violence.

ANSWERS

1. **B**, Page 364. The rape-trauma syndrome is common in victims of rape, even in individuals who are in good mental health. It may take a long time to resolve the fear and distrust engendered by the rape event, even if no significant physical injury occurred.
2. **C**, Pages 367-368. Although some rape victims will be extremely calm and controlled after the assault, they should always have the benefit of a knowledgeable

person for counseling and support. Regardless of the victim's apparent calmness and control of the situation, they should not leave the health care facility without having a known and accessible support system available.

3. **E,** Page 364. The story is very suggestive of the silent rape reaction, manifested by a victim of sexual assault who has been psychologically traumatized, but who has not admitted, or resolved, the episode and is unwilling to tell you about it. She would probably tell you of a recent loss of a loved one, as such an occurrence carries no social stigma. Pelvic inflammatory disease should not be diagnosed without some objective confirmation. AIDS-related complex is a rare diagnosis in a low risk, apparently healthy woman in whom a drug reaction is also unlikely. The latter can usually be resolved by history.
4. **D,** Page 369. One should consider rape, incest, or drug abuse whenever you encounter a sudden change in the behavior of a teenager. Obviously, many other factors could be responsible, but you should always ask straightforward questions about rape, incest, or drug abuse without moralizing.
5. **C,** Pages 367-368. Many rape victims struggle with feelings that they are to blame and somehow caused the episode. They should be supported and counseled that they are the victim and not responsible for the attacker's behavior. Many of the victims need time and consistent support to overcome feelings of guilt and self-blame.
6. **E,** Pages 366-367. In alleged rape cases it is important to record the findings and not make judgments either for or against rape. The patient's record is a medical-legal one and speculation has no place—including speculation on the possibility that the assailant used a condom or was azospermic. Sperm can "live" in midcycle cervical mucus for 3 to 5 days although they usually "die" rapidly in vaginal secretions. Therefore, it is important to get specimens from the cervical mucus.
7. **D,** Page 369. Most incestuous contacts appear to be of short duration, with only about 27% lasting more than a year. Approximately one third of the children who have an incestuous experience feel it was detrimental. An equal number feel that it was neither positive nor neutral. Generally, the more trusted the family member with whom it occurred, the more damaging the experience, but in most cases the impact fades with time. In any individual case, however, the effect is difficult to predict.
8. **E,** Pages 366-367. When examining a patient for alleged rape, the facts should be entered in the record, but the ***diagnosis of rape*** is a legal statement (rather than a medical term) that should be decided in the courts.
9. **D,** Page 371. Studies have documented that up to 25% of injured women seen in emergency departments are victims of domestic violence. Interestingly, physicians treating these injured women made a diagnosis of domestic battering in only 3% of cases. They were often treated with pain medications or psychiatric referrals only.
10. **C,** Page 372. The physician not only should arrange for appropriate involvement of the community resources, but also should follow the family to be sure that appropriate action is and continues to be taken.
11. **E,** Page 367. No test can absolutely prove a given individual committed a sexual assault, but DNAtyping can prove that a given individual did not do it.
12. **E,** Page 367; Table 12-1. The presence of motile or nonmotile sperm documents ejaculation. If motile sperm are found in the vagina, the ejaculation occurred within hours. Motile sperm may survive for several days in the endocervix.
13. **E,** Page 367. A verifiable trail of responsible and secure transmission of forensic evidence is desirable for it to be accepted in a court without question. Such material should not be left unattended in an accessible area. Receipts for delivery should be obtained. Many emergency departments have a protocol for the transmission of such material, and one should follow the specified procedures. If there is no protocol, it would be wise to suggest that one be developed after consulting the statutes of the state in which you reside.
14. **C,** Page 366. A single random, unprotected coital exposure by a healthy woman will result in a 2% to 4% pregnancy rate. A major factor influencing the rate is the time of exposure during the menstrual cycle. Still, most women will not accept even a small possibility of pregnancy and wish to have prophylaxis to protect themselves from becoming pregnant.
15. **E,** Page 363. Rape is legally defined by the states, so you should be familiar with

TABLE 12-1. Survival Time of Sperm

Source	Motile Sperm	Sperm	Acid Phosphatase
Vagina	Up to 8 hr	Up to 7-9 days	Variable (Up to 48 hr)
Pharynx	6 hr	Unknown	100 IU*
Rectum	Undetermined	20 to 24 hr	100 IU*
Cervix	Up to 5 days	Up to 17 days	Similar to vagina

From Anderson S: Sexual assault—medical-legal aspects, an unpublished training packet for pediatric house staff, Harborview Medical Center. Seattle, Wash. 1980.
*Minimum detectable.

the specific definition in your locale. However, it generally is defined as sexual intimacy without consent, with or without penetration, and with or without force. The inability to give appropriate consent by virtue of age or mental condition is deemed to be lack of appropriate consent. The presence of semen is not necessary.

16. **E,** Page 364. If a rape victim has the rape-trauma syndrome, the resolution phase involves long-term adjustment and reorganization of her (or his) life. This usually takes several months, and if not adequately addressed, it can persist for years. It should be considered when patients manifest unexplained anxieties, particularly insexual areas.
17. **A,** Page 365. Although up to 40% of rape victims will have minor bruises, only a small number will have serious injury. However, it is important to document any bruising, even though it is minor, as this evidence is fleeting and may not be present at a revisit in 1 or 2 weeks. To outline epithelial injury painlessly, that is not easily noted otherwise, one can apply gentian violet to the vulva and remove the excess with K-Y jelly. Fissures or breaks in the epithelium will retain the dye and become easily visible. This application and removal do not cause pain.
18. **D,** Pages 365-366. Prophylactic antibiotic treatment is given after an alleged rape in an attempt to avoid infection with gonorrhea, chlamydia, or treponema pallidum. According to the 1989 sexually transmitted disease (STD) treatment guidelines, the prophylactic treatment recommended after rape is ceftriaxone, 250 IM followed by doxycycline, 100 mg b.i.d. for 7 days, or tetracycline, 500 mg 4 times a day. Ampicillin, 3.5 g and 1 g of probenicid can be given to patients allergic to tetracycline or to pregnant women. Either regimen may result in some antibiotic side effects. Often an antifungal preparation is beneficial in preventing vaginal yeast infection. Benzathine penicillin should not be used.
19. **E,** Pages 303-305. Women worry greatly about pregnancy and sexually transmitted diseases after a rape. The efficacy of "morning after" therapy for pregnancy prevention is good. The side effects are least from the *dl*-norgestrel 0.5 mg (Ovral), 2 tablets 12 hours apart for 2 doses. This treatment has a high rate of efficacy. Ethinyl estradiol and diethylstilbesterol (DES) cause a great deal of nausea. Diethylstilbesterol (DES) has a known teratogenic effect if a pregnancy does occur and is not interrupted. There is no reason to traumatize a rape victim further by a IUD insertion or a D&C.
20. **A,** Page 373. Abuse of aging adults is becoming increasingly common and may be either physical or emotional abuse. The most common abuser is an adult child with whom the elderly person lives. If such a situation is suspected, community resources should be involved to remove the victim and counsel the abuser.

21-23. 21, **A;** 22, **B;** 23, **B,** Pages 365-366. *Chlamydia* trachomatis is an obligate intracellular bacteria that must be grown on cell culture. It lacks the energy systems to survive on its own. Syphilis can be diagnosed by serology or dark field examination. Immediately after rape neither will be positive as it takes more than 10 days to develop a lesion that will yield treponema that can be seen on dark field examination. Positive serology develops in 4 to 6 weeks. However, it is best to document that the victim has a negative serology at the time of the incident. Serology should be repeated 6 to 12 weeks later. Hepatitis screening is done to document seronegativity. The development of positive serology takes 1 to 3 months.

24. **B** (1, 2), Page 364. Burgess and Holstrom

(1974) described the rape-trauma syndrome. Their report was based on the response of 92 victims of forcible rape. Reactions were divided into two phases. The first is acute, or immediate, and lasts for hours or days. It is associated with disorganization of usual behavior patterns as well as emotional and somatic symptoms. Fear is common in both phases. The second phase is one of reorganization with a general decrease in symptoms and a return toward a normal function. During this phase, nightmares and fears of normal situations are common and may be difficult to resolve. Major lifestyle changes may be instituted, such as change of job or residence.

25. **B** (1, 2), Page 364. Rape is done primarily to assert power, rather than to fulfill a sexual urge. People who are relatively helpless are therefore at higher risk. Rape occurs regardless of any provocation or inducement on the part of the victim. Although (and perhaps because) many victims know their assailants, rapes often are not reported, due to shame, guilt, fear of reprisal, or uncertainty how to proceed.
26. **A** (1, 2, 3), Page 367. Sperm die and disintegrate rapidly in vaginal secretions. Therefore, cervical mucus sampling should always be done. Careful scrutiny of a pap smear may reveal sperm if any are present. Men with vasectomy will not deposit sperm, but will ejaculate acid phosphatase secretions from the prostate and seminal vesicles. ABO typing may be useful if an ABO type is found that is other than the victim's. It would prove exposure to a different antigen, and may also be useful in determining identity of the assailant. DNA typing can also be used.
27. **A** (1, 2, 3), Pages 365-367. A general history and physical examination should always be done as it may reveal serious injury (in approximately 1% of rapes) and minor injuries (in up to 40% of rapes). Preexisting conditions should be determined and documented. Obtain cultures, a serologic test for syphilis, and a a-HCG to exclude the possibility of preexisting sexually transmitted diseases or pregnancy. A review of evidence for coitus will be important if the victim intends to prosecute the perpetrator. The recognition of trauma is also valuable.
28. **A** (1, 2, 3), Page 371. Marital abuse is more common than generally recognized. It frequently involves many family members, especially if it has gone on for a long time. Often the woman stays in the relationship because she does not recognize how abnormal it is, and she is more afraid of being alone than remaining in the relationship. The spouse may need help in developing an exit plan with clothing, money, identification, and financial records as well as specific place to go.
29. **E** (3), Page 371. If the sores are bizarre and not on pressure points or over areas of decreased blood supply or dermatomes, one should think of self-inflicted trauma or domestic violence. In this setting the 82-year-old woman may be receiving punishment for urinary soiling.

CHAPTER

13 Breast Diseases

DIRECTIONS for questions 1 - 13: Select the one best answer or completion.

1. Which factor associated with benign breast disease is more closely associated with an increased risk of developing breast cancer? The
   A. degree of pain
   B. amount of nipple discharge
   C. size of the mass
   D. degree of epithelial hyperplasia seen microscopically on a biopsy specimen
   E. presence of a palpable axillary node
2. The most commonly encountered cancer of the breast is
   A. lobular carcinoma in situ
   B. lobular infiltrating carcinoma
   C. ductal carcinoma in situ
   D. ductal infiltrating carcinoma
   E. inflammatory carcinoma
3. The clearest indication for open breast biopsy in a woman with known fibrocystic breast disease occurs when there is
   A. a persistent, dominant three-dimensional mass on breast examination
   B. blood-tinged fluid on cyst aspiration
   C. lack of pain relief to premenstrual diuretic therapy
   D. spontaneous, unilateral nipple discharge
   E. multiple cystic areas seen on breast ultrasound
4. A 52-year-old woman presents with persistent, unilateral, spontaneous bloody nipple discharge and a cluster of microcalcifications by xeroradiography 3 cm deep under the nipple of the left breast. The next step in her management should be
   A. needle aspiration under ultrasound guidance
   B. repeat mammography in 3 months
   C. submission of the bloody discharge for cytologic examination
   D. open biopsy of the left breast as an outpatient
   E. computer tomography (CT) examination of the breast and ipsilateral axillary nodes
5. The drug showing the most efficacy in treating severe symptomatic fibrocystic disease is
   A. tamoxifen
   B. danazol
   C. bromocriptine
   D. hydrochlorothiazide
   E. medroxyprogesterone acetate
6. All of the following are important variables in the treatment selection of invasive breast cancer **EXCEPT**
   A. microscopic assessment of axillary nodes
   B. histologic aggressiveness
   C. receptor status
   D. patient age
   E. extent of disease on mammography
7. The lifetime risk for developing breast carcinoma in the future in a woman who has had a subcutaneous mastectomy for severe symptomatic fibrocystic breast disease
   A. is increased five-fold
   B. is increased two-fold
   C. is decreased two-fold
   D. is decreased five-fold
   E. does not change
8. Women have a two to four-fold greater risk of developing breast carcinoma if they have been treated for all of the following carcinomas **EXCEPT**
   A. pancreatic carcinoma
   B. stomach carcinoma
   C. ovarian carcinoma
   D. endometrial carcinoma
   E. colon carcinoma
9. The greatest lifetime risk for the development of breast cancer is associated with a(n)
   A. early menarche
   B. late menopause
   C. history of oral contraceptive use greater than 10 years
   D. history of postmenopausal estrogen use greater than 10 years
   E. first degree relative with breast cancer
10. All of the following are disadvantages to the use of magnetic resonance imaging in

the detection of breast carcinoma **EXCEPT**
A. the time required to perform an exam
B. the inability to identify microcalcifications
C. the loss of image quality with respiratory movements
D. the expense
E. its inability to differentiate cystic from solid masses

11. The main advantage of a fine needle aspiration of a breast mass (biopsy) is it
A. reduces the need for an open breast biopsy
B. reassures the patient if the biopsy is negative
C. differentiates between non-invasive from invasive disease
D. assists in determining the extent of in situ disease

12. The single best treatment for a 52 year old woman with a unilateral 2 cm infiltrating carcinoma of the right breast is
A. a right radical mastectomy
B. a right modified radical mastectomy
C. a bilateral modified mastectomy
D. a right lumpectomy plus radiation
E. unknown

13. The most significant factor in the prediction of systemic disease in a patient with breast carcinoma is
A. an initial tumor greater than 2 cm
B. a high mitotic index
C. a low thymidine labelling index
D. the DNA content
E. the absence of estrogen receptors

DIRECTIONS for questions 14 - 23: For each numbered item, select the one heading most closely associated with it. Each lettered heading may be used once, more than once, or not at all.

14-17. Match the diagnostic procedure with the statement
(A) digital radiography
(B) ultrasound
(C) thermography
(D) computed tomography
(E) magnetic resonance imaging

14. best used in differentiating a cystic breast mass form a solid mass
15. can best differentiate benign from malignant tissue
16. radiation exposure one tenth that of conventional mammographic equipment
17. published clinical studies suggest low sensitivity and poor specificity

18-20. Match the disease with the description
(A) fibrocystic breast disease
(B) fibroadenoma
(C) cystosarcoma phyllodes
(D) intraductal papilloma

18. rapidly growing breast tumor occurring primarily in the fifth decade accounting for 1% of breast malignancies
19. predominant symptom is spontaneous, unilateral nipple discharge in perimenopausal women
20. most common breast tumor in adolescents

21-23. Match the phases of fibrocystic breast disease with the description.
(A) hyperplastic
(B) mazoplastic
(C) adenosis
(D) cystic

Usually occurs in women

21. in their 40s and includes cysts of up to 5 cm in size
22. in their 20s and characterized by pain in axillary tails
23. in their 30s with a histologic picture showing marked ductal hyperplasia

DIRECTIONS for questions 24 - 30: For each of the questions below, ONE or MORE of the responses is correct. Select the best answer based on the following
A if 1, 2, and 3 are correct
B if only 1 and 2 are correct
C if only 2 and 3 are correct
D if only 1 is correct
E if only 3 is correct

24. On breast examination you find a 3 cm cystic mass in the upper outer quadrant of the left breast of a 38 year old woman. You plan to aspirate this cyst in the office. You should also
1. tell the patient there is probably a malignancy if the fluid if bloody
2. routinely submit the fluid for cytologic examination
3. do nothing more if the fluid is clear and the mass disappears after aspiration

25. A 2 cm lesion is found by a woman of 54 years who has been doing self breast examination (SBE) at monthly intervals for the past four years. Assuming the presence of breast cancer, true statements regarding this tumor include
1. it takes six to eight years to reach the size of 1 cm
2. there is a greater than 35% chance that this represents a clinical stage I cancer
3. the average breast cancer will double in diameter in six months

26. True statements about fibrocystic breast disease include
1. cyclic enlargement of the axillary nodes is a common finding

2. clinical evidence is palpated in approximately one third of all premenopausal women
3. it represents an exaggerated response to cyclic ovarian hormones

27. A 48 year-old has had a screening mammogram (xeroradiography). The report states that there is an area of microcalcification. In discussing these results with a medical student, you would acknowledge that
    1. a microcalcific cluster is better seen by xerography than by the screen film technique
    2. a breast biopsy is indicated
    3. microcalcific clusters are more likely to be associated with breast cancer than with benign breast disease
28. A 35-year old has just learned that her mother has breast cancer. She is both concerned about her mother and at the same time worried about the possibility that she will develop the disease. You should tell this woman that
    1. risk factors are additive
    2. risk factors identify only 25% of women who will eventually develop breast cancer
    3. a specific pattern of genetic inheritance has been worked out
29. The American Cancer Society guidelines regarding screening mammograms read
    1. mammogram should be scheduled twice annually for women with first-degree relatives with breast cancer
    2. obtain a mammogram at 1 or 2 year intervals between the age of 40 and 49 years
    3. annual mammogram are indicated for women 50 years or older
30. Cyclic changes in breast tissue include
    1. parenchymal ductal proliferation
    2. increase in breast volume
    3. differentiation of alveolar cells into secretory cells

ANSWERS

1. **D,** Page 381. Symptomatology and physical findings may be similar in both benign breast disease and in breast cancer. Pain and tenderness, a mass, and nipple discharge are characteristics of both. Numerous epidemiologic studies have found that the risk of developing breast cancer is increased in women with benign breast disease with associated epithelial hyperplasia. Although the presence of a palpable axillary node in a patient with breast cancer worsens the prognosis, this finding alone, with no known malignant disease of the breast, does not indicate an increased risk for the future development of breast cancer.
2. **D,** Pages 397-398. There are numerous classifications of breast cancer that contain both clinical and pathologic subgroups. In general, this tumor is similar to other adenocarcinomas found in other female reproductive organs. It originates most often in the epithelium of the collecting ducts and less often in the terminal lobular ducts. Ductal infiltrating carcinoma is by far the most common cancer (80%) with infiltrating lobular carcinoma occurring in approximately 9% of patients. In situ ductal carcinoma is limited to the surface of the ductal epithelium with invasive cancer developing from this disease within 10 years of diagnosis in 35% of patients. Both variants of lobular carcinoma occur in a young age group, are less virulent, and have a longer latency period. Inflammatory carcinomas comprise approximately 2% of breast cancers. This type is recognized clinically as a rapidly growing, highly malignant carcinoma. Infiltration of malignant cells into the lymphatics of the skin produces a clinical picture that simulates a skin infection. There is not a specific histologic type.
3. **A,** Pages 382, 395. Although most symptomatic patients with fibrocystic breast disease respond to medical treatment, the presence of a dominant, three-dimensional mass that does not change mandates biopsy. When blood-tinged fluid is aspirated, it should be sent for histologic analysis. Biopsy is indicated if the histology is positive or if the mass does not disappear with aspiration. The approach would be similar for cysts seen on breast ultrasound. Spontaneousdischarge alone does not necessarily warrant biopsy until further diagnostic assessments (such as mammography) are made. Lack of response to diuretic treatment of premenstrual pain symptoms likewise does not by itself warrant biopsy.
4. **D,** Pages 395-396. This patient has two indications for open breast biopsy—the presence of a spontaneous bloody nipple discharge and the presence of microcalcification (cluster) on xeroradiography. The cluster itself creates approximately a 25% chance of cancer that needs to be evaluated by thorough tissue evaluation. A positive needle biopsy alone is acceptable in certain centers, but open biopsy is still

procedure of choice in most centers in the U.S. because a needle biopsy has a **false negative** rate of approximately 20%. Additional imaging studies would not be useful in this patient prior to histologic evaluation.

5. **B,** Page 383. Danazol relieves breast symptoms **and** reduces nodularity in approximately 90% of patients. Depending on the age of the patients, this effect may last for several months following discontinuation of danazol, although symptoms eventually reappear. Tamoxifen, synthetic progestins, or bromocriptine may be beneficial in patients not responding to danazol. Diuretic therapy is often used for symptomatic treatment of women with mild to moderate premenstrual complaints associated with water retention. Some data indicate efficacy when using tamoxifen as adjunctive treatment for breast cancer. This medication may be used in situations where positive estrogen receptors are identified in malignant breast tissue.
6. **E,** Page 398. The three most important variables to consider when planning breast cancer treatment are the inherent histologic aggressiveness of the tumor, the presence of histologically positive nodes, and the receptor status (as another indicator of cell maturation). Microscopic metastatic disease occurs early via both hematogenous and lymphatic routes with approximately one third of women having positive histologic involvement of the nodes without gross adenopathy. It should be understood that breast cancer is to be considered a systemic disease at the time of diagnosis regardless of the initialclinical presentation. In general, hormone receptor positive tumors are better differentiated and exhibit less aggressive clinical behavior with a 60% to 80% response rate to adjunctive hormonal manipulation when both estrogen and progesterone receptors are positive. Older women are likely to be in poorer health and thus less likely to be candidates for some of the treatment options. Because breast cancer should be considered a systemic disease, findings on mammography generally do not predict the type of treatment that patients should receive. This technique does not identify involvement of disease outside of the involved breast.
7. **E,** Page 383. On rare occasions, a woman with severe fibrocystic change is treated surgically by either total mastectomy which removes all of the breast tissue, or by subcutaneous mastectomy which produces a better cosmetic result. This is usually followed by insertion of prosthetics. However, subcutaneous mastectomy does not remove all of the breast tissue so that if surgery is being performed prophylactically the patient should understand the risk of breast cancer remains about the same. These risk factors are contingent primarily on other risk factors for the development of carcinoma—in particular, family history.
8. **A,** Page 387. Once the patient has developed carcinoma in one breast, the risk is approximately 1% per year of developing cancer in the other breast. The extent of epithelial hyperplasia and atypia in women with benign breast disease determines magnitude of risk for developing carcinoma. Women with ovarian, endometrial, or colon carcinoma have a two to four-fold greater risk of developing breast carcinoma.
9. **E,** Pages 384-385; Table 13-2. Of the risk factors described, a first degree relative with breast cancer confers the greatest risk. Early menarche and late menopause are less important but still increase the risk slightly. Estrogens are considered tumor promoters in respect to the pathophysiology of breast carcinoma rather than inducers or initiators of carcinoma. Thus, any adverse effects should be increased with duration of use and a dose response curve should be recognized. Recently reported epidemiologic studies have found an elevated risk for subsets of women under the age of 45. However, there was no consistent evidence of an increase in breast cancer risk in middle aged women even long term oral contraceptive users.
10. **E,** Pages 394-395. Experience with magnetic resonance imaging (MRI) for the detection of breast carcinoma is limited. Because of cost, this modality should not be used as a screening test. Other limitations that reduce its efficacy in identifying breast masses is the time the exam requires (it takes approximately 45-60 minutes), and its inability to identify microcalcifications. Other restrictions include the loss of image quality with respiratory movements. A MRI may be of help in differentiating solid from cystic masses and may have some use in preoperative staging.

11. **A,** Page 395. When a fine needle aspiration or biopsy is positive, this technique reduces the incidence of open biopsy. However, a negative test is non-diagnostic and an open biopsy must be performed subsequently. Other drawbacks of fine needle aspiration are that it does not differentiate noninvasive from invasive carcinoma nor does it delineate the extent of an in situ ductal carcinoma.
12. **E,** Page 401. Until approximately 20 years ago radical mastectomy was the standard operation for carcinoma of the breast. With a better understanding of cancer of the breast as a systemic disease, there has been a change in therapeutic emphasis to less radical surgery and an increase in the use of radiotherapy and chemotherapy. Recently concluded randomized prospective studies have found no difference in the therapeutic results contrasting conservative surgery and postoperative radiation versus radical surgery for stage I or stage II breast carcinoma. It is important to offer every woman alternatives in the treatment of this disease, including a discussion of cosmetic results and patient concerns regarding body image.
13. **A,** Pages 401-402. The two major factors in predicting the likelihood of systemic spread in a breast carcinoma patient are the diameter of the primary tumor and the number of positive axillary nodes. Women whose initial tumor is less than 2 cmin diameter with negative axillary tumors have a five year survival rate of over 90%. Other factors such as mitotic index, the thymidine labelling index, DNA content and presence or absence of estrogen and progesterone receptors are also predictors of an extended disease free interval, but are less important than size of the initial lesion.

14-17. 14, **B**; 15, **E**; 16, **A**; 17, **C**; Pages 393-395. Certain characteristics of numerous screening and diagnostic tests available limit their usefulness and application to large-scale use. **Ultrasound** may be useful when there is a need to differentiate a cystic mass from a solid mass, especially when an attempt to aspirate the mass has failed. However, it is limited by not being able to reliably identify microcalcifications or lesions smaller than 2 mm. **Thermography** is both insensitive and nonspecific, so it is not recommended. **Digital radiography** is the technique by which X-ray photons are detected after passing though the breast tissue. It will probably be the screening modality of the future, for it reduces radiation exposure to one tenth that of other radiographic techniques. **Magnetic resonance imaging** is too cumbersome to be considered an effective screening measure, but it can differentiate benign from malignant tissue. It may prove effective as a diagnostic test in certain cases, such as predicting the extent of disease and recurrence.

18-20. 18, **C**; 19, **D**; 20, **B**; Page 383. Cystosarcoma phyllodes are fibroepithelial tumors that usually arise from fibroadenomas. They are rare, but as they are malignant approximately 25% of the time, they constitute the most common type of breast sarcoma. This is in contrast to a fibroadenoma of the breast, which is often found in teenagers as an isolated painless lump. The treatment of a fibroadenoma is simple excision. An intraductal papilloma is usually small and treatment is not necessary if malignancy has been ruled out by excisional biopsy.

21-23. 21, **D**; 22, **B**; 23, **C**. Page 382. The three phases of clinical fibrocystic breast disease are mazoplasia, adenosis, and cystic. These phases correlate well with changes found in women in their third, fourth, and fifth decades of life. Each stage has associated histologic characteristics and symptomatology. The history of fibrocystic breast disease in general is characterized by proliferation and hyperplasia of the lobular, ductal, and acinar epithelium with accompanying fibrous tissue proliferation.

24. **E** (3 only), Page 395. Needle aspiration of breast pathology is a useful test intermediate between palpation of the breast and open biopsy. Although in young women mammography should be performed first because needle aspiration might cause hematoma formation that would obscure mammographic detail. Aspirated fluid need not be sent for cytology if it is clear. In this event, the aspiration completes the workup if the mass concomitantly disappears. Bloody fluid most often indicates a traumatic aspiration rather than the rare cystic carcinoma.
25. **B** (1, 2), Page 388. The kinetics of growth in breast carcinoma suggest that it doubles in volume every 3 months and doubles in diameter every year. It usually takes 6 to 8 years before reaching a diameter of 1

cm. It takes another year before reaching 2 cm, which is the mean diameter of a breast cancer found through regular monthly SBE. When found by this technique, the cancer will be clinical Stage I 38% of the time.

26. **C** (2, 3), Pages 381-382. Fibrocystic breast changes represent an exaggerated response of the breast tissue to cyclic ovarian hormone production, and clinical evidence of this entity can be found in approximately one third of American woman. Characteristic findings in these patients do not include demonstrable cyclic changes in the axillary nodes, although some women complain of pain radiating toward the axilla along the axillary tail of Spence. Some have postulated that fibrocystic changes occur in the response to increased daily prolactin production, although there is no documentation that fibrocystic change occurs more commonly in women with elevated serum prolactin levels.
27. **B** (1, 2), Page 392. The presence of five calcifications within the volume of one cubic centimeter is termed a **cluster.** Subsequent breast biopsies will find 25% of these to be associated with cancer and 75% with benign disease. Because of these observations, this finding should be more vigorously pursued by tissue confirmation. Because of better **edge enhancement** using xeromammography, microcalcifications are generally better seen using this technique. Microcalcifications are not seen well with ultrasound due to poor resolution of masses less than 2 mm.
28. **B** (1, 2), Page 385. Although there are a number of known risk factors for the development of breast cancer, the long latency period of the disease prior to clinical presentation makes the importance of identifying risk factors less helpful. Although there are limits in the clinical applicability of risk factors, women at increased risk should be screened at more frequent intervals. Many risk factors are additive. At best, knowledge of risk factors identifies only 25% of women who get the disease. In the United States approximately one in 11 (9%) women can be expected to develop breast cancer. Although familial tendencies have been noted, no specific genetic inheritance pattern has been identified.
29. **C** (2, 3), Pages 391-392. Based on large-scale studies regarding the efficacy of mammographic screening programs (Health Insurance Plan of New York; Breast Cancer Detection Demonstration Project), and the development of sensitive low dose radiation techniques, the American Cancer Society suggests a baseline mammographic examination between ages 35 and 40; mammography at least every other year between the ages of 40 and 50; and annual mammography for women age 50 and older. No specific guidelines were made for more frequent mammographic exams with available techniques because an analysis of the rate of tumor growth vs. sensitivity of current techniques did not support such recommendations.
30. **A** (1, 2, 3), Pages 378, 380. Breast tissue responds to the cyclic hormonal changes of estrogen and progesterone production. During the follicular phase, there is parenchymal proliferation of the ducts, followed by dilation of the ductal system and differentiation of the alveolar cells into secretory cells during the luteal phase. Premenstrual breast symptoms are thought to be secondary to increased blood flow, vascular engorgement, and water retention resulting in increased breast volume. Although the breast secretory cells are sensitive to prolactin, none is thought to be produced locally in the breast tissue.

CHAPTER

14 Problems of Prenatal DES Exposure

DIRECTIONS for questions 1 - 15: Select the one best answer or completion.

1. Clear cell adenocarcinoma appears to originate in a specific cell type within vaginal adenosis. This cell type is the
   A. endocervical cell
   B. tuboendometrial cell
   C. reserve cell
   D. underlying vaginal stroma cell
   E. underlying cervical stroma cell
2. The origin of vaginal adenosis is thought to be columnar epithelium derived from the
   A. metanephros
   B. yolk sac
   C. wolffian ducts
   D. vaginal plate
   E. müllerian ducts
3. A woman is known to have had an in utero exposure to DES. A cervical biopsy is taken from the most abnormal portion of the cervix as determined by colposcopic evaluation. Histologically, the area is reported as either active immature squamous metaplasia or dysplasia. Analysis of the DNA content of the lesion indicates aneuploidy. From these results you would assume the chromosomal number and histologic diagnosis to be
   A. Chromosomal number—triple the haploid number; histologic diagnosis—dysplasia.
   B. Chromosomal number—not an exact multiple of the diploid number; histologic diagnosis—dysplasia.
   C. Chromosomal number—double the haploid number; histologic diagnosis—dysplasia.
   D. Chromosomal number—less than the haploid number; histologic diagnosis—active immature squamous metaplasia
   E. Chromosomal number—not an exact multiple of the diploid number; histologic diagnosis—active immature squamous metaplasia.
4. Assuming a normal initial pelvic examination in a DES-exposed woman, follow-up examinations should be scheduled every
   A. month for a year, then every 3 months for a year, then every 6 months
   B. 3 months for 2 years, then every 6 months
   C. 6 months for 2 years, then every year
   D. 6 months
   E. year
5. The cervicovaginal abnormalities, such as vaginal adenosis, associated with DES-exposure are likely over time to
   A. remain stable
   B. become dysplastic
   C. develop into a clear cell adenocarcinoma
   D. develop into a squamous carcinoma
   E. regress
6. Diethylstilbestrol-associated clear cell adenocarcinoma is a time-limited disease since this medication can no longer be used during pregnancy because the FDA placed limitations on its use in
   A. 1941
   B. 1951
   C. 1961
   D. 1971
   E. 1981
7. A 30-year-old, whom you have been following with vaginal adenosis associated with in utero DES exposure, is planning to get pregnant. Before she becomes pregnant she should have
   A. a cerclage
   B. a hysterosalpingogram
   C. the adenosis ablated
   D. a laparoscopic examination
   E. none of the above
8. The risk of developing a clear cell adenocarcinoma of the vagina or cervix in a DES-exposed woman is
   A. 1/100
   B. 1/200
   C. 1/400
   D. 1/500
   E. 1/1000
9. A 32-year-old gravida 0 was examined by you for the first time 4 weeks ago. Be-

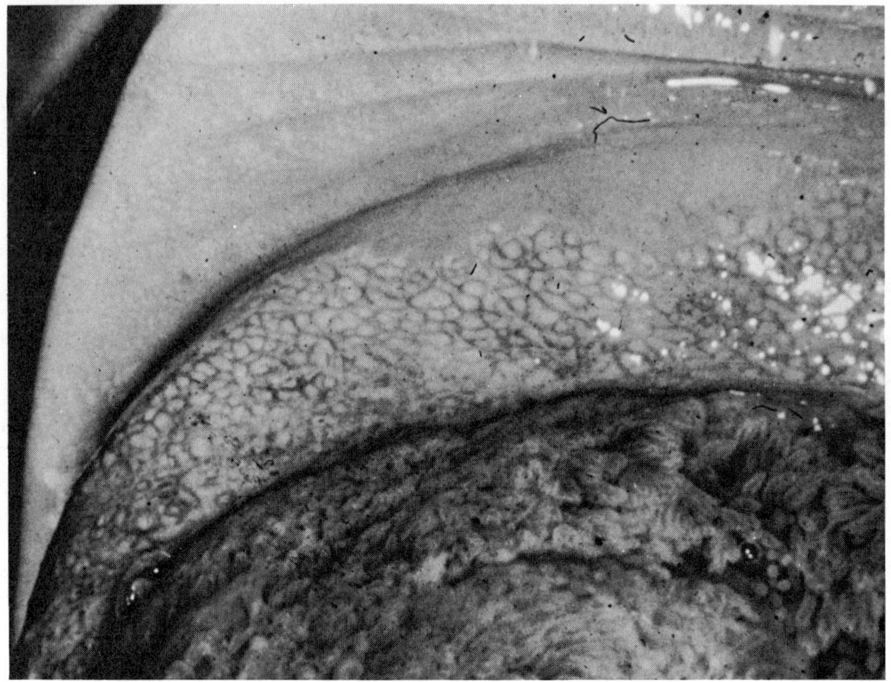

FIGURE 14-1.
(From DiSaia PJ, Creasman WT: Clinical gynecologic oncology, 2nd ed. St. Louis, The C.V. Mosby Co., 1984, p.58)

cause of the appearance of her cervix, you asked her to find out whether her mother had taken DES while "carrying her." Her mother's physician forwarded all the records. They indicate that 50 mg of DES per day had been prescribed from the 10th to the 20th week of pregnancy because your patient's mother had vaginal bleeding during early pregnancy.

The pap smear obtained 4 weeks ago is normal (Bethesda System). The patient states that she has had a pap every year for more than 5 years, and she has never had an abnormal one. Today, you use a colposcope and see the cervix as pictured in Figure 14-1.

You would recommend

A. a hysterectomy
B. a large loop excision of the transformation zone (LLETZ)
C. a laser conization
D. four quadrant biopsies
E. that the patient return in a year

10. The formula for Diethylstilbestrol is seen in
    A. Figure 14-2 A
    B. Figure 14-2 B
    C. Figure 14-2 C
    D. Figure 14-2 D
    E. Figure 14-2 E
11. Clear cell adenocarcinomas of the vagina and cervix associated with DES exposure are most likely to be diagnosed in patients in the age group
    A. under 9 years of age
    B. 9 to 14 years
    C. 15 to 21 years
    D. 22 to 28 years
    E. over 29 years
12. A 25-year-old gravida 0 DES-exposed female has a pap and biopsy diagnosis of CIN II of the cervix. The biopsies were obtained under colposcopic direction. Colposcopy was satisfactory. The appearance of the cervix is depicted in Figure 14-3.

    Acceptable care of this patient at this juncture is
    A. laser vaporization
    B. cryotherapy
    C. trachelectomy
    D. repeat pap smear in 6 months
    E. repeat colposcopy in 6 months
13. Abnormalities that have been *reported* to occur in the DES-exposed male include all of the following **EXCEPT**
    A. abnormalities in the semen analysis

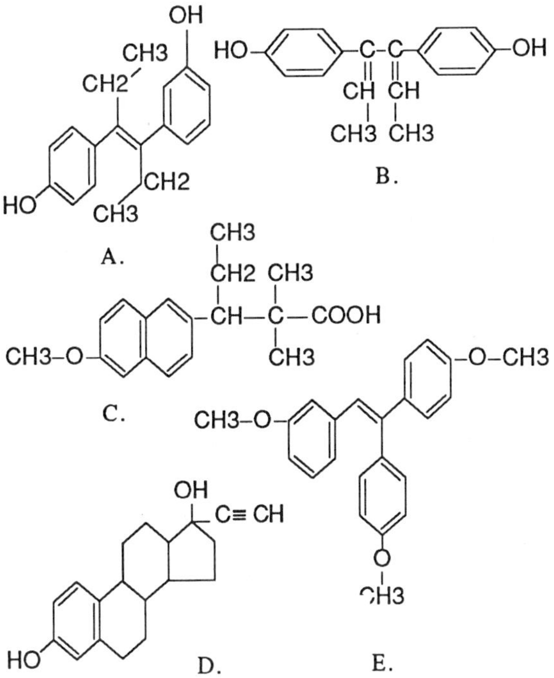

FIGURE 14-2.

B. cryptorchidism
C. epididymal cysts
D. carcinoma of the testis
E. hypoplasia of the testis

14. Examination of any DES-exposed woman should include all of the following **EXCEPT**
    A. cytologic evaluation of the ectocervix
    B. cytologic evaluation of the endocervix
    C. cytologic evaluation of the vaginal fornices
    D. colposcopy
    E. biopsies of non-iodine-staining areas of the vagina
15. A 25-year-old gravida 0 is referred to a rural health clinic with a complaint of heavy vaginal discharge. The history includes known in utero exposure to DES. Previous pap smears and colposcopy have been negative.

    On examination the cervix appears as pictured in Figure 14-4 A. A sample of the vaginal discharge is placed on a slide and allowed to dry. It is then stained, and is shown in Figure 14-4 B. Management should include
    A. laser vaporization
    B. cryotherapy
    C. a biopsy of the cervix at 7 o'clock
    D. prescribing an appropriate antibiotic therapy

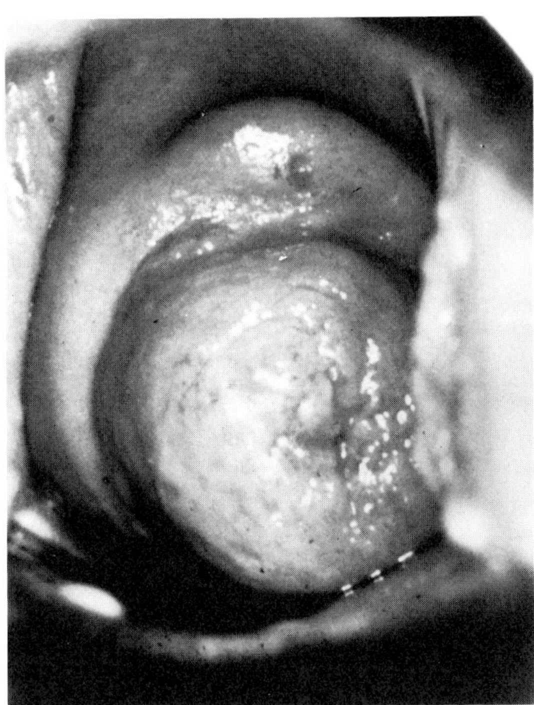

FIGURE 14-3.
(From Robboy SJ, Scully RE, Herbst, AL: J. Reprod. Med. 15:13, 1975)

    E. telling the patient that she has a 50% chance of developing adenosis

DIRECTIONS for questions 16 - 19: For each numbered item, select the one heading most closely associated with it. Each lettered heading may be used once, more than once, or not at all.

Given a patient with known intrauterine exposure to DES for each of the conditions listed in 16 - 19, there is

(A) a great increase in incidence (>25%)
(B) a moderate increase in incidence (>5% but <25%)
(C) a slight increase in incidence (<5%)
(D) a suspected increase in incidence based on clinical studies, but this has not been proven
(E) no data to support an increase in incidence

16. altered immune response
17. breast carcinoma
18. adenosis
19. ectopic pregnancy

DIRECTIONS For each numbered item 20 - 25, indicate whether it is associated with
A only (A)
B only (B)

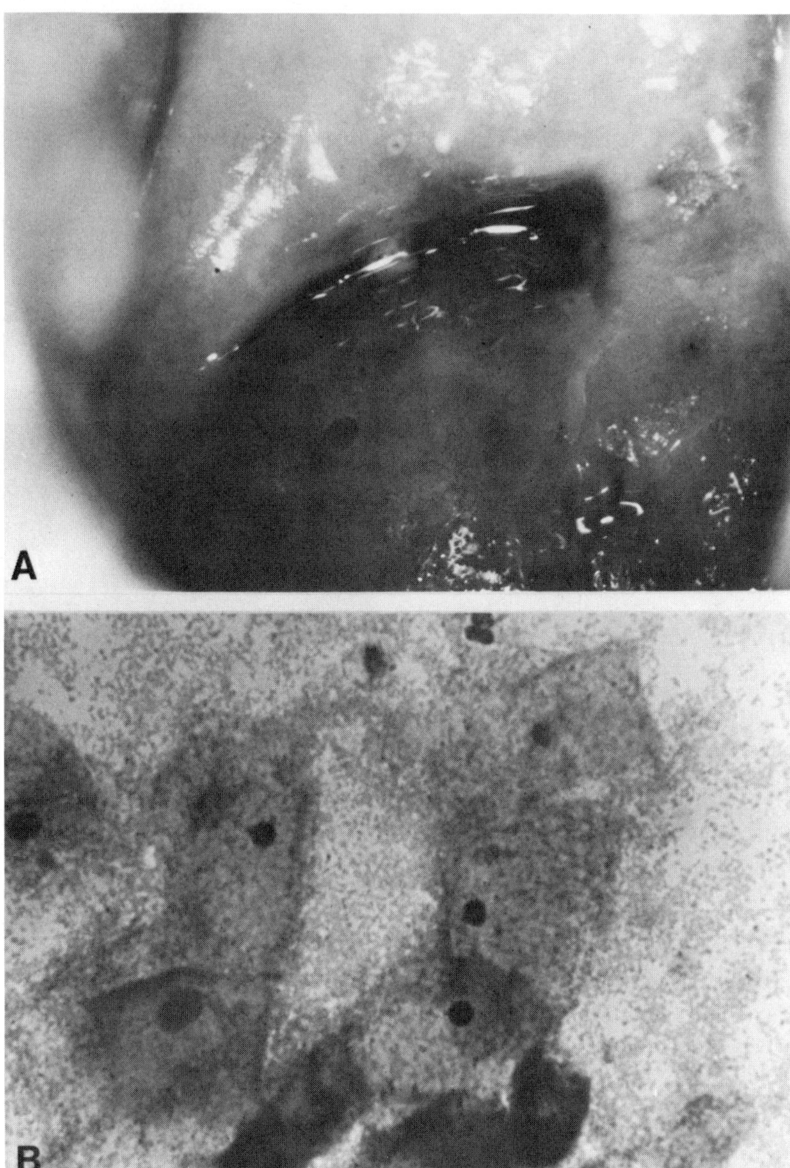

FIGURE 14-4.

C both (A) and (B)
D neither (A) nor (B)

Questions 20-22.

(A) Steroidal estrogen
(B) Stilbene-type estrogen
(C) Both
(D) Neither

20. Constriction rings near the entrance of the fallopian tube
21. Cervical collar
22. Neural tube defect

Questions 23-25.

(A) DES exposure at 25 weeks
(B) DES exposure at 10 weeks
(C) Both
(D) Neither

23. Duplication of a ureter
24. Smaller than normal endometrial cavity
25. T-shaped uterus

DIRECTIONS for questions 26 - 30: For each of the questions below, ONE or MORE of the responses is correct. Select the best answer based on the following

A if 1, 2, and 3 are correct
B if only 1 and 2 are correct
C if only 2 and 3 are correct
D if only 1 is correct
E if only 3 is correct

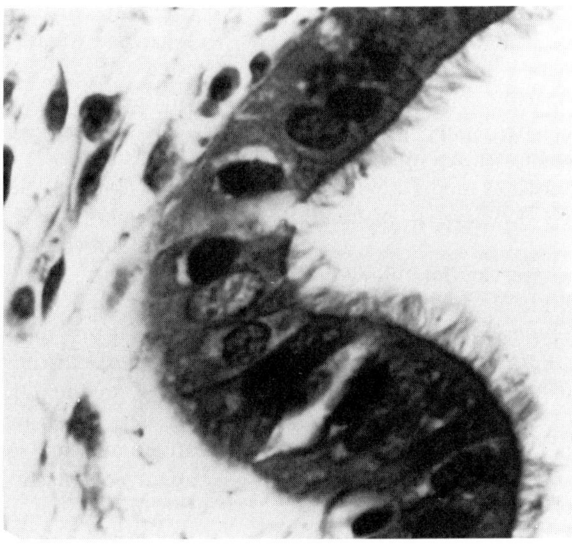

FIGURE 14-5.

(From Herbst AL, ed: Intrauterine exposure to diethylstilbestrol in the human. Washington, DC, American College of Obstetricians and Gynecologists, 1978)

26. Structural abnormalities of the cervix or vaginal fornices are not found in all women with an in utero exposure to Diethylstilbestrol. Factors that appear to increase the probability of a structural abnormality include a woman
    1. who had her menarche at age 15
    2. who has never been pregnant
    3. whose mother started taking Diethylstilbestrol at 22 weeks of pregnancy
27. A 27-year-old gravida 0, who has been followed with a cervicovaginal ridge associated with an in utero DES exposure, is planning to get pregnant and seeks information. It would be correct to tell her that statistically she has a greater chance of
    1. having an ectopic pregnancy
    2. not becoming pregnant
    3. delivering prematurely
28. Figure 14-5 is a photomicrograph of a biopsy specimen. It could have been taken from
    1. a fallopian tube
    2. the vagina of a DES-exposed woman
    3. the endometrial cavity
29. A 23-year-old gravida 0, who gives a history of in utero DES exposure, requests contraceptive advice. Proper counseling should include
    1. a diaphragm
    2. an intrauterine device
    3. oral contraceptives
30. Synonyms for a cervicovaginal ridge include
    1. Collar
    2. Hood
    3. Ectropion

ANSWERS

1. **B,** Page 410. It appears that the clear cell adenocarcinomas arise from the tuboendometrial cell.
2. **E,** Pages 418-419. Müllerian-derived columnar epithelium is replaced by a solid core of squamous epithelium that arises from the vaginal plate. The vaginal plate grows cephalad from the urogenital sinus, and the solid core of squamous epithelium ultimately canalizes to form the permanent lining of the vagina. In mice, when squamous transformation of columnar epithelium is arrested by estrogen treatment, persistence of müllerian-type columnar epithelium results in the upper vagina and cervix. In utero exposure to DES in humans may have a similar effect, that is, a DES-induced persistence of glandular epithelium in the vagina leading to adenosis.
3. **B,** Page 414. Tissues having a normal diploid (2N) distribution are "euploid" and normal. Polyploidy refers to the nuclear DNA measurement being increased by multiples of the diploid amount. Aneuploidy occurs when the DNA content reveals a wide distribution of intermediate

modal values that differ from the diploid or polyploid ranges, and often a wide range of intermediate values are encountered. Metaplasia usually contains diploid values and occasionally some polyploid values. Tissues showing an aneuploid distribution usually consist of moderate or severe dysplasia, (CIN II, CIN III), or frank malignancy.

4. **E,** Page 414. The intervals for follow-up examinations depend on the findings as well as the completeness of the initial examination. Yearly intervals are adequate for most individuals.
5. **E,** Pages 418, 422. Adenosis, ectropion, and cervicovaginal ridges heal spontaneously in many but not all DES-exposed females. The risk of developing cancer in the DES-exposed female is less than 1 cancer per 1000 exposed women.
6. **D,** Page 418. Insofar as clear cell adenocarcinomas developed in the DES-exposed females through their 20s and early 30s, the cancers will continue to be diagnosed for a number of years, since DES usage in pregnancy is known to have continued, albeit on a limited basis, until 1971.
7. **E,** Pages 416-418. Cerclage is not indicated as an interval procedure. In fact, it only should be considered during pregnancy in patients who have undergone midtrimester losses. Indications for cerclage are no different than if the woman had not been exposed to DES. Although there may be an increased risk for an unfavorable outcome in DES-exposed females with an abnormal hysterosalpingogram, the results of the examination have not been correlated with any individual or specific adverse pregnancy outcome. Routine hysterographic evaluation of DES-exposed females is, therefore, not warranted. Ablation of the adenosis could destroy a large portion of the reproductive tract. Unless it is associated with dysplasia or malignancy, it is not indicated. In view of the higher rates of ectopic pregnancy among the exposed, some structural or functional alteration of the fallopian tubes appears likely. This is generally not recognized by laparoscopic examination.
8. **E,** Pages 418, 422. The risk of clear cell adenocarcinoma of the vagina and cervix is increased in DES-exposed women, but these tumors occur in less than 1 per 1000 exposed.
9. **E,** Page 413-414. This woman's age places her at low risk for DES-associated changes. Figure 14-1 depicts a heavy mosaic pattern (histologically proven metaplasia) in a hood surrounding the cervix of a DES-exposed offspring (from DiSaia PJ, Creasman WT: Clinical gynecologic oncology, 2nd ed. St. Louis, the C.V. Mosby Company, 1984, p.58). Squamous metaplasia may give rise to an atypical-appearing transformation with areas of "mosaicism" and "punctation," findings that often suggest the presence of intraepithelial neoplasia in the unexposed female. However, in the DES-exposed offspring such changes often indicate the presence of active immature squamous metaplasia rather than a dysplastic process. Colposcopy does allow for the careful evaluation of the transformation zone in the DES-exposed woman and provides a guide for biopsy sites in individuals whose pap smears indicate atypia of the squamous cells. In this case, with known negative pap smears for 5 years, it would be reasonable to do nothing and see the patient in 1 year.
10. **A,** Page 410. Both A, diethylstilbestrol and B, dienestrol are members of the stilbene group and differ only in the location of double bonds. Vallestril, C, is a napthalene. D is TACE, chlorotrianisene, and E is ethinyl estradiol.
11. **C,** Page 418. Clear cell adenocarcinomas are extraordinarily rare before age 14. Then there is a rapid rise in the age-incidence curve that plateaus at about age 19, followed by a drop to lower levels through the 20s.
12. **A,** Pages 211, 414-415. Figure 14-3 depicts a vaginal hood (from Robboy SJ, Scully RE, Herbst, AL: J. Reprod. Med. 15:13, 1975). Local destruction of the entire area of intraepithelial neoplasia is important. In the cervix, laser treatment can be utilized, and occasionally local surgical therapy in the form of conization is indicated. Although cryotherapy has been used extensively and successfully to treat intraepithelial neoplasia of the cervix in the unexposed woman, it has been reported to be followed by cervical stenosis in many DES-exposed women. For that reason, this modality of therapy should be avoided if possible. Trachelectomy, cervicectomy, is unwarranted in a young woman without any children. It represents under treatment for a malignant process and over treatment for a benign one.
13. **D,** Page 421. Cryptorchidism, hypoplasia

of the testis, and more frequently epididymal cysts, as well as abnormalities in semen analyses, have been described in DES-exposed males. The testicular and semen changes have not been verified by some studies. An increased incidence of testicular cancer has not yet been reported. If cryptorchidism is verified, however, one would expect an increased incidence of carcinoma since cryptorchidism is a risk factor.

14. **E,** Pages 413-414. When examining a DES-exposed woman, cytologic samples are obtained from the vagina, including the fornices, as well as from the ectocervix and the endocervical canal. Colposcopy permits a detailed assessment of the cervicovaginal epithelium (transformation zone). Biopsies should be performed of any suspicious nodular areas or from the most abnormal parts of the transformation zone if there is an **atypical** Pap smear. Staining the vagina and cervix with an iodine containing solution identifies the normal glycogen-containing squamous epithelium and provides the examiner with a useful marker of the boundary between normal squamous epithelium and nonglycogenated areas of metaplasia, adenosis, and ectropion.
15. **D,** Pages 412, 421. Figure 14-4 depicts a normal cervix. The smear contains clue cells. Thus, the patient should be treated. There is no area to ablate with laser or cryotherapy. Vaginal adenosis occurs in about one third not one half of DES-exposed females.

16-19. 16, **D;** 17, **E;** 18, **A;** 19, **B;** Pages 415, 421, 410-411, 416, Table 14-2. There has been concern based on experimental animal studies that DES-exposed offsprings may have an altered immune state and be subject to an increased frequency of autoimmune disease. While not establishing a definitive clinical association, these data do raise concern of a possibility of altered immune function in the DES-females. The answer to question 17 is tricky. Because of the high doses of estrogen taken during pregnancy by DES mothers, there have been concerns of an increased risk of estrogen-sensitive tumors in this group. The question, however, addressed the in utero exposed woman, not the woman actually ingesting DES. Thus, the answer is E, not D. Adenosis has been reported to occur in 30% to 90% of DES-exposed subjects. However, data from case-control studies that are not influenced by the potential bias of self-selection or physician referral suggest the overall prevalence is of the order of 30% to 40%. Unfavorable pregnancy outcomes, including premature live birth, ectopic pregnancy, and nonviable birth, have been reported more commonly among DES-exposed females. The most reliable source of data to evaluate these outcome comes from case-control studies that have calculated the outcome of first pregnancies. Seven percent of exposed women experienced ectopic pregnancy.

20-22. 20, **B;** 21 **B;** 22, **D;** Page 421. A constriction ring near the entrance of the fallopian tube and a cervical collar have been associated with DES exposure. Ingestion of steroidal estrogens during pregnancy has not been reported to be associated with such changes. Neither DES nor steroidal estrogen use has been reported to increase the incidence of a neural tube defect.

23-25. 23, **D;** 24, **B;** 25, **B;** Page 415. DES exposure does not appear to cause anatomic abnormalities of the urinary tract. Various types of abnormalities of the shape and size of the endometrial cavity have been identified on hysterosalpingograms performed on DES-exposed women. These associations appear in part to be related to the increased risk for uterine changes in individuals whose mothers began DES treatment in early pregnancy.

26. **B** (1, 2), Page 412; see Jeffries JA, Robboy SJ, O'Brien PC, et al: "Structural anomalies of the cervix and vagina in women enrolled in the Diethylstilbestrol Adenosis (DESAD) Project." Am J Obstet Gynecol 148:59, 1984. Factors that appear to increase the frequency of structural changes of the cervix and vagina include nulligravidity and a late menarche. The dosage of DES and time started during pregnancy are important interrelated factors. A larger dosage of the drug or initiation of treatment early in pregnancy, i.e. before the 18th week, leads to a greater risk of adenosis.
27. **A** (1, 2, 3), Pages 416, 422. Unfavorable pregnancy outcomes, including premature live birth, ectopic pregnancy, and nonviable birth, have been reported more commonly among DES-exposed females. Although reproductive performance in DES progeny has been associated with an increased proportion of unfavorable outcomes, over 80% of DES women who de-

sire pregnancy have delivered at least one live-born infant. Primary infertility is more frequent in DES females and tubal factors appear to be a contributory cause.

28. **A** (1, 2, 3), Pages 410-411. Figure 14-5 is a photomicrograph of vaginal adenosis (from Herbst AL,ed: Intrauterine exposure to diethylstilbestrol in the human. Washington, DC, American College of Obstetricians and Gynecologists, 1978). The columnar epithelium of vaginal adenosis usually contains various cell types. One type resembles the epithelium of the endocervix, another contains cells that are similar to the epithelium of the endometrium and/or fallopian tube.
29. **A** (1, 2, 3), Page 415. No data indicate that any contraceptive method, including oral contraceptive steroids, is contraindicated in the DES-exposed female. There has been concern regarding the potential increased risk of endocrine-related tumors. In spite of these concerns, no current evidence indicates increased risk of these types of malignancies associated with the use of estrogen-containing compounds. Also, there has been concern about prescribing an intrauterine device because of the abnormal contours of the endometrial cavity that have been demonstrated on hysterosalpingogram. It has not yet been demonstrated, however, that the intrauterine device causes excessive risk for the DES-exposed female.
30. **B** (1, 2), Page 410. A cervicovaginal ridge is a structural change in the cervix and/or upper vagina of DES-exposed females. It is also called a hood, cockscomb, pseudopolyp, or collar. Ectropion is the presence of glandular (columnar) epithelium on the ectocervix (portio of the cervix).

CHAPTER 15 Abortion

DIRECTIONS for questions 1 - 19: Select the one best answer or completion.

1. A 23-year-old gravida 4, para 1, ab 3, registered for prenatal care. The patient's first pregnancy, 5 years ago, went to term. She delivered a 3800 g male. This was followed by spontaneous abortions at 18, 16, and 14 weeks. The patient is again pregnant and according to her last menstrual period is 14 weeks pregnant. An ultrasound examination was requested and is depicted in Figure 15-1. The next step in management should be
   A. a dilatation and curettage
   B. an amniocentesis for karyotype
   C. a progestational agent
   D. a cerclage
   E. bed rest
2. An immunologic etiology for repetitive abortions is
   A. suggested by the fact that couples with repetitive abortions have less sharing of more than one HLA at the A, B, and DR locus than a control population
   B. suggested by the observation that this population has an increased amount of maternal blocking factor
   C. highly unlikely because of the protective effect of progesterone
   D. controversial. Some studies support such an etiology and others refute findings in the supporting study
3. A gravida 3, para 0, ab 3, has just had a hysterosalpingogram which is shown in Figure 15-2. While discussing this finding, you are told that the patient had an in utero DES exposure.

   Appropriate management should include
   A. Strassman metroplasty
   B. Jones metroplasty
   C. Tompkins metroplasty
   D. uterine cerclage
   E. none of the above
4. A 31 year-old gravida 2, para 1, is 9 weeks pregnant by dates. She reports having bled for 2 days last week. An ultrasound is obtained and is depicted in Figure 15-3.

   Given these findings, it would be accurate to tell the patient that she has a
   A. 50% chance of aborting
   B. slightly increased likelihood of an anomalous infant
   C. marked increased likelihood of having a preterm birth
   D. placenta previa
   E. nonviable fetus
5. The most common genetic cause of fetal loss is due to errors in
   A. maternal gametogenesis
   B. paternal gametogenesis
   C. fertilization
   D. zygote division
   E. implantation
6. A 25 year-old unsensitized Rh negative, gravida 4, para 1, ab 2, whose last menstrual period was 10 weeks ago has just passed some products of conception. This women states that she has always had regular periods

   Of the following all are indicated **EXCEPT**
   A. Oxytocin
   B. Curettage
   C. Iron sulfate
   D. Anti-D gamma globulin
   E. HLA typing of husband and wife
7. An 18-year-old and her 20-year-old husband want an explanation for the fact that they have no live-born children. She has a history of two previous spontaneous abortions at 8 and 10 weeks. The last abortus was submitted for karyotype and was 45X. You would be correct in telling this couple that
   A. the survival rate of 45X conceptions is about 1 in 300
   B. this is a rare chromosomal abnormality found in abortus material
   C. the karyotype of this abortus is associated with an older maternal age
   D. another abortus with this karyotype is likely
   E. there is a greater than 75% chance

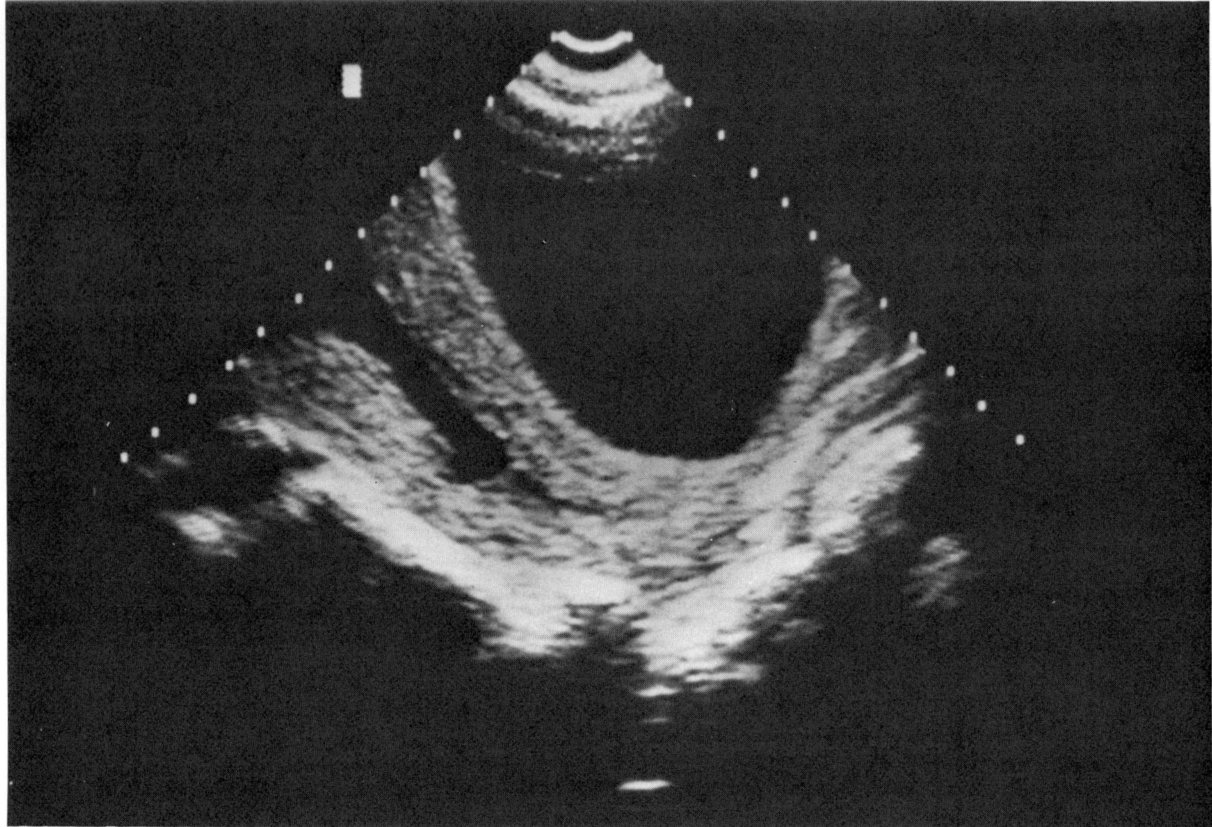

FIGURE 15-1.

that one of them has a chromosomal abnormality

8. Women who have repetitive abortions and have had no living children are more likely than individuals who have aborted once to
   A. abort before rather than after 12 weeks' gestation
   B. have a chromosomally abnormal abortus
   C. have a uterine or cervical etiology
   D. feel little or no emotional trauma after the abortion
   E. have a greater than 50% chance of having a term infant in the next pregnancy
9. An 18-year-old gravida 1, para 0, on examination is noted to have blood coming through her closed cervix. Her LMP was 8 weeks ago, and the uterus is 6 weeks size. A β-HCG is positive. To her knowledge, she has not passed any tissue. This constitutes
   A. an incomplete abortion
   B. an inevitable abortion
   C. a threatened abortion
   D. a septic abortion
   E. a missed abortion
10. A 30-year-old moved to the United States from India 5 years ago. She has never had a live-born infant, and she has tried to become pregnant for 8 years. She thinks she aborted on at least two occasions 6 years ago when she was 4 to 6 weeks late for her period. She showed her doctor the material she passed, and he assured her that she had aborted, but there was no histologic proof. For the last 5 years, her periods have been very scant and infrequent. She denies pelvic pain or dysmenorrhea. She does have premenstrual tension, but it is not severe enough to require medication.

    Her physical exam is completely normal. Her pelvic exam is also normal. The uterus is normal sized, anterior, and smooth. The ovaries are easily palpated. There is no pain.

    The procedure *most* likely to establish the diagnosis is

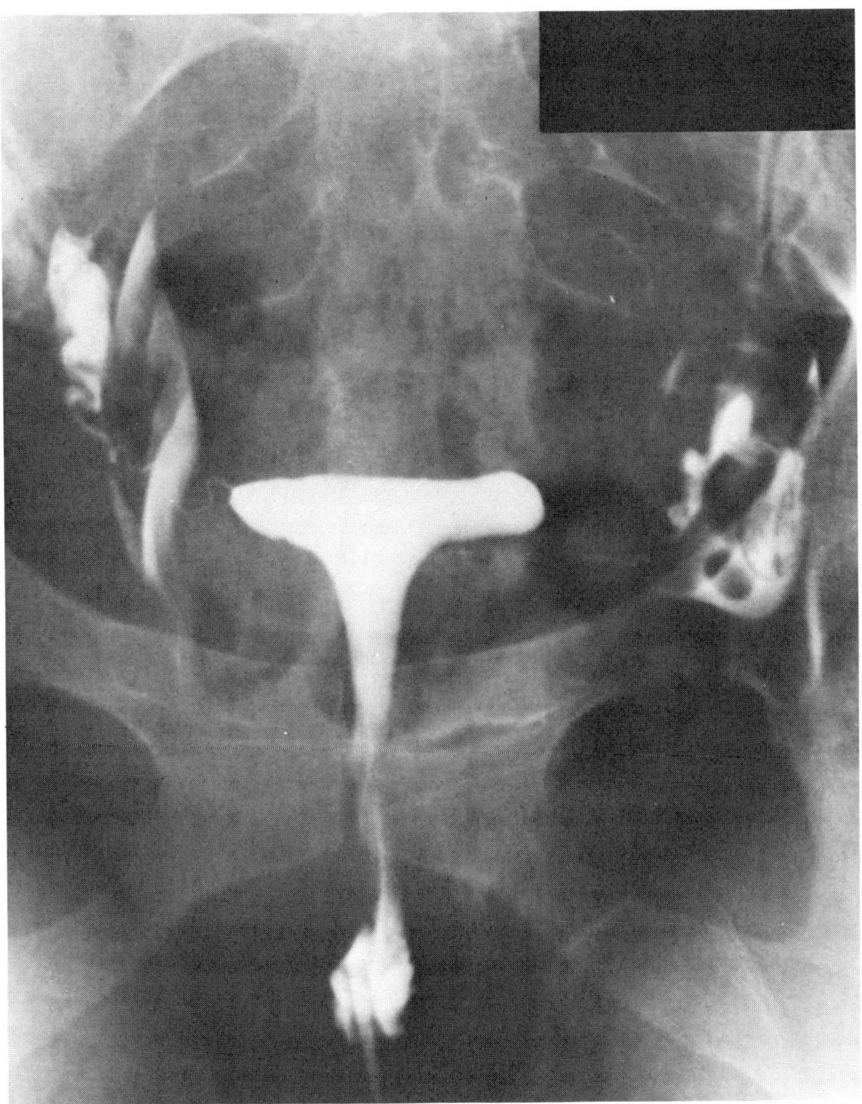

FIGURE 15-2.

A. a hysterosalpingogram
B. dilatation and curettage
C. hysteroscopy
D. laparoscopy
E. laparotomy

11. Patients with systemic lupus erythematosus who have circulating lupus anticoagulant have an increased likelihood of aborting. It is postulated that this immunoglobulin is responsible for the abortion by
A. promoting the activation of prothrombin
B. decreasing platelet adhesiveness
C. causing complete fetal heart block
D. decreasing prostacyclin formation
E. interfering with the maternal blocking factor

12. Luteal insufficiency is an entity that has been associated with repetitive pregnancy loss. This diagnosis can be associated with all of the following **EXCEPT**
A. low levels of HCG
B. normal levels of serum progesterone
C. administration of a synthetic progestin
D. low levels of serum progesterone
E. an endometrium histologically one day less than expected

13. A 26-year-old gravida 2, para 1, is 14 weeks pregnant by dates. On pelvic examination the uterus felt smaller than you would have anticipated. A representative

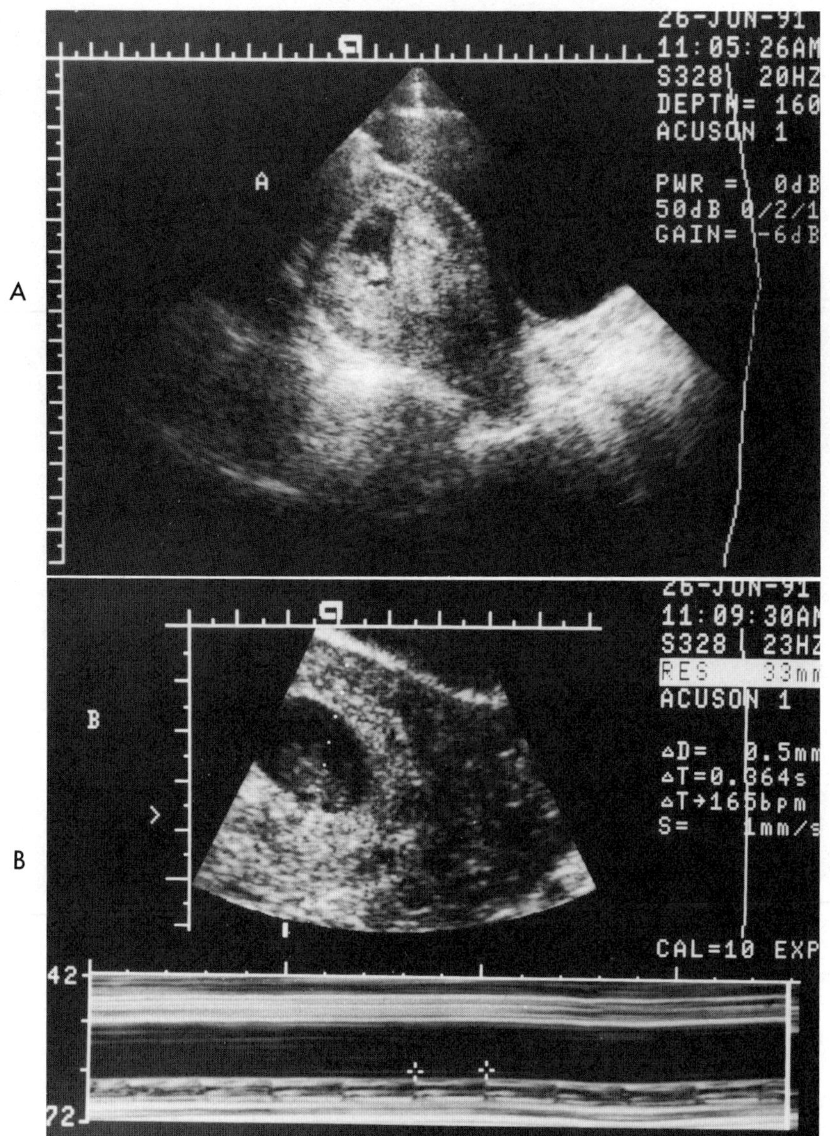

FIGURE 15-3.

image of the ultrasound that you ordered is depicted in Figure 15-4. This patient should have

A. an immediate determination of her serum fibrinogen level
B. her karyotype determined
C. a quantitative serum β-HCG level.
D. an immediate suction dilatation and curettage
E. a culdocentesis

14. The management of a patient with a septic threatened abortion not in shock should include
    A. single agent antibiotics
    B. an intraarterial line
    C. corticosteroids
    D. digitalis
    E. uterine evacuation
15. A 33-year-old gravida 4, para 0, ab 4, is now 8 weeks pregnant. On ultrasound a gestational sac containing a fetus of appropriate size is visualized. Cardiac activity is recorded at 140 beats/minute. Although the patient has bled for 3 days, a source is not seen on this scan. A serum β-HCG level is at the mean for 8 weeks. The patient states that she is currently staining 6 to 7 pads a day. She doesn't have any cramps.

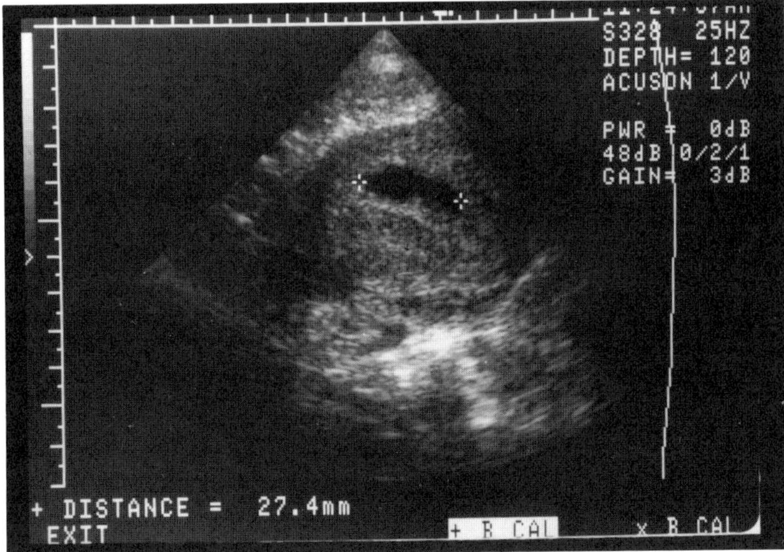

FIGURE 15-4.

Your management would include
- A. thyroid replacement
- B. iron replacement
- C. absolute bed rest
- D. progesterone suppositories
- E. aspirin

16. You are counselling a young couple with a history of repetitive abortions. A correct statement which you might include in your discussion would be that
    - A. the likelihood that either has an abnormal karyotype is greater than 20%
    - B. the paternal rather than the maternal karyotype is most apt to be abnormal
    - C. an X chromosome mosaicism of the father, rather than the mother, is apt to be revealed
    - D. the abnormality is most likely to be a Robertsonian translocation
    - E. if a translocation is found in 1 parent about 10% of their pregnancies will abort
17. The most frequent chromosomal trisomy found in abortuses is
    - A. 13, 15
    - B. 16
    - C. 18
    - D. 21
    - E. 22
18. The patient is a 35 year-old gravida 4, para 0, who is interested in attempting another pregnancy. You would suggest all of the following tests for her **EXCEPT** a
    - A. serum TSH
    - B. mid luteal serum progesterone
    - C. test for lupus anticoagulant activity
    - D. hysterosalpingogram
    - E. culture for *Chlamydia trachomatis*

DIRECTIONS for questions 19 - 23: For each numbered item, select the one heading most closely associated with it. Each lettered heading may be used once, more than once, or not at all.

19-21. Incidence of embryonic loss

- (A) 1% to 2%
- (B) 15% to 20%
- (C) 40%
- (D) 70%
- (E) 80%

19. Clinically recognized abortions
20. Total human pregnancy loss
21. Percent of abortions occurring in the first trimester

22-23. In answering questions 22 and 23 consider Figure 15-5.

- (A) Figure 15-5 A
- (B) Figure 15-5 B
- (C) Figure 15-5 C
- (D) Figure 15-5 D

22. Greatest incidence of spontaneous abortion
23. Metroplasty by the Strassman technique

DIRECTIONS For each numbered item 24 - 26, indicate whether it is associated with

A only (A)
B only (B)
C both (A) and (B)
D neither (A) nor (B)

- (A) Increased likelihood of abortion of chromosomally normal fetus

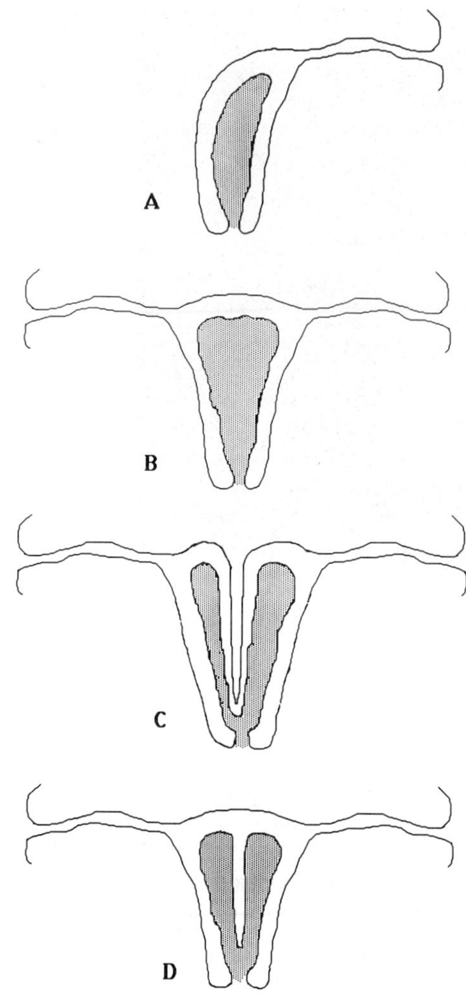

FIGURE 15-5.

(B) Increased likelihood of abortion of chromosomally abnormal fetus
(C) Both
(D) Neither

24. A woman who smokes 2 packs per day
25. A woman who has had GI series and IVP at about the time of implantation
26. A woman who imbibes an alcoholic beverage on an average of 3 times a week

DIRECTIONS for questions 27 - 32: For each of the questions below, ONE or MORE of the responses is correct. Select the best answer based on the following

A if 1, 2, and 3 are correct
B if only 1 and 2 are correct
C if only 2 and 3 are correct
D if only 1 is correct
E if only 3 is correct

Questions 27-29

27. Antiphospholipid antibodies have been found in the circulation of women with
    1. recurrent abortions
    2. a variety of collagen vascular diseases
    3. a history of recurrent thrombotic episodes
28. A 23-year-old is 5 weeks late for her menstrual period. She started spotting 8 days ago. You obtained a serum β-HCG 7 days ago that was 3770 mIU/ml and a second β-HCG yesterday that was 4500 mIU/ml. The differential diagnosis at this point includes
    1. an ectopic pregnancy
    2. a threatened abortion
    3. a normal pregnancy
29. Which organisms are associated with septic abortion?
    1. *Escherichia coli*
    2. *Bacteroides* species
    3. *Clostridium perfringens*

Questions 30-32

30. In counseling a woman about the possibility of a spontaneous abortion in a subsequent pregnancy, it would be important to know that she
    1. has had 3 previous abortions
    2. is 35 years of age
    3. has one living child
31. In order to determine the relative risk of another abortion and suggest management options, it also would be important to know that she
    1. is a controlled insulin-dependent diabetic
    2. is married to a 55-year-old
    3. aborted 1 month ago
32. Assume all six of the above statements were true. With this information, you should
    1. ask her to delay her attempt to get pregnant for 3 months
    2. obtain a serum thyroxine
    3. obtain a serum progesterone 3 days before the expected period

ANSWERS

1. **D,** Pages 425, 435-436, 443, 445-446. The ultrasound depicted in Figure 15-1 is a longitudinal view through the pelvis. One can see a well-filled bladder and the lower uterine segment and cervix. Since there is fluid in the cervical canal itself, the diagnosis is highly suggestive of an incompetent cervix. The best treatment of cervical incompetence is placement of a concentric nonabsorbable silk or Mersilene suture at the level of the internal os (cerclage), utilizing either the technique described by Shirodkar or McDonald. This ultrasound

does not show the fetus. For a dilatation and curettage to be indicated either the history or the ultrasound should have suggested an anembryonic pregnancy, an inevitable or incomplete abortion, or intrauterine fetal death. There is nothing in the history to suggest a threatened abortion. Besides, although some physicians recommend that patients with threatened abortion restrict their physical activities or stay at bed rest, there is no evidence that these measures or any active medical therapy improves the prognosis of the threatened abortion. Treatment with progestins was previously advocated, but there is no evidence that such therapy improves the prognosis.

2. **D,** Pages 432, 439. An immunologic etiology for repetitive abortions is not well established. There are conflicting studies. Some suggest greater sharing of more than one HLA antigen at the A, B, and DR locus. An immunologic etiology would be supported by a decreased rather than an increased maternal blocking factor. This factor, the circulating IgG antibody, coats the foreign fetal antigens and prevents the fetus from being rejected. Some protection of the fetus from an immunologic effect is provided by progesterone. This neither supports nor refutes the immunologic etiology.
3. **E,** Page 435. No therapy has been shown to be beneficial in lowering the abortion rate in women exposed to DES who have abnormalities of the uterine cavity (as illustrated in Figure 15-4) and recurrent abortion.
4. **B,** Pages 443-445. This sonogram depicts a 7 week viable pregnancy as evidenced by the normal fetal heart rate seen in Figure 15-3 B. The placenta is not clearly visualized in Figure 15-3 A. Besides, even if the placenta appeared to be near the internal os, a diagnosis of placenta previa should not be made with certainty during the first or second trimester since differential growth may change its position relative to the internal os at the time of labor. It had been quoted that there was a 50% chance of aborting if a patient bled prior to 20 weeks. The recent literature suggests that the risk of abortion is greater among those women who bleed for 3 or more days, 24%, than those who bleed only 1 or 2 days, 7%. Sonographic studies reveal that in groups of women with threatened abortion with a live fetus about 85% of these fetuses subsequently deliver and survive. There is no evidence that women with gestational bleeding who do not abort have an increased incidence of complications of pregnancy, but they may have a slightly increased incidence of fetal anomalies and preterm birth.
5. **A,** Page 429. Twenty-six percent of all fetal loss is due to errors of maternal gametogenesis, 5 to errors of paternal gametogenesis, 4 to errors of fertilization, and 4 to errors of zygote division.
6. **E,** Pages 445-446, 449. A complete abortion usually occurs before 6 weeks' and after 14 weeks' gestation. In this question it is fair to assume that the abortion is incomplete. A patient with an inevitable or incomplete abortion may receive intravenous oxytocin. The uterus should be emptied by gentle, complete sharp or suction curettage. This can often be done on an outpatient basis. It is important not to be too vigorous since intrauterine adhesions are a possible complication. The evacuation should be complete to minimize the chance of a septic abortion. Since there is always loss of a significant amount of blood, these patients should receive iron supplementation following the curettage. If the patient is Rh negative and the father Rh positive or Rh unknown, the woman should receive 50 micrograms of anti-D gamma globulin. Some physicians will place the patient on a 2 or 3 day regimen of ergonovine maleate after the D & C. In cases of recurrent abortion the value of obtaining HLA typing of husband and wife is controversial and does not appear to be cost effective.
7. **A,** Pages 429-430. The survival rate of 45X conceptions is about 1 in 300. This is the most common single chromosomal abnormality found in abortus material. The most common type of chromosomal abnormality is an autosomal trisomy. There is evidence that monosomy 45X is associated with a younger maternal age than other aneuploid or euploid abortions. Karyotypes of abortuses of women who have had more than one abortion tend to be similar to the first if the first abortus was either normal or an autosomal trisomy. Chromosome abnormalities in the parents are an infrequent cause of abortions, as more than 95% of couples who have two or more spontaneous abortions are chromosomally normal.
8. **C,** Page 447. Women with recurrent abortions have a tendency to abort later in gestation, with two thirds of such abortions

occurring beyond 12 weeks of gestation. The abortuses of women who have three or more abortions are more likely to be chromosomally normal (80% to 90%) than those of women with a single spontaneous abortion. If the cause of repetitive abortion is found, it is likely to be associated with a uterine or cervical problem such as a fusion anomaly, leiomyomata, intrauterine adhesions, or cervical incompetence. With recurrent abortion the emotional trauma is magnified, and the physician needs to express sympathy and understanding as counseling is performed and a diagnostic regimen is outlined. If a woman has had no live births and three abortions, she has about a 50% chance of having a term gestation in her next pregnancy, and if she has had one live birth this chance is increased to about 70%.

9. **C**, Page 425. An incomplete abortion is the passage of some but not all fetal or placental tissue through the cervix before 20 weeks' gestation. An inevitable abortion is uterine bleeding from a gestation of less than 20 weeks accompanied by cervical dilation but without expulsion of any placental or fetal tissue through the cervix. A threatened abortion is the presence of any uterine bleeding from a gestation of less than 20 weeks without any cervical dilation or effacement. A septic abortion is any type of abortion that is accompanied by uterine infection. A missed abortion is fetal death before 20 weeks' gestation without expulsion of any fetal or maternal tissue for at least 8 weeks thereafter.
10. **C**, Pages 436-437. This woman has a history that is compatible with intrauterine adhesions. The cause is not clear, but perhaps she contracted genital tuberculosis, which is still encountered in India. Adhesions in the uterine cavity can cause partial or complete obliteration of the endometrium, leading to menstrual abnormalities and amenorrhea as well as being a cause of abortion. The best means of diagnosis is hysteroscopy. The problem may be strongly suspected at the time of D&C and can be recognized by hysterosalpingogram. On occasion adhesions will be missed on hysterosalpingogram. A laparotomy and laparoscopy would not be helpful.
11. **D**, Pages 437-438. It is thought that abortion occurs because of thrombosis in the placental blood supply. Abortions associated with this disease often occur during the second trimester. The antibody interferes with prostacyclin formation, leading to a relative excess of thromboxane, thus causing a thrombotic tendency. There is interference with the activation of prothrombin by the prothrombin activator complex. Decreased platelet adhesiveness is a feature of von Willebrand's disease and is implicated in bleeding, not abortion. The fetus of a mother with systemic lupus erythematosus not infrequently has a complete heart block. It is unlikely that this is the cause of the increased rate of spontaneous abortion in patients with systemic lupus erythematosus. It has been hypothesized that a maternal blocking factor coats the foreign fetal antigens and prevents the fetus from being rejected. This concept is still theoretical and no evidence has been presented to suggest that the lupus anticoagulant in any way interferes.
12. **E**, Pages 437-438. Some investigators have reported luteal deficiency to occur in as many as one third of women with recurrent abortion, whereas others have reported it to be an infrequent cause of abortion. Maintenance of the endometrium for the first 7 weeks of gestation depends on progesterone produced by the corpus luteum. The function of the latter depends on HCG produced by the trophoblast. When progesterone secretion from the corpus luteum is lower than normal or the endometrium has an inadequate response to normal circulating levels of progesterone, endometrial development may be inadequate to support the implanted blastocyst and may lead to spontaneous abortion. Synthetic progestins are luteolytic. There is no evidence that their administration corrects luteal insufficiency. It has even been suggested that their use may contribute to the problem. Diagnosis of luteal insufficiency as a cause of infertilityhas been made by performing a histologic examination of the endometrium and finding a discrepancy of three days or more between the expected and actual endometrial dating pattern in at least two menstrual cycles.
13. **D**, Pages 428, 443, 445. The ultrasound is diagnostic of a blighted ovum or a missed abortion. One can see a large gestational sac but not a fetal pole. There is no evidence of free fluid making a culdocentesis unnecessary since the diagnosis of a heterotropic pregnancy is extremely unlikely.

A quantitative β-HCG is unnecessary. Likewise, with only one pregnancy loss, a karyotype is not cost effective. The incidence of hypofibrinogenemia is uncommon in gestations of less than 14 weeks or duration of fetal death of less than 6 weeks.

14. **E**, Pages 440, 447. Patients with a septic abortion should receive combination antibiotics, including an agent that will be effective against anaerobic bacteria. Newer antibiotics such as Imipenem may become an exception to this rule. The uterine cavity should be evacuated to provide drainage of the infected material. This may be accomplished surgically or medically. An intraarterial line and digitalis may be considered if the patient develops septic shock, but is unnecessary in the case of a septic abortion without shock. Likewise, corticosteroids are not indicated in this patient and their use in septic shock is controversial.
15. **B**, Pages 437-438, 440, 446. Thyroid and progesterone have not proven effective in preventing an abortion. The presence of vaginal bleeding in some cases is the first sign of uterine evacuation of an already nonviable conceptus. The administration of a progestin may increase the probability of having a missed abortion. Iron replacement is indicated in women who are bleeding, especially when there is a good chance that there will be significant blood loss. There is no evidence that bed rest is of value. Should she abort, the longer the patient is in bed, the greater the emotional and possibly even the financial loss to the family. Both corticosteroids and aspirin, which inhibits platelet aggregation have been suggested for patients who have had recurrent abortions, not for patients with a threatened abortion.
16. **D**, Pages 430-431. A maternal and paternal karyotype is an accepted part of the work-up of a couple with repetitive abortions. The yield is not large, however. More than 90% of couples in this category are chromosomally normal. Abnormalities occur in the female parent about twice as frequently as the male. About half of all chromosomic abnormalities are balanced reciprocal translocations, and one-fourth Robertsonian translocations. If the karyotype is abnormal, mosaicism in one of the parents (usually X chromosome mosaicism of the mother) is a frequent finding. If a translocation is found in 1 parent, about 80% of their pregnancies will abort.
17. **B**; Page 429. In most surveys of chromosomal anomalies of abortuses the relative frequency of the types of anomalies is similar. The most frequent type is autosomal trisomy, which accounts for about half the abnormal karyotypes. Trisomies of all autosomes except for autosome 1 have been reported after karyotyping of abortions, with trisomy 16 being the most frequent. About one third of all autosomal trisomies in abortuses are trisomy 16, with trisomy 13, 15, 21, and 22 being the next most frequent.
18. **E**, Pages 441, 447, 449. Numerous infectious agents present in the cervix, uterine cavity, or seminal fluid have been postulated to be etiologic factors for abortion. *Chlamydia trachomatis* is a common sexually transmitted pathogen, but there is no evidence that it causes abortion in asymptomatic women. The work-up for a couple with a history of recurrent abortion should include a history and physical examination with pertinent questions regarding cervical incompetence. It should also incorporate a complete blood count, a serum TSH, and a midluteal serum progesterone measurement. A hysterogram should be performed. If no abnormalities are found, a karyotype of the husband and wife should be done. The value of HLA typing does not appear to be cost effective. Tests to detect lupus anticoagulant should be included.

19-21. 19, **B**; 20, **D**; 21, **E**; Pages 426, 450. About 15% to 20% of all known human pregnancies terminate in clinically recognized abortion. However, the incidence of total human embryonic loss is estimated to be much higher. The rate of human pregnancy loss is estimated to be as high as 70%. About 80% of abortions occur in the first trimester, with the incidence decreasing with increasing gestational age.

22-23. 22, **A**; 23, **C**; Page 433. Figure 15-5 A is a unicornuate uterus, B is a normal uterus, C is a bicornuate uterus, and D is a septate uterus. The unicornuate uterus is associated with the greatest incidence of spontaneous abortion, about 50. This is higher than the 25 to 30 reported with either a septate or bicornuate uterus. A bicornuate uterus can be unified using the Strassman technique. Either a transfundal metroplasty, as described by Jones or Tompkins, or a transcervical hysteroscopic resection of the uterine septum are the methods used to correct a septate uterus.

Surgical corrections should not be considered if the woman has never aborted and should not be performed until other causes of abortion have been ruled out.

24-26. 24, **A;** 25, **D;** 26, A; Pages 441-443. In one study, for women who smoked more than 14 cigarettes per day, the risk of having an abortion was 1.7 times greater than for women who did not smoke. There was no increased risk of an aneuploid abortion in smokers. There is little likelihood that irradiation of less than 5 rads (several times greater than the amount used in all diagnostic procedures listed) will cause an abortion in the human, even if it is administered during the time of implantation. The risk of abortion is threefold normal with daily ingestions of alcohol, and twofold greater in women who drink at least 2 days a week. Just as with smokers, the risk of abortion is confined to chromosomally normal embryos.

27. **A** (1, 2, 3), Page 440. Lupus anticoagulant and Antiphospholipid antibodies have been found in women with systemic lupus erythematosus as well as in those with other connective tissue diseases. It has been found in women with a history of recurrent thrombotic episodes as well as in women with no other disease process. About 50% of women with lupus anticoagulant have a false positive serologic test for syphilis. Lupus anticoagulant is found in a subset of women with recurrent abortions.

28. **B** (1, 2), Pages 443-445, 449. A β-HCG of 3770 mIU/ml is not compatible with a pregnancy of 8 to 9 weeks. In normal gestations the level of HCG double about every 2 days, and the rate of increase in a particular patient can be compared with the expected normal rate of increase. The patient could have an unruptured tubal pregnancy. By definition this cannot be called a normal pregnancy because the patient is bleeding. The finding that the β-HCG is not rising as expected strongly suggests that this pregnancy will not go to term. If this is not a tubal pregnancy, the patient will probably abort.

29. **A** (1, 2, 3), Page 446. A septic abortion, is usually polymicrobial, with *Escherichia coli* and aerobic gram-negative rods frequently involved. Group B beta-hemolytic streptococci, anaerobic streptococci, *Bacteroides* species, and on occasion *Clostridium perfringens* are other organisms that can cause this problem.

30. **A** (1, 2, 3), Pages 426, 428, 450. See answer 31.

31. **C** (2, 3), Pages 426-428, Figure 15-3, 438-439. When talking to a woman contemplating pregnancy, it is important to know facts about previous pregnancies. In this case the woman has a history of repeated pregnancy wastage. The risk of a pregnancy terminating in a spontaneous abortion increases with increasing maternal and paternal age. For women with no live births and a reproductive history of three prior pregnancies terminating in abortion, the chance of having an abortion in a subsequent pregnancy is about 50%, whereas women with at least one live birth and three spontaneous abortions only have a 30% chance that the next pregnancy will terminate in abortion. In the last 25 years, the incidence of a spontaneous abortion in a diabetic, when she is controlled either by diet or by insulin, is the same as the general population. If conception occurs within 3 months after a prior live birth, the incidence of abortion is increased compared to the relatively stable rate if conception occurs later than 3 months.

32. **D** (1 only), Pages 426, 430, 437-438. If conception occurs within 3 months after a prior live birth, the incidence of abortion is increased compared to the relatively stable rate if conception occurs after 3 months. Although older studies indicate that hypothyroidism may be a cause of abortion, there is no definitive evidence that hypothyroidism is a cause of abortion in humans. Furthermore, a better screening test is a serum TSH. Some 90% of couples who have two or more spontaneous abortions are chromosomally normal. That means that obtaining both maternal and paternal chromosomes in cases of repetitive abortion will be fruitful in roughly 10% of cases. Several investigators have reported that in conception cycles the midluteal peak progesterone levels in the circulation are always greater than 9 ng/ml. Serum progesterone 3 days before menses will be close to the nadir for that cycle.

CHAPTER

16 Ectopic Pregnancy

DIRECTIONS for questions 1 - 14: Select the one best answer or completion.

1. An 18 year-old is seen in the emergency room. She is 5 weeks late for her period. She is sexually active and has used foam irregularly for contraception. At the time you see her, her BP is 90/60 and her pulse 110. She is receiving Ringer's lactate. The intern has performed a culdocentesis and obtained 15 ml of non-clotting blood. A pregnancy test is negative. You would
   A. admit and observe
   B. obtain a sonogram
   C. repeat the culdocentesis
   D. obtain a radioimmunoassay for β-hCG
   E. perform a laparotomy
2. The overall subsequent conception rate for women who have had an ectopic pregnancy is
   A. 30%
   B. 40%
   C. 50%
   D. 60%
   E. 70%
3. Of women with an ectopic pregnancy the number who have a subsequent live birth is about
   A. 1/4
   B. 1/3
   C. 1/2
   D. 2/3
   E. 3/4
4. At the time of diagnosis, in patients with a ruptured tubal pregnancy
   A. less than half will have blood in the peritoneal cavity
   B. the culdocentesis will be positive 40% to 50% of the time
   C. blood obtained by culdocentesis has previously clotted and thus will not clot
   D. blood obtained by culdocentesis will have a hematocrit of less than 15%
   E. most of the blood found in the peritoneal cavity is of fetal origin
5. Women with ectopic pregnancies should receive Rh(D) immunoglobulin if they are
   A. Rh negative, antibody negative
   B. Rh negative, antibody positive
   C. Rh positive, antibody negative
   D. Rh positive, antibody positive
   E. Du positive, antibody negative
6. In cases where a salpingectomy is the treatment of choice for a ruptured tubal pregnancy
   A. the ipsilateral ovary should also be removed
   B. the contralateral ovary should also be removed
   C. both ovaries should be removed
   D. both ovaries should be preserved if at all possible
   E. a wedge excision of the ipsilateral ovary should be performed
7. With currently available equipment for abdominal ultrasonography, the visualization of a "fetal pole" or embryonic sac in the oviduct can be accomplished in what percentage of patients with tubal pregnancies?
   A. ≥75%
   B. 66-75%
   C. 46-65%
   D. 26-45%
   E. ≤25%
8. According to current epidemiologic data, the single largest factor contributing to the five fold increase in the number of women diagnosed with ectopic pregnancy is
   A. an increase in fertility rate
   B. an increase in the number of adolescents becoming pregnant
   C. Gamete Intrafallopian Transfer (GIFT)
   D. an increase in the incidence of salpingitis
   E. a decrease in the use of barrier contraception
9. Although the overall death to case rate ratio of ectopic pregnancy has decreased seven fold since 1970, the annual percentage of all maternal deaths in the United States that are a result of ectopic pregnancy has nearly doubled. The main reason for this is
   A. an increase in pregnancy rates among unmarried women

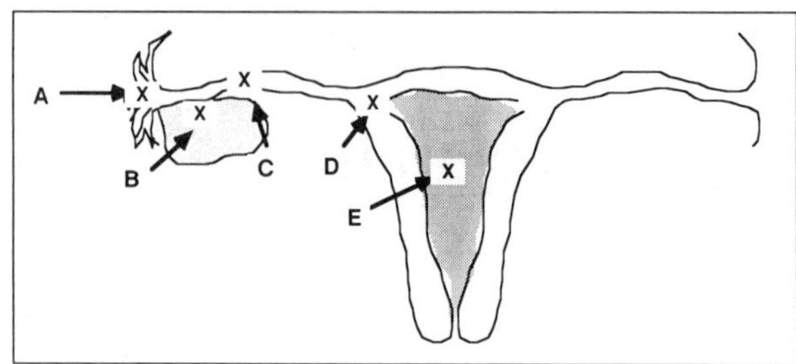

FIGURE 16-1.
Sites of implantation.

B. a death to case rate ratio in black women which has increased three fold
C. a decrease in maternal mortality associated with term pregnancy
D. a decrease in the rate of complications from legal abortion

10. The greatest risk for development of a subsequent ectopic pregnancy follows
    A. one induced abortion
    B. two induced abortions
    C. prior postpartum endometritis
    D. previous pelvic surgery
    E. a previous ectopic pregnancy
11. The following observations about a tubal ectopic pregnancy are true **EXCEPT**
    A. there is a predictable rise in β-hCG
    B. trophoblastic growth is limited to the long axis of the tube
    C. the patient experiences episodic lower quadrant abdominal pain
    D. there is a hemoperitoneum
    E. inflammatory cells are visualized within the walls of the surgically removed oviduct
12. The most consistent symptom of ectopic pregnancy is
    A. amenorrhea
    B. vaginal bleeding
    C. subjective symptoms of pregnancy
    D. abdominal pain
    E. passage of tissue
13. The main advantage of not removing the oviduct at the time of surgery for an unruptured tubal pregnancy is
    A. an increase in subsequent live birth rate
    B. decreased repeat ectopic pregnancy rate
    C. a reduction in overall maternal mortality
    D. a decreased incidence of future anovulatory bleeding
14. The chemotherapeutic agent under investigation in the United States for the medical treatment of an ectopic pregnancy is
    A. adriamycin
    B. RU486
    C. cytoxan
    D. methotrexate
    E. chlorambucil

DIRECTIONS for questions 15 - 20: For each numbered item, select the one heading most closely associated with it. Each lettered heading in Figure 16-1 may be used once, more than once, or not at all.

15. associated with the highest morbidity
16. most common location of ectopic gestations
17. location of less than 1% of ectopic gestations
18. most common location for implantation in women wearing IUDs
19. most common location for implantation for a conception following an ectopic pregnancy
20. associated with a "tubal abortion"

DIRECTIONS For each numbered item 21 - 27, indicate whether it is associated with
A only (A)
B only (B)
C both (A) and (B)
D neither (A) nor (B)

21-24. Match the hormones with the statements
(A) β-hCG
(B) progesterone
(C) both
(D) neither

21. responsible for the decidual change in the endometrium
22. generally reduced in ectopic as compared to intrauterine pregnancies at 8 weeks
23. doubles about every 2 or 3 days in early intrauterine gestations
24. responsible for the Arias-Stella reaction

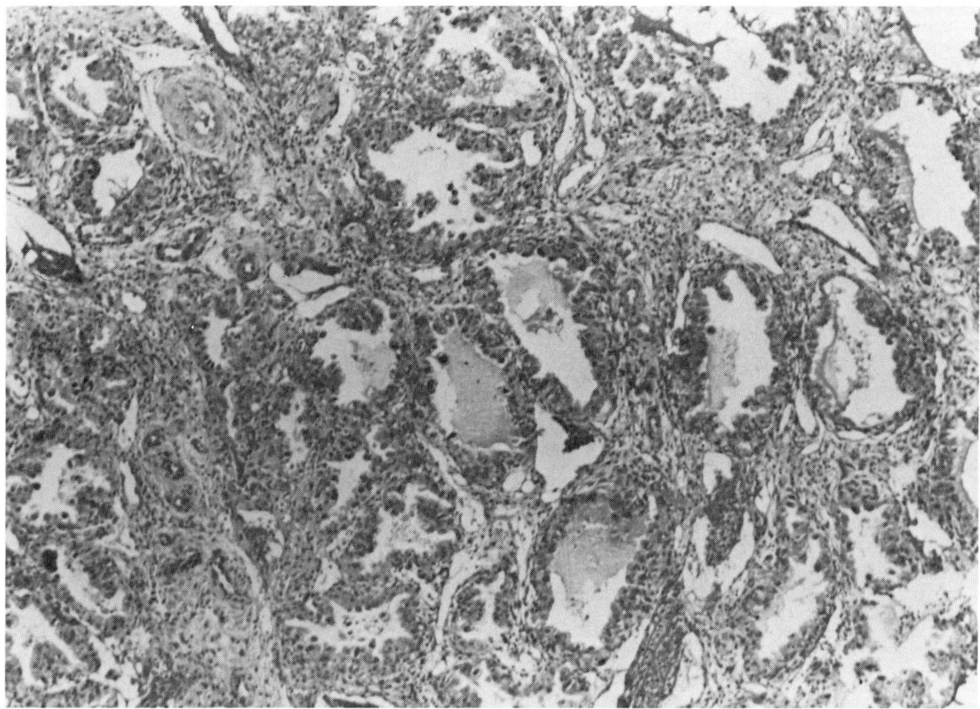

FIGURE 16-2.

25-27. Match the possible location of the pregnancy with the histologic picture
(A) an intrauterine pregnancy
(B) an extrauterine pregnancy
(C) both
(D) neither

25. See Figure 16-2
26. See Figure 16-3
27. See Figure 16-4

DIRECTIONS for questions 28 - 30: For each of the questions below, ONE or MORE of the responses is correct. Select the best answer based on the following

A if 1, 2, and 3 are correct
B if only 1 and 2 are correct
C if only 2 and 3 are correct
D if only 1 is correct
E if only 3 is correct

28. An assay for a-hCG is obtained and reported to be 800 mIU/ml. A second test is performed 72 hours later. This time the value is 1200 mIU/ml. A sonogram is repeated. The picture is not changed. The patient sees you a day later, 96 hours after the first visit. Your updated differential diagnosis is
    1. an ectopic pregnancy
    2. a blighted ovum
    3. an early intrauterine pregnancy
29. Factors that contribute to or cause death from ectopic pregnancy in more than half of the cases include
    1. physician delay and misdiagnosis
    2. blood loss
    3. anesthetic complications
30. You are an expert witness. The plaintiff, a 35-year-old woman, claims that she no longer can become pregnant as a result of the defendant's mismanagement. The plaintiff has been under the defendant's care for several years during which time he hospitalized her for acute pelvic inflammatory disease and the surgical removal of the organ depicted in Figure 16-5, a picture of which is the defendant's Exhibit A.
    On the witness stand you might emphasize that
    1. the physician did an inadequate surgical procedure
    2. the initial cervical cytology should have suggested the diagnosis
    3. loss of fertility is usually a consequence of this clinical occurrence

ANSWERS

1. **E**, Pages 473-474. This patient appears to be in shock and should receive immediate attention. Both a sonogram and a radioimmunoassay would delay definitive treat-

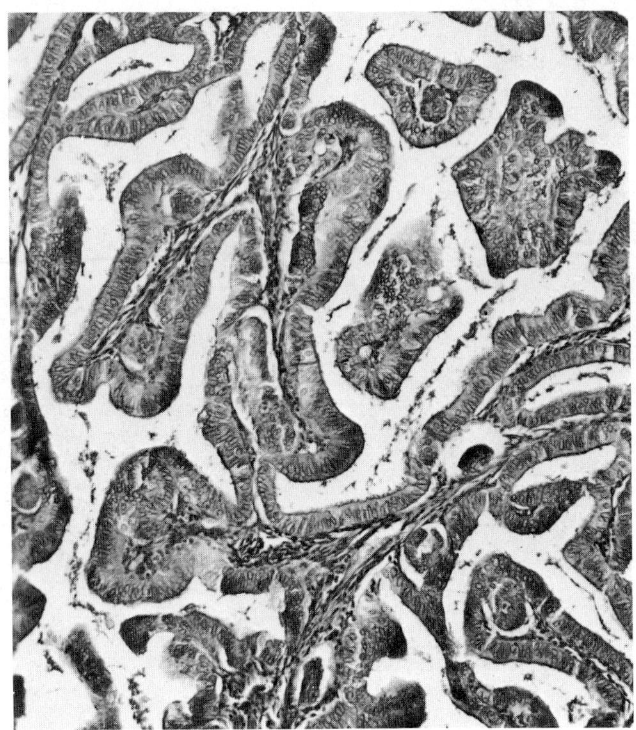

FIGURE 16-3.

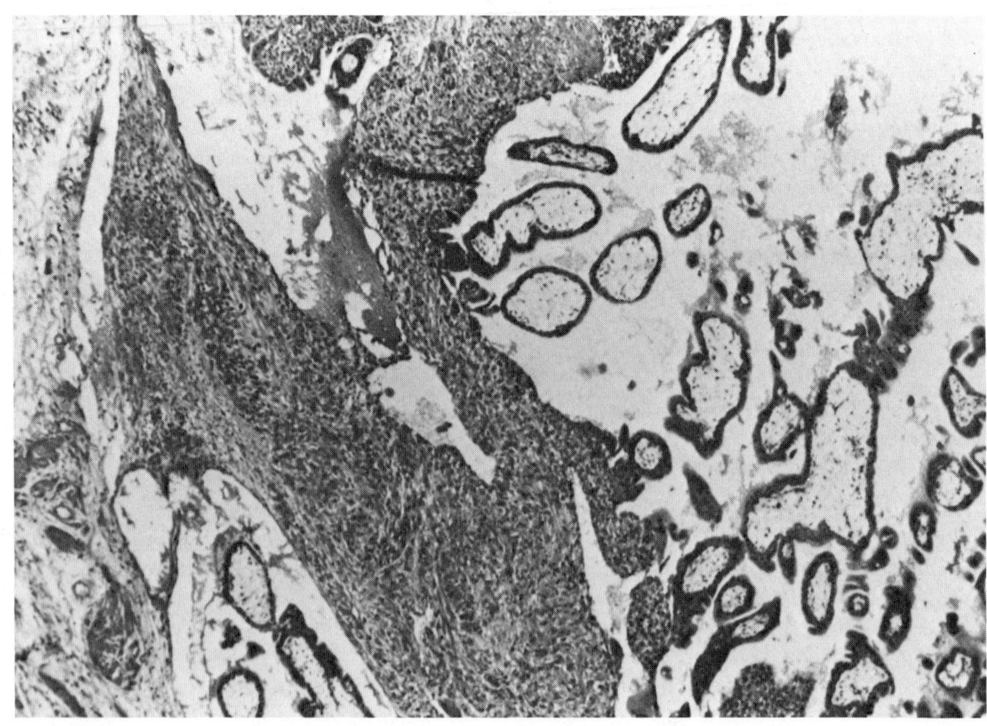

FIGURE 16-4.

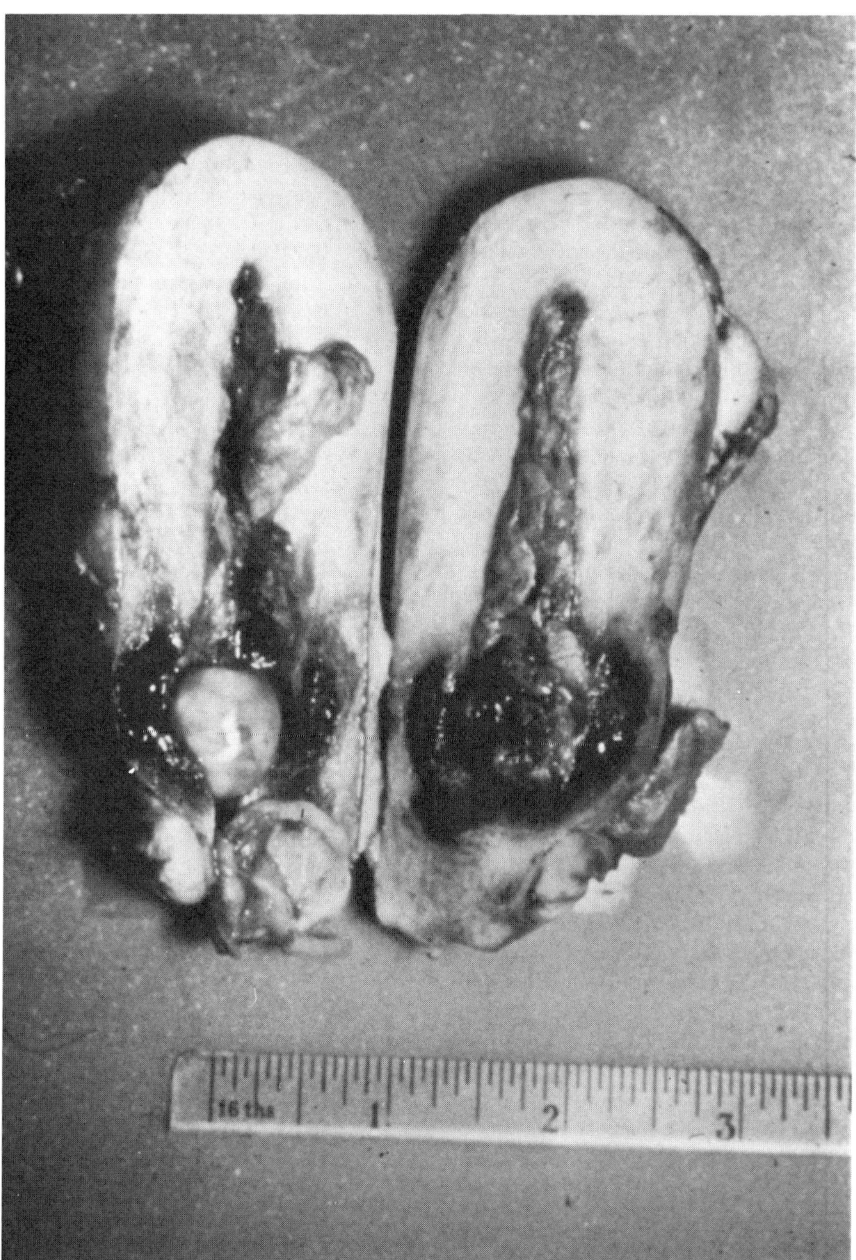

FIGURE 16-5.

ment. A radioimmunoassay may be more sensitive, but the diagnosis is a hemoperitoneum. In this case, the most likely diagnosis is a ruptured corpus luteum. On occasion, an arteriole in the ovary is bleeding and requires suturing.

2. **D,** Page 484. The overall subsequent conception rate for women with an ectopic pregnancy is about 60%. Also see the comment for Answer 16-3.

3. **B,** Pages 484-485. A little less than half of pregnancies subsequent to an ectopic pregnancy terminate in another ectopic gestation or spontaneous abortion. Since the conception rate for these women is 60%, this means that only about one third will have a subsequent live birth. However, these general figures are modified by several factors, particularly age, parity, evidence of contralateral tubal disease,

and whether the tube containing the ectopic was or was not ruptured.

4. **C,** Pages 472, 473-474. Blood is almost always found in the peritoneal cavity in patients with ruptured ectopic pregnancies of any location except cervical implantations. As we begin to make the diagnosis prior to rupture, the number of patients with blood in the peritoneal cavity is likely to fall. The blood is from the mother. It is able to clot and does so in the same way that peripheral blood does. Following clotting, this blood undergoes lysis to yield the non-clotting blood found on culdocentesis. In patients with rapid catastrophic blood loss, the blood obtained by culdocentesis may clot on occasion because it has not had time to undergo lysis. Blood obtained by culdocentesis generally will have a hematocrit of greater than15%. In the presence of a ruptured tubal pregnancy, a culdocentesis is positive over 90% of the time.
5. **A,** Page 484. While the risk of Rh sensitization of an Rh negative mother by an ectopic pregnancy is low, all Rh negative patients who are not already sensitized should receive Rh(D) immunoglobulin. A person who is classified as RhDu positive rarely develops antibodies when challenged by Rho(D) antigen.
6. **D,** Page 479. While data concerning the removal of the ipsilateral ovary is conflicting, most authors agree that there should be as little as possible done to or around the ovary in order to preserve future fertility options.
7. **E,** Page 478. In 1987, using abdominal scanning techniques, the visualization of an ectopic gestation occurs in only about 25% or less of patients. Transvaginal scanning techniques eventually may raise this rate to 50% or better. Improvements in imaging are occurring at such a rapid rate that it is difficult to predict their efficacy in the future. Visualization of an intrauterine gestational sac containing a fetal pole is possible at 5 to 7 weeks of gestational age (menstrual dates).
8. **D,** Pages 458-459. The Centers for Disease Control reported a marked increase in ectopic pregnancy in the United States between 1970-1987. During this time there was a five fold increase in the annual number of women hospitalized for ectopic pregnancies (from 17,800 to 88,000); there was a tripling of the rate reported per 1,000 pregnancies. The increased incidence of ectopic pregnancies is thought to be mainly the result of an increased incidence of salpingitis, which is a major risk factor for ectopic pregnancy. The improvement in diagnostic techniques may also contribute to this reported increase.
9. **B,** Pages 459-460. About 40-50 deaths from ectopic pregnancy occur annually. Even though the percentage of maternal deaths has risen from 8% in 1970 to 14% in 1980, the percent ofectopics becoming fatal has decreased. The overall death to case rate of ectopic pregnancy has decreased seven fold in all women with ectopic pregnancy and is similar in all age groups, but is about three times higher in black women. Because the incidence of ectopic pregnancy is also higher in blacks in the United States, a pregnant black woman is about five times more likely to die of ectopic pregnancy than a white woman. Ectopic pregnancy is the most common single cause of all maternal deaths among black women causing about one fifth of such deaths.
10. **E,** Page 466; Table 16-6. Although some studies have suggested that prior induced abortion increases the risk of ectopic pregnancy, it has been shown that when techniques are used to control the effects of other risk factors, the history of one prior induced abortion does not significantly increase the risk of an ectopic pregnancy. Another study suggests that two or more prior induced abortions do not increase the risk of an ectopic pregnancy. Previous pelvic surgery and previous pelvic infection transmit an extra risk, but not the same as a prior ectopic pregnancy which confers a relative risk of 7.7.
11. **A,** Pages 469, 471. Items regarding histopathology of ectopic pregnancy are important in understanding the natural history of the disease. Because of limited space or inadequate nourishment the trophoblastic tissue of most ectopic pregnancies does not grow as rapidly as that of pregnancies within the uterine cavity resulting in an unpredictable rise in β-hCG. Trophoblastic growth occurs in both the parallel axis as well as the circumferential axis of the fallopian tube. The patient does experience episodic lower quadrant abdominal pain. A hemoperitoneum is nearly always present in cases of an ectopic preg-

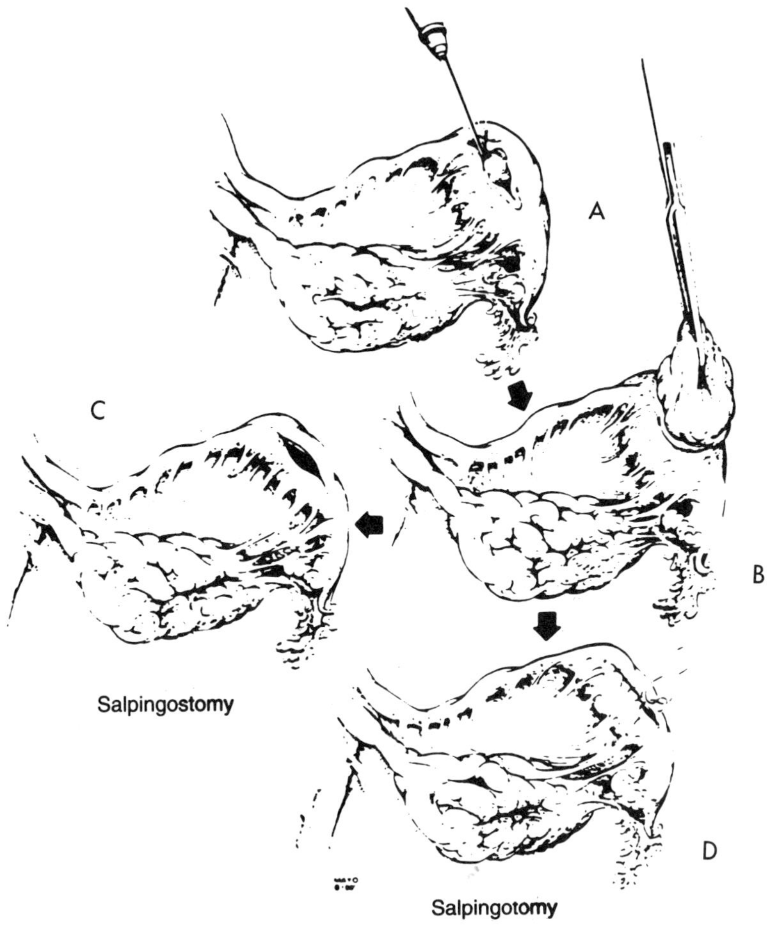

FIGURE 16-6.

A, Incision is made nto the antimesenteric border of the fallopian tube. **B,** Ectopic pregnancy is gently removed from within the fallopian tube. **C,** Salpingostomy site is allowed to heal by secondary intention. **D,** Salpingotomy is completed by primary closure.

(From Leach RE and Ory SJ: J Reprod Med 34:325, 1989.)

nancy involving the fallopian tube. When the oviduct is removed and examined histologically, inflammatory cells are nearly always seen including plasma cells, lymphocytes, and histiocytes.

12. **D,** Page 472; Table 16-7. The most common symptoms associated with an ectopic pregnancy are abdominal pain, absence of a menstrual bleed, and irregular bleeding. Pain is nearly a universal symptom but is nottype-specific. Before rupture the pain may be only a vague soreness or colicky type of pain. Its location may be generalized, unilateral, or bilateral. Shoulder pain occurs in about one fourth of patients with an ectopic as a result of diaphragmatic irritation from a hemoperitoneum.

13. **A,** Pages 479-481. With increasing frequency, conservative management (not removing the oviduct) of an unruptured ectopic pregnancy is the preferred surgical choice for a woman who desires future fertility. When conservative surgery is correctly performed, the repeat ectopic pregnancy rate is not increased in comparison with salpingectomy. Furthermore, the subsequent live birth rate is increased. Current operations appear to have an inappreciable effect on overall maternal mortality, and there is little information about the effects of these operations on regular cyclic bleeding. The best results of conservative operation occur after salpingotomy or salpingostomy, the latter being used more frequently in the United States.

14. **D,** Pages 481-482. After initial reports of the successful treatment of ectopic pregnancies with methotrexate in 1982, a number of studies have evolved analyzing critically this treatment alternative. These protocols prescribed methotrexate over a five day course of treatment in doses ranging from 60-300 mg intramuscularly. Current investigations center around the use of oral methotrexate. Although RU486 shows promise for similar purposes, its use in this country is currently limited. The other chemotherapeutic agents are not efficacious in treating trophoblastic disorders. Preliminary results indicate the disadvantages of methotrexate treatment include the need for subsequent laparotomy for bleeding, and the unacceptable toxic side effects of the drug.

15-20. 15, **D;** 16, **C;** 17, **B;** 18, **E;** 19, **E;** 20, **A.** Pages 459-460, 466-467; Figure 16-7 from Droegemueller W, Herbst AL, Mishell DR, Stenchever MA: Comprehensive gynecology, St. Louis, The C.V. Mosby Co, 1987. While most ectopic gestations implant in the mid to distal portion of the tube, the area of implantation associated with the greatest morbidity and mortality is the interstitial portion due to the catastrophic consequences of a rupture in that area. Implantations at or near the fimbrial end of the tube may abort without causing tubal rupture. Less than 1% of ectopic pregnancies are found implanted in the ovary. About 2% of all ectopic pregnancies are interstitial. Most pregnancies after previous ectopic pregnancy or while wearing an IUD are intrauterine.

21-24. 21, **B;** 22, **C;** 23, **A;** 24, **B.** Pages 474, 476. Both progesterone and β-hCG are generally lower in ectopic pregnancies in comparison to normal intrauterine pregnancies. The rate of increase in β-hCG is much slower in ectopic pregnancies. Normally it doubles in 48 to 72 hours. The progesterone produced by the corpus luteum is responsible for both the decidual and the Arias-Stella reaction.

25. **C,** Page 471. Sometimes the secretory cells of the endometrial glands become hypertrophied with hyperchromatism, pleomorphism, and increased mitotic activity (Figure 16-2). This is known as the Arias-Stella reaction, and it can be confused with neoplasia. It is not unique for an ectopic pregnancy; it can occur with an intrauterine pregnancy as well as following stimulation with clomiphene.

26. **D,** Page 907. Figure 16-3 is a microscopic section of a grade I endometrial adenocarcinoma. There is glandular atypia. The glands are closely packed. They are not uniform in size or shape. In some areas the glands are stratified with beginning tufting and papillae. The cells are irregular in size and shape.

27. **B,** Page 462. Figure 16-4 is a photomicrograph of a tubal pregnancy. Chorionic villi can be identified on the right. A well-developed myometrium is not seen. Instead, adipose tissue (on the left) is seen in close proximity to the villi.

28. **B,** (1, 2). Page 474. The β-hCG has increased 40% in 72 hours. This indicates an abnormal pregnancy, either a blighted ovum or an ectopic. In a normal pregnancy the β-hCG should be at least 66% higher than the initial value in 48 hours.

29. **B,** (1, 2). Page 460. Over half of all deaths from ectopic pregnancy occur as a result of blood loss and physician delays or misdiagnosis. Anesthetic complications account for less than 2% of all ectopic pregnancy deaths.

30. **E,** (3 only). Page, 469. This is a hysterectomy specimen from a cervical pregnancy. Most cervical pregnancies occur after sharp uterine curettage. More than half the patients with cervical pregnancy require hysterectomy for treatment. Even if a hysterectomy is not performed, the prognosis for future fertility is poor.

CHAPTER

17 Benign Gynecologic Lesions

DIRECTIONS for questions 1 - 23: Select the one best answer or completion.

1. A 28 year-old gravida 1, para 0 at 24 weeks gestation with a known history of leiomyomata presents with severe uterine pain. The fetal status is normal. On palpation a 6 cm. tender area is noted and thought to be on the uterus. The examination is otherwise unremarkable. The most likely diagnosis is
   A. a ruptured uterus
   B. a placental abruption
   C. hyaline degeneration of a myoma
   D. carneous degeneration of a myoma
   E. premature labor
2. Of the dermatologic diseases of the vulva listed below, the one best treated by wide excision is
   A. contact dermatitis
   B. psoriasis
   C. lichen planus
   D. hidradenitis suppurative
   E. seborrheic dermatitis
3. A 32 year-old patient has a six month history of dyspareunia, dysuria, and dribbling of urine. A palpable, tender mass is apparent in the anterior vagina. The most likely diagnosis is
   A. a Skene's gland cyst
   B. chronic cystitis
   C. a vaginal inclusion cyst
   D. a Gartner's duct cyst
   E. a urethral diverticulum
4. During a routine gynecologic examination of an asymptomatic, sexually active, 28 year-old, a 3 cm sausage-shaped cystic mass is found protruding from the anterolateral wall of the upper vagina. The treatment of choice is
   A. expectant management
   B. oral antibiotics
   C. laparoscopy and cystoscopy
   D. marsupialization of cyst
   E. excision of cyst
5. A 25 year-old gravida 1, para 1, who is six weeks postpartum and breast feeding, comes to the Emergency Department with heavy vaginal bleeding since having intercourse two hours ago. This was the first time in several months she had attempted coitus. Although the examination is difficult, a one centimeter transverse bleeding laceration of the posterior fornix is identified. The proper management is
   A. vaginal estrogen cream
   B. vaginal packing
   C. suturing the laceration
   D. hospitalization for observation
   E. discharge to be followed in the office in the AM
6. A 37 year-old patient complains of intermenstrual and postcoital spotting. The findings on speculum examination are illustrated in Figure. 17-1. Appropriate therapy for this patient's condition is
   A. hysterectomy
   B. fractional dilatation and curettage
   C. removal of mass in the office
   D. laser conization
   E. vaginal estrogen cream
7. An asymptomatic 25 year-old gravida 5, para 5 who has had a tubal ligation, presents with a 20 week, irregular pelvic mass which you suspect is uterine myomata. The next step in management should be
   A. magnetic resonance imaging
   B. ultrasound
   C. CT Scan
   D. hysteroscopy
   E. hysterectomy
8. A 47 year-old asymptomatic patient is found to have an 8 week size irregular myomatous uterus. Appropriate management should be
   A. re-evaluation in 6-12 months
   B. administration of GnRH analogues
   C. fractional dilatation and curettage
   D. myomectomy
   E. hysterectomy
9. A 23 year-old graduate student is found to have an asymptomatic 4 cm ovarian cyst. Her menstrual periods are regular. She is not sexually active and does not use oral contraceptives. The cyst is freely mobile

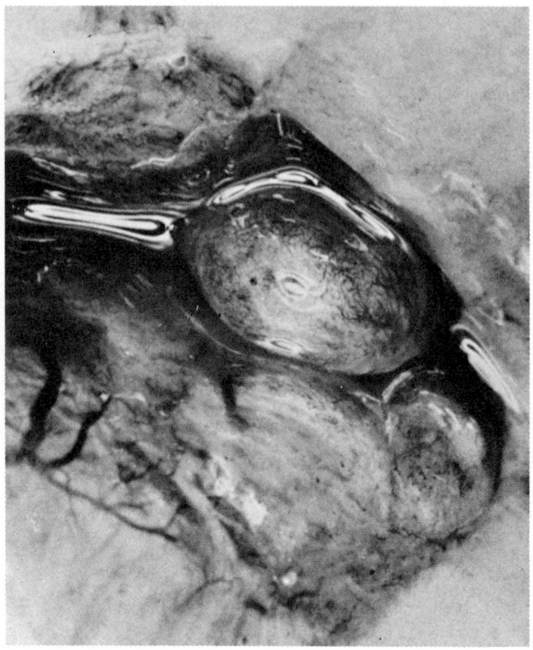

FIGURE 17-1.
(From Kolstad P, Stafl A, eds: Atlas of colposcopy, 2nd ed. Baltimore, University Part Press, 1977, p. 66.)

and non-tender to palpation. The treatment of choice is
A. re-examination in 6 weeks
B. oral contraceptives
C. needle aspiration under ultrasound
D. laparoscopy
E. laparotomy

10. A 28 year-old gravida 0 whose last normal menstrual period was 6 weeks ago presents with a one week history of left lower quadrant pain. She uses a diaphragm for contraception. Her previous menstrual history was normal. She denies any history of pelvic inflammatory disease. Abdominal examination is normal. On pelvic examination, there is a tender 3 cm left adnexal mass. The Hct. is 38%, WBC is 6,000 and serum pregnancy test is negative. The most likely diagnosis is
A. ectopic pregnancy
B. tubo-ovarian abscess
C. salpingitis
D. endometriosis
E. corpus luteum cyst

11. After the delivery of twins at term by cesarean section, and closing the uterine incision, bilateral ovarian masses similar to those in figure 17-2 are found. Your next step would be to
A. perform a total abdominal hysterectomy with bilateral salpingo-oophorectomy.
B. perform a bilateral oophorectomy
C. perform a bilateral wedge resection
D. aspirate the cysts
E. close the abdomen

12. The most common complication of a cystic teratoma is
A. infection
B. torsion
C. rupture
D. hemorrhage
E. malignant degeneration

13. A 25 year-old on birth control pills whose last normal menstrual period was one week ago complains of a sudden onset of severe left lower quadrant pain, which awoke her from sleeping. She had several milder episodes over the last week for which she did not seek medical care. She is nauseated and has vomited three times.
On physical examination, her temperature is 100°F. There is tenderness in the left lower abdominal quadrant and there is an exquisitely tender 5 cm left adnexal mass. A β-hCG is negative. The most appropriate action is to
A. administer parenteral broad spectrum antibiotics
B. perform IVP
C. perform a barium enema
D. perform laparoscopy or laparotomy
E. perform culdocentesis

14. A 25 year-old gravida 1, para 1, complains of pain during intercourse. This has been a problem for three months and is noted primarily on entry. Physical examination is normal except for several punctate ulcers in the vestibule, which are primarily located around the Bartholin's glands. They are exquisitely tender when touched by an cotton tip applicator stick. The complaint is most likely due to
A. contact dermatitis
B. vulvar vestibulitis
C. psoriasis
D. hidradenitis suppurativa
E. syringoma

15. During pregnancy, most myoma
A. grow
B. shrink
C. enlarge and undergo degeneration
D. shrink and undergo degeneration
E. remain the same size and do not undergo degeneration

16. The most common type of degeneration to occur within a myoma is
A. calcific
B. red

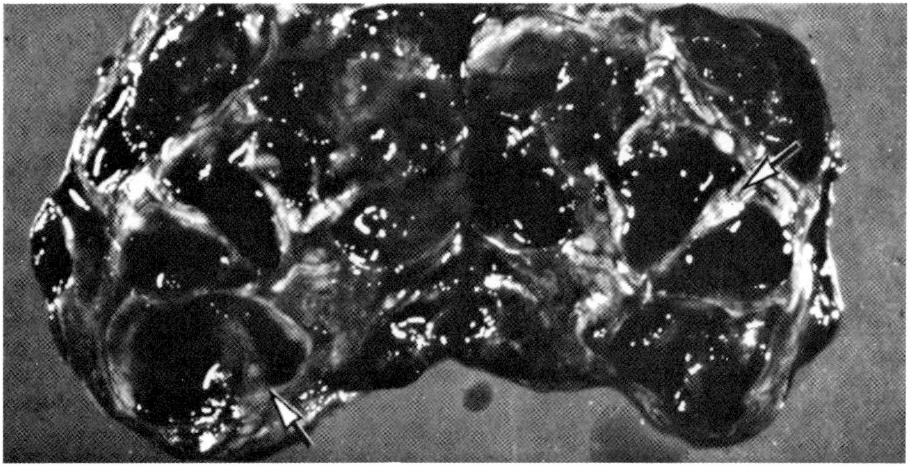

FIGURE 17-2.
(From Blaustein A: In Blaustein A, ed: Pathology of the female genital tract. New York, Springer-Verlag, 1977, p. 397.)

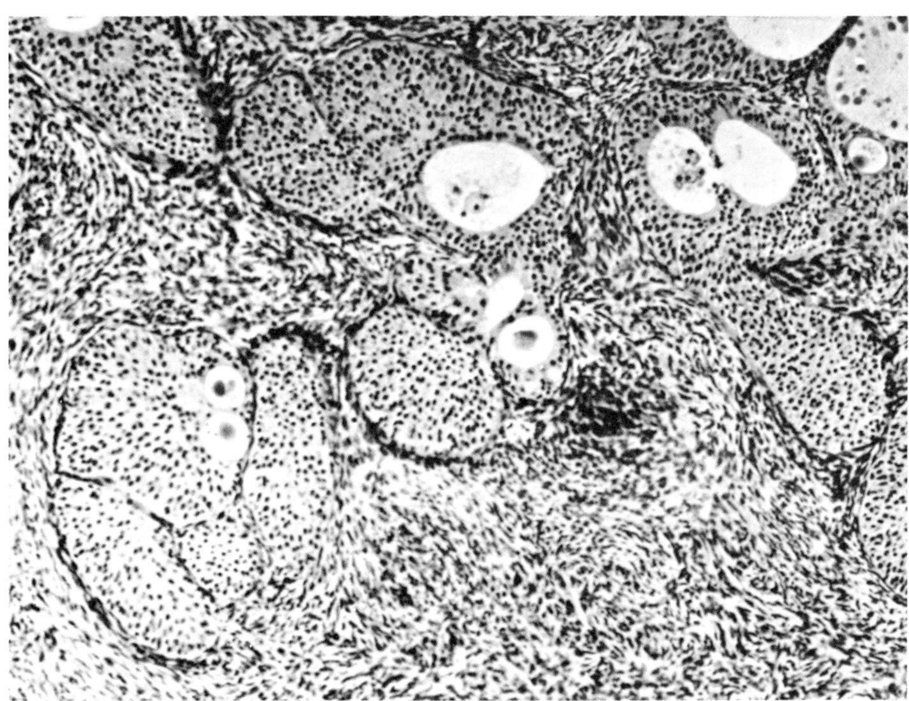

FIGURE 17-3.

C. hyaline
D. myxomatous
E. sarcomatous

17. Medical treatment of myomata is best accomplished with
A. danazol
B. depo-provera (medroxyprogesterone)
C. GnRH analogues
D. estrogens
E. testosterone

18. A 35 year-old gravida 0 is undergoing surgery for a solid left ovarian mass. The frozen section of the ovary is pictured in Figure 17-3. The pelvis is otherwise normal. Based on this histological picture, the patient should have a
A. total abdominal hysterectomy with bilateral salpingo-oophorectomy
B. total abdominal hysterectomy with left salpingo-oophorectomy

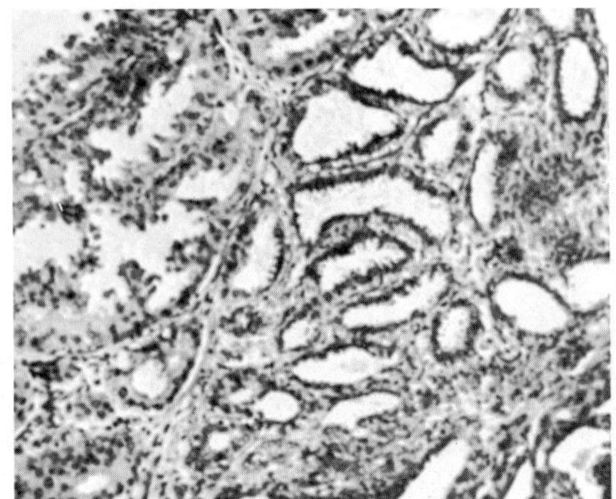

FIGURE 17-4.

C. bilateral salpingo-oophorectomy
D. left salpingo-oophorectomy
E. left oophorectomy

19. Optimal therapy for the lesion pictured in Figure 17-4 is
    A. vulvectomy
    B. excisional biopsy
    C. irradiation
    D. 5-fluorouracil
    E. methotrexate
20. The most common large cyst of the vulva is a
    A. epidermal inclusion cyst
    B. Bartholin's duct cyst
    C. Gartner's duct cyst
    D. nabothian cyst
    E. sebaceous cyst
21. A 72 year-old patient asks about several 1 mm dark blue lesions on the vulva which have appeared since her last annual visit. The most likely diagnosis is a
    A. pyogenic granuloma
    B. cherry angioma
    C. angiokeratoma
    D. strawberry hemangioma
    E. nevus
22. A 55 year-old patient presents with the lesion in Figure 17-5. She complains of mild dysuria. The initial therapy for this condition is
    A. topical estrogen
    B. operation excision
    C. laser ablation
    D. fulguration
    E. cryosurgery
23. The chromosomal makeup of benign cystic teratomas is
    A. 46,XX
    B. 46,XY

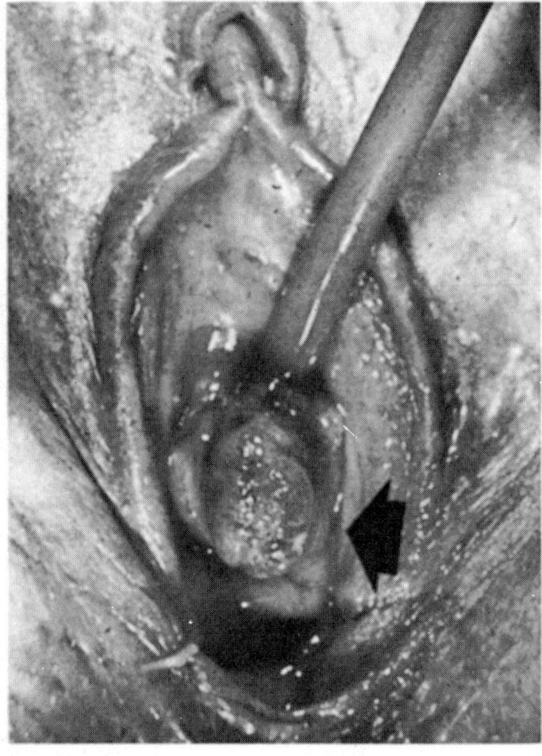

FIGURE 17-5.

C. 45,X
D. 47,XXX
E. 47,XXY

DIRECTIONS for questions 24 - 29: For each numbered item, select the one heading most closely associated with it. Each lettered heading may be used once, more than once, or not at all.

24-26. Match the description with the most closely associated vulvar lesion

(A) fibroma
(B) lipoma
(C) hidradenoma
(D) granular cell myoblastoma
(E) Bowen's disease

24. most commonly benign solid vulvar tumor
25. arise from neutral sheath cells
26. histologically similar to adenocarcinoma

27-29. Match the association with the ovarian neoplasm

(A) cystic teratoma
(B) fibroma
(C) serous cystadenoma
(D) dysgerminoma
(E) endometrioma

27. tubercle of Rokitansky
28. Meig's syndrome
29. Brenner tumor

DIRECTIONS For each numbered item 30 - 35, indicate whether it is associated with
A only (A)
B only (B)
C both (A) and (B)
D neither (A) nor (B)

30-32. Match the conditions with the statements below

(A) hematometra
(B) pyometra
(C) both
(D) neither

30. result of cervical stenosis
31. associated with amenorrhea
32. associated with endometriosis

33-35. Match the statements with the tubal pathology

(A) leiomyoma of oviduct
(B) paratubal cyst
(C) both
(D) neither

33. may undergo torsion
34. mesonephric duct origin
35. salpingectomy indicated

DIRECTIONS for questions 36 - 42: For each of the questions below, ONE or MORE of the responses is correct. Select the best answer based on the following
A if 1, 2, and 3 are correct
B if only 1 and 2 are correct
C if only 2 and 3 are correct
D if only 1 is correct
E if only 3 is correct

36. Indications for a surgical management of an adnexal mass include a
    1. solid tumor
    2. prepubertal patient
    3. cystic mass greater than 8 cm.
37. A hysterectomy should be performed if a myomatous uterus
    1. is the size of a 14 week gestation
    2. appears to be enlarging and the patient is menopausal
    3. on ultrasound evaluation is found to contain echogenic areas thought to be calcium deposits
38. Clinical features of an early malignant melanoma include
    1. a smooth border
    2. asymmetry
    3. variation of the color
39. Symptoms associated with cervical myomas include
    1. urinary urgency
    2. dyspareunia
    3. abnormal bleeding
40. A 65 year-old patient is undergoing office endometrial sampling because of vaginal spotting. With difficulty, a 1 mm dilator is passed into the endometrial cavity resulting in the discharge of pus from the cervical os. This patient should have
    1. intravenous broad spectrum antibiotics
    2. a pelvic ultrasound
    3. a fractional dilatation and curettage at a later date
41. A 28 year-old patient is concerned about of a growth on her labia. The significant pelvic examination finding is shown in Figure 17-6. The differential diagnosis encompasses a
    1. fibroma
    2. lipoma
    3. Bartholin's duct cyst
42. A 35 year-old patient notes that her left labia majora is enlarged and somewhat tender. The clinical diagnosis is a vulvar hematoma. It is likely that this woman
    1. is pregnant
    2. delivered 5 days ago over an intact perineum
    3. has strenuously exercised in the last several hours

ANSWERS

1. **D,** Pages 511, 515. The blood supply to myomas is less than to a similar sized area of normal myometrium. Therefore, as a myoma grows, it outgrows its blood supply resulting in degeneration. The most acute form of degeneration is red or carneous degeneration typified by the rapidly growing myoma during the midtrimester of pregnancy. The sudden muscular infarction causes pain and localized peritonitis. Treatment should be medical since surgical intervention in a pregnant patient results in profuse blood loss. Placental abruption at 24 weeks is unusual and the uterus would be expected to be diffusely tender.
2. **D,** Pages 501-502. Hidradenitis suppurative is a chronic refractory infection of the skin and subcutaneous tissue. It may progress from subcutaneous nodules to draining abscesses and sinuses. The treatment of choice is early, aggressive wide excision. Dermatologic conditions such as contact dermatitis, psoriasis, lichen planus, and seborrheic dermatitis can all be treated with a topical steroid.
3. **E,** Pages 502-503. The most common symptoms associated with a urethral diverticulum are urinary urgency, frequency, and dysuria. Dyspareunia and dribbling after micturition have also been reported by the 80% of patients with a urethral di-

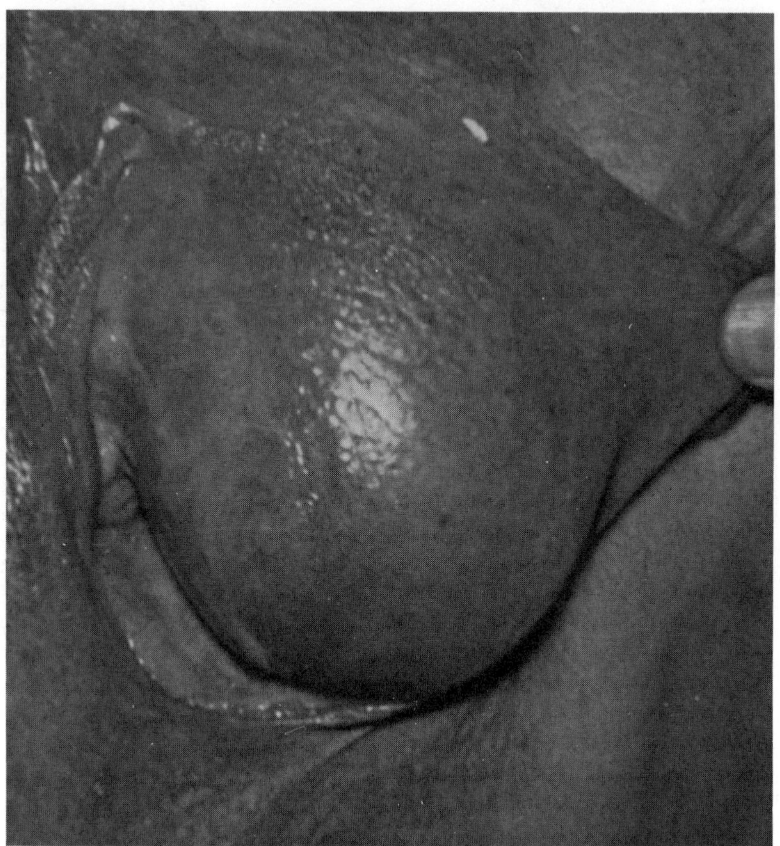

FIGURE 17-6.

verticulum who are symptomatic. The diagnosis may be confirmed by several techniques including urethrography, cystourethroscopy, and positive pressure urethrography using a Davis catheter.

4. **A,** Page 504. Gartner's duct cysts are dysontogenetic cysts of mesonephric origin, usually found in the upper half of the vagina. They occur in approximately one out of two hundred women and are usually asymptomatic. Unless symptoms such as vaginal pain, dyspareunia, difficulty with urination or a large palpable mass occur, they may be followed conservatively.
5. **C,** Page 505. Coitus is the most frequent cause of trauma to the lower genital tract of adult women. Predisposing factors include virginity, pregnancy, postpartum, postmenopausal vagina epithelium, prolonged abstinence, hysterectomy, and inebriation. The most prominent symptom of a coital vaginal laceration is profuse or prolonged vaginal bleeding. Many women who develop a laceration experience sharp pain during intercourse, and about 25% note persistent abdominal pain. The most troublesome, but extremely rare complication of a vaginal laceration, is vaginal evisceration. Management includes suturing the laceration under adequate anesthesia. It should be noted that patients such as the one described have vaginas that show little estrogen effect and are thereby at greater risk for trauma.
6. **C,** Pages 505-507. A patient with intermenstrual and postcoital spotting has symptoms suggestive of a cervical polyp. The differential diagnosis for the lesion in figure 17-1 includes an endocervical or endometrial polyp, a prolapsed myoma, a squamous papilloma, products of conception, sarcoma, and a cervical malignancy. In most instances, an endocervical polyp can be removed by twisting it off its base using a surgical clamp. This can usually be done in the office. If the intermenstrual and postcoital spotting continue after removal of

polyp, endometrial sampling is indicated to identify an endometrial lesion whose symptoms mimicked those of a polyp.

7. **E,** Page 518. This question raises several issues. First, what is most cost effective? The diagnosis of uterine myomas is usually confirmed by palpation of an enlarged, firm, irregular uterus during pelvic examination. In experienced hands, further verification is unnecessary. Hysterectomy would be the logical surgical procedure. Thus, the answer given. In difficult cases, concentric calcifications on abdominal x-ray or characteristics findings on ultrasound, CT scan, and magnetic resonance imaging may aid in the diagnosis. Ultrasound remains the most cost-effective single imaging technique. Submucous myomas may be observed during hysteroscopy. They also appear as filling defects on hysterosalpingogram. The second issue is the availability of expert assistance if an ovarian malignancy is encountered at laparotomy. In communities without an oncologist, ultrasound should be employed if there is doubt about the diagnosis. The third issue is that medical therapy is also an option for this patient if myomas are confirmed. At this patient's age, and given the size of the myomata, medical therapy will provide only a short term response. If the patient does not desire surgery, frequent follow-up is mandatory.
8. **A,** Page 518. Most women with uterine myomas do not require surgery. This is particularly true for asymptomatic, perimenopausal patients since the condition tends to improve with declining levels of circulating estrogen. Re-examination allows determination of the rate of growth. Symptomatic patients must be evaluated appropriately with therapy ultimately depending on severity and persistence of symptoms, age, parity,and reproductive plans. Dilatation and curettage would be warranted in cases of abnormal bleeding. Myomectomy, both transabdominal and hysteroscopic, is reserved for symptomatic women who have not completed childbearing. A few small series of cases using Danazol, GnRH analogues or medroxyprogesterone have reported reduction in tumor size. Myomas tend to return after the medication is discontinued.
9. **A,** Page 522. The initial management of a suspected functional ovarian cyst is observation. Since most follicular cysts reabsorb spontaneously or silently rupture in 4-8 weeks, re-evaluation in 6 weeks would be acceptable. A 6 week rather than 4 week interval is preferable so that the patient may be examined at a different point in her cycle. Oral contraceptives remove any influence by pituitary gonadotrophins and may be prescribed for a short term trial. Recent data demonstrate that oral contraceptives do not bring about the disappearance of functional ovarian cysts better than observation alone. Surgical intervention is not warranted in the asymptomatic patient initially.
10. **E,** Page 524. Halban's syndrome describes a persistently functioning corpus luteum cyst which clinically mimics an ectopic pregnancy. This triad includes a delay in normal menses with subsequent spotting, unilateral pelvic pain, and a small tender adnexal mass. With the advent of rapid, sensitive pregnancy tests that measure β-hCG, the distinction between ectopic pregnancy and persistent corpus luteum cyst is made more easily because the pregnancy test is almost always positive in the presence of an ectopic pregnancy.
11. **E,** Pages 525-526. Pregnancies producing large placentas, such as those associated with twins, diabetes, and Rh sensitization, are more likely to be associated with theca lutein cysts. The ovaries should be handled delicately to avoid cyst rupture and hemorrhage. No further surgery is warranted since the cysts will regress as the gonadotrophin stimulation disappears.
12. **B,** Page 528. The most frequent complication of a cystic teratoma is torsion, which occurs in approximately 11% of patients. The overall incidence of rupture is less than 5%, occurring more commonly in pregnancy and the puerperium with resultant leakage and incitement of a chemical peritonitis. Infection, hemorrhage and-malignant degeneration are all unusual complications, occurring is less than 1% in patients
13. **D,** Page 537. The differential diagnosis includes an ectopic, pelvic inflammatory disease (PID), and ovarian torsion. A pregnancy test is negative and the last menstrual period was one week ago. This makes the diagnosis of an ectopic unlikely. This patient is obviously sick and has a low grade fever. PID is unlikely. Most patients with adnexal torsion, like the one

described, are ill enough to warrant operative intervention. In cases where the diagnosis is in doubt, laparoscopy may be needed to rule out conditions such as abscess and a ruptured corpus luteum. In selected cases of partial torsion, it is acceptable to untwist the pedicle, perform a cystectomy, and then stabilize the ovary. This does carry the risk of releasing venous thrombi. In cases of vascular compromise, unilateral salpingo-oophorectomy is the operation of choice.

14. **B,** Page 500. Vulvar vestibulitis presents as vulvar burning and pain at the introitus. Typical signs include focal ulceration and inflammation of the vestibular mucosa with punctate 3 mm to 10 mm lesions particularly between the two Bartholin glands. It spontaneously remits in one third of patients and is usually treated conservatively initially with anesthetics. Only if refractory should laser surgery or surgical excision be contemplated. Contact dermatitis is due to either true allergies or a contact irritant. Psoriasis usually affects intertriginous areas and is manifest by red-yellow papules. Hydradenitis suppurativa is a chronic infection of the skin and subcutaneous tissue which typically progresses to draining abscesses and sinuses. Syringoma is a rare, benign tumor of the exocrine sweat glands. It starts as small subcutaneous papules and may coalesce to form cords of tissue.
15. **E,** Page 516. Serial ultrasound examinations have shown that 80% of myomas do not change size during pregnancy. If the myoma does change size, there is usually no associated pain. The most acute form of degeneration is red or carneous infarction, which occurs in approximately 5-10% of pregnant women with myomas.
16. **C,** Page 516. Ultimately, most myomas outgrow their blood supply resulting in some type of cellular degeneration. The most common form of degeneration of a myoma is hyaline degeneration. On a cellular level, the smooth muscle cells are replaced by fibrous connective tissue. It occurs in 65% of cases. The other extreme is malignant degeneration, which is known to occur in 0.3% to 0.7% of cases.
17. **C,** Page 518. Myomas can be medically treated by decreasing the circulating level of estrogens. GnRH analogues are successful in reducing the size of myomas in as many as 80-100% of patients. In some there is as much as a 90% diminution in size. Maximum reduction occurs within eight months. Unfortunately, after the therapy is discontinued, most myomas return to their pretreatment size within six months. Thus, GnRH agonist have been used most successfully preoperatively to reduce the size of the myomas—to reduce blood loss at the time of surgery. Since myomata tend to get smaller after patients are climacteric, the perimenopausal use of a GnRH agonist will alleviate the need for a hysterectomy in selected patients.
18. **E,** Page 534; Figure 17-3 from Czernobilsky. In Blaustein A, ed: Pathology of the female genital tract. New York, Springer-Verlag, 1977, p.490. The ovarian tumor in Figure 17-3 is a Brenner tumor, a smooth, solid ovarian tumor that is usually asymptomatic. Typically, they occur in women age 40-60 years with 90% of these neoplasms discovered as an incidental finding during a gynecologic procedure. Histologically, the Brenner tumor is identified by solid masses or nests or epithelial cells with a surrounding fibrous stroma. The appropriate management of a Brenner tumor is simple excision.
19. **B,** Page 497; Figure 17-4 from Kaufman RH,: Cystic tumors. In Gardner HL, Kaufman RH, eds: Benign diseases of the vulva and vagina, 2nd ed. Boston, G.K. Hall, 1981, p. 101. Reproduced with permission. Although possibly mistaken for an adenocarcinoma, the lesion pictured in Figure 17-4 is a hidradenoma, a small, benign vulva tumor which originates in the apocrine sweat glands in the inner surface of the labia majora. The therapy for hidradenomas is excisional biopsy. No medical therapy is indicated, and vulvectomy is a surgical excision which is far too great in scope.
20. **B,** Page 494. The most common large cyst of the vulva is a cystic dilation of an obstructed Bartholin's duct. Treatment is not necessary unless it becomes infected or symptomatic. Sebaceous and inclusion cysts are the most common small vulvar cysts. Sebaceous cyst are typically multiple, freely mobile and found in the anterior half of the labia majora. Inclusion cysts may develop following traumatic injury. Gartner's duct cysts are found in the vagina while nabothian cysts are found on the cervix.
21. **B,** Page 495. Senile or cherry angiomas are commonly-found small lesions arising on the labia majora of post menopausal

women. They are typically less than 3 mm in diameter, multiple in number and dark-blue or red-brown in color. Pyogenic granulomas are an overgrowth of inflamed granulation tissue and are usually approximately 1 cm. in diameter. They may be clinically mistaken for nevi or vulvar condylomas or cancer. Angiokeratomas are purple, twice the size of cherry angiomas, and typically occur in patients between ages 30-50. They tend to grow rapidly and may bleed during strenuous exercise. Strawberry or cavernous hemangiomas are congenital defects usually found in young children.

22. **A,** Pages 492-493; Figure 17-4 from Marshall FC, Uson AC, Melicow MM: Surg Gynecol Obstet 110:724, 1960. By permission of Surgery, Gynecology & Obstetrics. A urethral caruncle is a fleshy outgrowth from the edge of the urethra. They are most commonly found in postmenopausal women and may respond to topical or oral estrogen. If it does not regress or is symptomatic, therapeutic modalities include operative excision, laser ablation, fulguration or cryosurgery.

23. **A,** Pages 526-528. Benign cystic teratomas contain elements from all 3 germ cell layers, ectodermal tissue being predominant. Malignant transformation of a benign cystic teratoma occurs in no more than 1-2% of cases, usually in patients over 40. The malignant component is usually a squamous carcinoma. Benign teratomas are bilateral 10-15% of the time. The chromosomal makeup is 46,XX. In a series of experiments using chromosome banding techniques and electrophoretic variance, it has been discovered that the chromosomes of dermoids are different than the chromosomes of the host. It has been postulated that dermoids begin by parthenogenesis from secondary oocytes. An alternative hypothesis is that the dermoid results from fusion of the second polar body with the oocyte.

24-26. 24, **A**; 25, **D**; 26, **C**; Pages 496-498. Fibromas are the most common solid tumor of the vulva; lipomas are the other common benign tumor of mesenchymal origin. Both are slow-growing, have a low grade malignant potential and are typically excised to establish the diagnosis. Granular cell myoblastomas arise from neutral sheath (Schwann) cells and are sometimes called Schwannomas. These rare, slow-growing, solid tumors are painless and benign but infiltrate surrounding tissue. If the initial excision is not wide enough, these tumors tend to recur. A hidradenoma may be mistaken histologically for adenocarcinoma because of its hyperplastic, adenomatous pattern. There is, however, a lack of mitotic figures and nuclear pleomorphism. The tumor arises from apocrine sweat glands and may be solid or cystic. It typically occurs in Caucasian women between the ages of 30-70. The treatment of choice is excisional biopsy.

27-29. 27, **A**; 28, **B**; 29, **C**; Pages 526-534. Most of the solid elements in a cystic teratoma are contained in a nipple of the cyst wall termed the protuberance or tubercle of Rokitansky. Meig's syndrome is the association of an ovarian fibroma with ascites and hydrothorax. Both the ascites and hydrothorax resolve when the tumor is removed. Although classically described with an ovarian fibroma, these clinical features are also found with other ovarian tumors. Thirty percent of Brenner tumors are found in association with a serous or mucinous cystadenoma of the ipsilateral ovary.

30-32. 30, **C**; 31, **C**; 32, **A**; Pages 508-511. Both a pyometra and a hematometra may be the result of cervical stenosis. A hematometra is the consequence of complete genital tract obstruction in a reproductive age woman, who has an intact hypothalamic-pituitary axis. Postmenopausal women develop pyometra and are usually asymptomatic. Retrograde menstruation in a patient with a hematometra is commonly associated with endometriosis.

33-35. 33, **C**; 34, **B**; 35, **D**; Pages 519-521. Both tubal myomas and paratubal cysts may undergo acute torsion resulting in acute lower abdominal and pelvic pain. Most cases of paratubal cyst torsion are associated with pregnancy or the puerperium. Tubal myomas arise from smooth muscle cells as do the commonly coexistent uterine myomas. Paratubal cysts may be of mesonephric, paramesonephric, or mesothelial origin. Both tubal myomas and paratubal cysts may mimic an ovarian tumor. The former simulates a solid tumor while the latter is often indistinguishable from a cystic ovarian mass. The treatment of a tubal myoma is excision of the myoma in cases when it is symptomatic. Similarly, paratubal cysts are excised and do not require salpingectomy unless tubal torsion has occurred.

36. **A** (1, 2, 3), Page 522. Any adnexal mass that is noted prior to puberty or after the menopause requires surgical intervention. It should be noted that approximately 50% of ovarian cysts in prepubertal girls are follicle cysts. Similarly, a solid adnexal mass of any size, or a cystic mass larger than 8 cm warrants surgery. A 5-8 cm cystic mass which persists several months despite either oral contraceptive suppression or normal menstruation should also be evaluated surgically. Increasingly, simple cysts in young women are likely managed through the laparoscope.
37. **B** (1, 2), Page 518. In addition to symptomatic myomas, there are situations in which asymptomatic uterine myomas may be removed. Myomas larger than the size of a 12-14 week gestation are expected to eventually produce symptoms and may obscure the palpation of the adnexa. The growth of myomata after menopause is the classic finding in cases of leiomyosarcoma. Myomas which expand into the broad ligament may compress the ureter, resulting in hydroureter and possibly even renal compromise. Calcium deposits within a myoma are indicative of benign degeneration and are not an indication for hysterectomy.
38. **C** (2,3), Page 495. Although vulvar nevi are usually asymptomatic, it should be recalled that approximately 30% of malignant melanoma arise from a pre-existing nevus. Since a disproportionate number of malignant melanomas (5-10%) arise in the vulvar area, all vulvar nevi should be excised and examined histologically. Characteristic clinical features of an early malignant melanoma may be remembered by thinking of "ABCD" as described by Friedman: asymmetry, border irregularity, color variegation, and a diameter greater than 6 mm.
39. **A** (1, 2, 3), Pages 507-508. Cervical myomas constitute up to 8% of all myomas. Symptoms depend upon the direction in which the myomas expand, such that urinary difficulty, pain with intercourse and painful menses are all possible symptoms. Prolapsed cervical myomas may also become ulcerated and infected resulting in abnormal bleeding.
40. **E** (3 only), Pages 508-509. Cervical stenosis that results in a pyometra in a postmenopausal patient may be caused by a previous operation, radiation, infection, neoplasia, or atrophic changes. A pyometra in a postmenopausal patient usually does not require antibiotics since the primary goal of therapy is achieved with transcervical drainage. Ultrasound would have no diagnostic or therapeutic value at this time. After the acute infection has subsided, however, a fractional dilatation and curettage should be performed to rule out carcinoma of the endometrium.
41. **A** (1, 2, 3), Pages 494-496; Figure 17-6 from Friedrich EG, ed: Vulvar disease, 2nd ed. Philadelphia, W.B. Saunders Co., 1983, p.233. The lesion visualized in Figure 17-6 could be any of the three diagnoses listed. Since a Bartholin's duct cyst is the most common large cyst found within the vulvar and a fibroma is the most common benign solid tumor of the vulvar, these would be the two most likely diagnoses. A lipoma, the other common benign solid tumor of the vulva, is softer and usually larger than a fibroma. For a symptomatic patient, surgical management is indicated. Fibromas and lipomas are surgically excised while a Bartholin's duct cyst can be excised or marsupialized.
42. **B** (1,2), Page 499. Hematomas of the vulva are usually due to trauma, such as a straddle injury from some type of fall. Spontaneous hematomas are rare and typically are a result of rupture of a varicose vein during pregnancy or the postpartum period. Traumatic injuries resulting in vulvar hematomas have been related to sexual assault or recreational activities such as bicycling, sledding, skiing, and amusement park rides. The management of vulvar hematomas is usually conservative, utilizing controlled direct pressure. Application of ice is also helpful. Surgery is indicated only if the hematoma expands despite conservative measures.

CHAPTER

18 Endometriosis and Adenomyosis

DIRECTIONS for questions 1 - 13: Select the one best answer or completion.

1. Of the following side effects of GnRH agonist therapy, the least common is
   A. hot flashes
   B. hot flushes
   C. insomnia
   D. reduced bone mineral content
   E. vaginal dryness
2. In a 25 year-old with pelvic pain, endometriosis is best confirmed by
   A. the initial history
   B. a repeat pelvic exam on first day of menstrual flow
   C. laparoscopic visualization and biopsy
   D. speculum visualization
   E. hysterosalpingogram
3. The most common site for endometriosis is the
   A. rectosigmoid
   B. ovary
   C. appendix
   D. uterosacral ligament
   E. fallopian tube
4. A 22 year-old gravida 0 undergoes laparoscopy for progressive dysmenorrhea and chronic pelvic pain. She is found to have minimal endometriosis. She is not sexually active, uses no contraception, but does plan to marry in 6 months. She and her fiance look forward to having children someday. Optimal therapy for this woman would be
   A. conception
   B. oral contraceptives
   C. danazol therapy
   D. GnRH agonist
   E. laparotomy and resection of the endometriosis
5. At laparoscopy performed for progressive dysmenorrhea and dyspareunia, a 42 year-old gravida 3, para 3, is found to have endometriosis with extensive ovarian involvement. The recommended therapy should be
   A. danazol
   B. oral contraceptives
   C. laparotomy and resection of endometriotic lesions
   D. total abdominal hysterectomy
   E. total abdominal hysterectomy, bilateral salpingo-oophorectomy
6. The chemical structure of danazol is depicted in
   A. figure 18-1, A
   B. figure 18-1, B
   C. figure 18-1, C
   D. figure 18-1, D
   E. figure 18-1, E
7. Of the 5 photomicrographs shown in the figures listed below, the one diagnostic of endometriosis is
   A. figure 18-2
   B. figure 18-3
   C. figure 18-4
   D. figure 18-5
   E. figure 18-6
8. Of the 5 photomicrographs shown in the figures listed below, the one diagnostic of adenomyosis is
   A. figure 18-2
   B. figure 18-3
   C. figure 18-4
   D. figure 18-5
   E. figure 18-6
9. A 42 year-old gravida 4, para 4, has bothersome dysmenorrhea and menorrhagia. On pelvic examination the uterus is globular, tender, boggy, and approximately twice normal size. The most likely diagnosis is
   A. endometriosis
   B. adenomyosis
   C. leiomyomata Uteri
   D. leiomyosarcoma
   E. endometrial carcinoma
10. In a patient with endometriosis after 6 months treatment with a GnRH agonist, ovarian function will generally return within
    A. 1-2 weeks
    B. 3-5 weeks
    C. 6-12 weeks
    D. 14-20 weeks
    E. 24-30 weeks

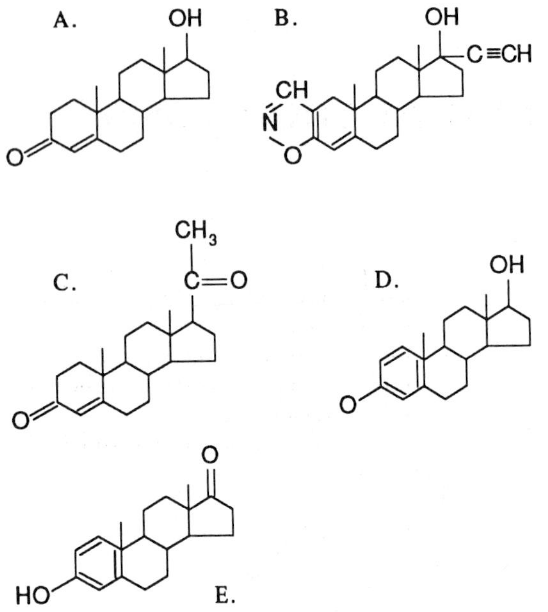

A. OH

B. OH C≡CH CH N O

C. CH_3 C=O O

D. OH O

E. O HO

FIGURE 18-1.

11. Of the following, the *least common* symptom associated with endometriosis involving the GI tract is
    A. abdominal cramping
    B. lower abdominal pain
    C. pain with defecation
    D. constipation
    E. intermittent rectal bleeding
12. A 30 year-old has completed her childbearing. She has mild endometriosis confirmed by laparoscopy a year ago. Since that procedure, the patient's dyspareunia and dysmenorrhea have gotten worse. The most reasonable operative procedure at this point is a
    A. dilatation and curettage
    B. uterine suspension
    C. total abdominal hysterectomy
    D. presacral neurectomy
    E. resection of the uterosacral ligaments
13. A 29 year-old patient has documented mild endometriosis and chooses high dose continuous progestin therapy over the alternative medical treatments offered. She should be informed that her chances of

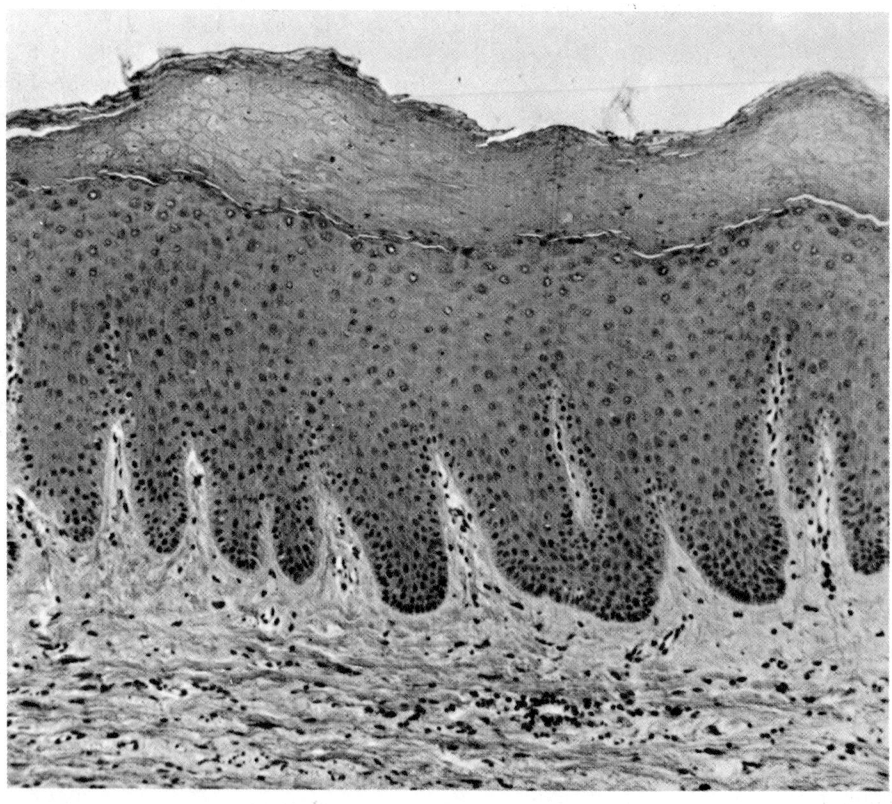

FIGURE 18-2.

(From Friedrich EG, Wilkinson EJ: The vulva. In Blaustein A, ed: Pathology of the female genital tract, 2nd ed. New York, Springer-Verlag, 1982.)

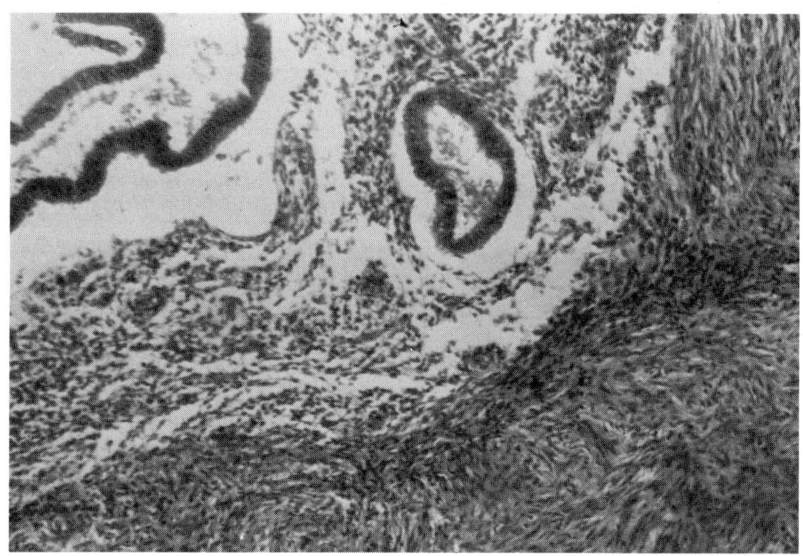

FIGURE 18-3.

(From Droegemueller W, Herbst AL, Mishell Dr, Stenchever MA: Comprehensive Gynecology, St. Louis, The C.V. Mosby Co., 1987.)

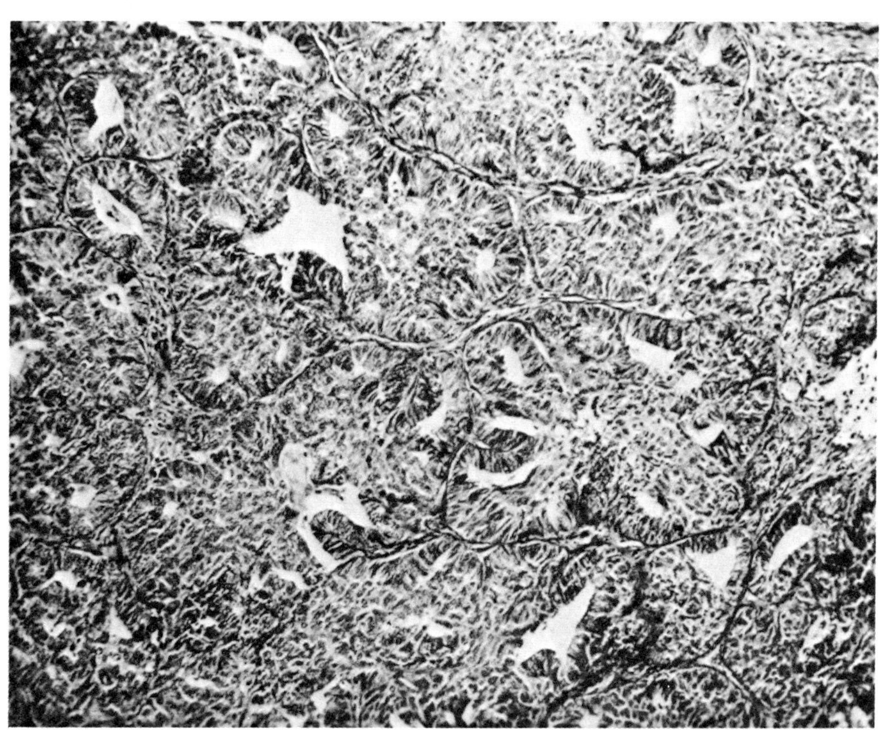

FIGURE 18-4.

(From Kurman RJ, Norris HJ: In Blaustein A, ed: Pathology of the female genital tract, 2nd ed. New York, Springer-Verlag, 1982.)

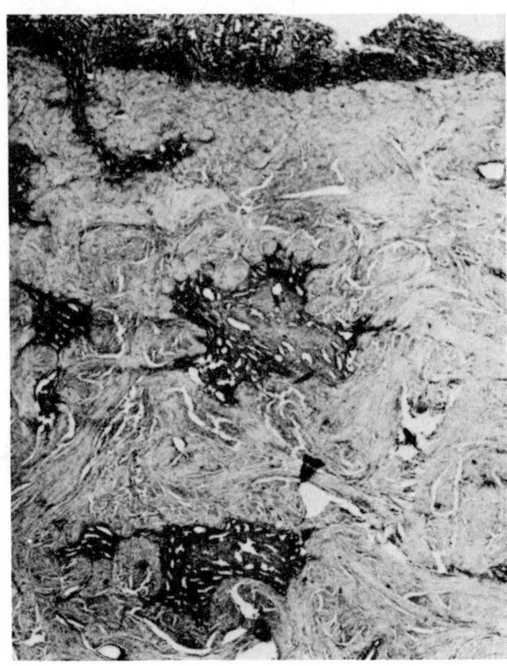

FIGURE 18-5.

(From Janovski NA, Dubranszky V: Atlas of gynecologic and obstetric diagnostic histopathology. New York, McGraw-Hill, 1967, p. 217.)

having abnormal bleeding on progestin therapy is approximately

A. 5%
B. 10%
C. 20%
D. 40%
E. 60%

DIRECTIONS: For each numbered item 14 - 21, indicate whether it is associated with

A only (A)
B only (B)
C both (A) and (B)
D neither (A) nor (B)

14-18. Match the effects with the hormonal therapy for endometriosis

(A) GnRH agonist
(B) danazol
(C) both
(D) neither

14. decreased FSH
15. decreased LH
16. altered immunologic function
17. amenorrhea
18. decreased HDL

19-21. Match the timing of the hormonal therapy for endometriosis with the effect

(A) GnRH therapy begun in follicular phase

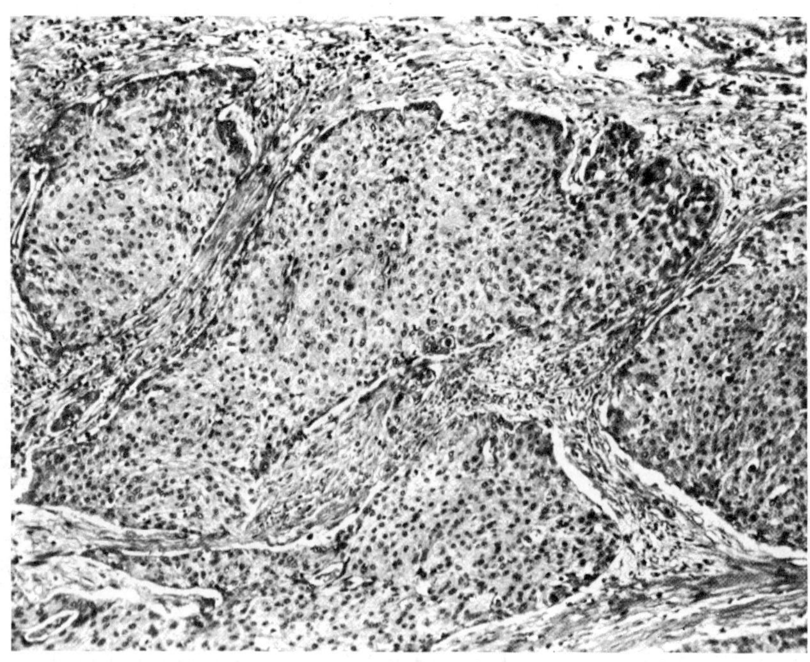

FIGURE 18-6.

(From Clement PB, Scully RE: Semin Oncol 9:251, 1982.)

(B) GnRH therapy begun in luteal phase
(C) both
(D) neither

19. amenorrhea within 5 weeks
20. estradiol at levels of castrated female within 2 weeks
21. initial LH surge intact

DIRECTIONS for questions 22 - 37: For each of the questions below, ONE or MORE of the responses is correct. Select the best answer based on the following

A if 1, 2, and 3 are correct
B if only 1 and 2 are correct
C if only 2 and 3 are correct
D if only 1 is correct
E if only 3 is correct

22. Laser systems appropriate for the surgical management of endometriosis include the
    1. $C0_2$ laser
    2. potassium-titanyl-phosphate (KTP) laser
    3. neodymium: yttrium-aluminum-garnet (Nd:YAG) laser
23. Endometriosis is associated with
    1. anovulation
    2. pain
    3. first trimester abortion
24. Clinical descriptors of young women at a higher risk of having endometriosis encompass a
    1. 13 year-old girl with imperforate hymen
    2. 22 year-old woman with regular menses lasting 8 days
    3. 20 year-old woman with irregular menses lasting 3 days
25. In an effort to explain the etiology of endometriosis, it has been postulated that
    1. endometriosis is due to implantation of endometrial cells shed as a result of retrograde menstruation
    2. cells of müllerian duct, derived from coelomic epithelium, undergo metaplasia to form endometrial tissue
    3. endometrial tissue can be transplanted via both lymphatic and vascular systems
26. At the time of laparoscopy for pelvic pain several lesions are seen. Those that should be biopsied to confirm a diagnosis of endometriosis include a
    1. 0.5 cm blood-filled cyst
    2. power burn area
    3. clear vesicle
27. The classic signs of endometriosis embrace
    1. tender nodularity of the uterosacral ligaments
    2. a fixed retroverted uterus
    3. bilateral symmetric adnexal enlargement
28. According to the staging of endometriosis of Puleo and Hammond used to follow patients with pain, the criteria for mild disease include
    1. tubal obstruction
    2. no significant adhesions
    3. superficial ovarian implants
29. Indications for treatment with danazol include
    1. hereditary angioneurotic edema
    2. benign cystic mastitis
    3. endometriosis
30. The therapy effect of danazol is due to the fact that it
    1. binds to progesterone receptors
    2. binds to estrogen receptors
    3. activates steroidogenesis in ovary
31. A 26 year-old is started on danazol for the treatment of moderate endometriosis. She should be instructed to
    1. take 200 mg twice a day, the most effective regimen
    2. take each pill on an empty stomach
    3. start treatment on the first day of the menstrual cycle.
32. A 29 year-old gravida 0, presents with a chief complaint of progressive dysmenorrhea for 2 years. She has had dyspareunia for 12 months, the duration of her marriage. She has never used contraception. Her underlying problem is probably due to
    1. adenomyosis
    2. chronic pelvic inflammatory disease
    3. endometriosis
33. Surgery is mandatory in the treatment of endometriosis for cases in which there is
    1. ureteral obstruction
    2. compromise of large bowel function
    3. an 8 cm ovarian endometrioma
34. The glands and stroma of adenomyosis are
    1. derived from aberrant glands of the basalis layer of the endometrium
    2. relatively deficient in estrogen and progesterone receptors in comparison with glands and stroma of the endometrium
    3. primarily confined to that part of the myometrium nearest the endometrium
35. Steroid hormone therapy after definitive surgical treatment for endometriosis should be employed to manage
    1. menopausal symptoms
    2. residual macroscopic endometriosis
    3. suspected microscopic endometriosis

36. GnRH agonist therapy for endometriosis is effective when there is
    1. severe adhesive disease
    2. only one endometrioma which is <4 cm in diameter
    3. all lesions are <1 cm in diameter
37. The side effects of GnRH agonists can be made more tolerable with the addition of
    1. danazol
    2. low dose estrogen
    3. progestins

ANSWERS

1. **D**, Page 560. Side effects of GnRH agonist therapy are primarily those of estrogen deficiency, i.e. hot flashes, hot flushes, vaginal dryness, and insomnia. There are conflicting data about bone mineral content. Any decrease in bone density is, partially or completely, reversible.
2. **C**, Pages 553, 555. In most cases, the diagnosis of endometriosis is confirmed by direct laparoscopic visualization and biopsy. In many cases it is discovered during an infertility work-up. Some people feel that pelvic exam on the first day of the cycle allows evaluation at the time of maximal swelling and tenderness. As with the history, the pelvic examination does not confirm the diagnosis. Because vaginal implants are rare, confirmation via speculum exam is unlikely. Abnormalities found on hysterosalpingogram are not specific for the diagnosis of endometriosis. Endometriosis does not have a specific pattern on either ultrasound or magnetic resonance imaging. The specificity and sensitivity of magnetic resonance imaging for endometriosis is approximately 60%. Assays for CA-125 have a low specificity as they are also increased in other conditions, such as pelvic inflammatory disease and epithelial ovarian tumors. It is, however, elevated in a majority of patients with endometriosis and does tend to increase with advancing stages.
3. **B**, Pages 548-549. The ovaries are the most common site for endometriosis in 2 out of 3 patients.
4. **B**, Pages 556-564. For a symptomatic young patient with minimal endometriosis, medical suppression is a logical first step in therapy. Laparoscopic laser ablation is a surgical modality often used at the time of diagnosis and could have been done in this patient. Danazol and GnRH agonist are appropriate drugs for patients whose symptoms persist or disease progresses despite oral contraceptive. Laparotomy with resection of endometriotic lesions or hysterectomy with bilateral salpingo-oophorectomy are procedures reserved for more advanced or debilitating endometriosis. Recommending conception must be individualized to the patient's personal needs and circumstances, and carries with it an inherent paradox since infertility is more common in patients with endometriosis.
5. **E**, Page 564. In a 42 year-old multigravida, the most logical approach to ovarian endometriosis is to recommend hysterectomy with bilateral salpingo-oophorectomy. The extirpative procedure removes not only macroscopic disease, but removes the potential stimulus for future endometriosis, i.e., the ovaries. Although this is optimal treatment, the patient must share in the decision regarding oophorectomy. Any medical regimen would be considered less acceptable because of the patient's age and extent of disease. It should also be noted that with pelviscopic surgical techniques, even moderately advanced endometriosis can often be managed at the initial laparoscopic procedure utilizing laser vaporization.
6. **A**, Pages 556-557. Danazol is an attenuated, orally active, androgen. Chemically it is a synthetic steroid, the isoxasole derivative of ethisterone (17′-ethinyltestosterone). Choice B is testosterone, C is progesterone, D is estradiol, and E is estrone.
7. **B**, Page 550. The 3 cardinal histologic features of endometriosis are ectopic endometrial glands, ectopic endometrial stroma, and hemorrhage into adjacent tissue. In addition, previous hemorrhage can be discovered by identifying large macrophages filled with hemosiderin near the periphery of the lesion. It has been estimated that no specific pathologic diagnosis can be made in about one third of typical endometriosis cases. Figure 18-2 is hyperplastic dystrophy of the vulva. Figure 18-4 is adenocarcinoma of the endometrium. Figure 18-5 is adenomyosis. Figure 18-6 is squamous cell carcinoma of the cervix.
8. **D**, Pages 568-569. The standard criteria for the diagnosis of adenomyosis is the finding of endometrial glands and stroma more than one low power field (2.5 mm) from the basalis. The glands are typically inactive or proliferative. Cystic hyperplasia is seen occasionally, but secretory patterns are rare. The myometrium reacts to

the ectopic endometrium by undergoing both hypertrophy and hyperplasia, thus producing the globular enlargement of the uterus.

9. **B,** Page 569. Patients with adenomyosis are usually asymptomatic. Symptomatic adenomyosis usually presents in women between 35 and 50 years of age, often a parous women. The classic symptoms are menorrhagia, dysmenorrhea, and occasionally dyspareunia. The tender, boggy, and enlarged uterus described in this patient is typical. The degree of tenderness and the consistency of the uterus may vary, depending upon the time in the patient's menstrual cycle that she is examined.
10. **C,** Page 561. After six months of GnRH agonist therapy, ovarian function will return to normal within 6-12 weeks. The greatest advantage of a GnRH agonist over danazol appears to be the production of medical castration without androgenic side effects.
11. **E,** Pages 564, 566. Gastrointestinal involvement occurs in 5% of cases of endometriosis. Involvement of the small bowel is rare. Most cases of gastrointestinal endometriosis are asymptomatic. If they are symptomatic, however, rectal bleeding is less likely than cramping, lower abdominal pain, pain on defecation, or constipation.
12. **C,** Pages 563-564. No well-controlled studies have documented the benefit of dilatation and curettage or uterine suspension in endometriosis. Occasionally, presacral neurectomy or uterosacral resection is performed for midline pain. In women who have completed childbearing and are in their late 20's or early 30's, hysterectomy with ovarian preservation can be optimal. In 5-10% of women, the disease is subsequently progressive and a second operation, a bilateral oophorectomy is necessary.
13. **D,** Page 562. The most persistent side effect of progestin therapy for endometriosis is bleeding or spotting. It is reported that approximately 40% of patients who take high dose progestin therapy for endometriosis develop abnormal bleeding. This can be alleviated somewhat by adding small doses of oral estrogen.

14-18. 14, **C;** 15, **C;** 16, **B;** 17, **C;** 18, **B;** Pages 556-561. Both GnRH and danazol decrease the levels of follicle stimulating hormone (FSH) and luteinizing hormone (LH). Recent studies have also demonstrated that danazol may also modulate immunologic functions by way of affecting macrophages or T-lymphocytes. Both drugs induce amenorrhea and have been found to be effective in the treatment of endometriosis, with several double-blind trials demonstrating comparable efficacy. Danazol decreases high density lipoprotein levels and elevates low density lipoprotein levels, thereby having a potential effect on atherosclerotic disease. GnRH agonists have no effect on sex hormone binding globulin such that the androgenic side effects seen with danazol are not observed. This is due to an increase in free serum testosterone that results with decreased sex hormone binding globulin.

19-21. 19, **B;** 20, **B;** 21, **B;** Page 560. A patient's response to agonist therapy depends on when therapy is initiated. If during the **follicular** phase, estradiol levels rise for approximately three weeks, after which, they rapidly decline. There is no LH surge and amenorrhea is induced within 6-8 weeks. If, on the other hand, after insuring that the patient is not pregnant, agonist therapy is begun during the **luteal** phase, LH levels are elevated for one week, and estradiol levels are suppressed to those of a castrated female within two weeks. Amenorrhea is induced within 4-5 weeks.

22. **A** (1, 2, 3), Page 563. At the present time, various types of laser delivery systems have been used effectively in the surgical treatment of endometriosis. These include the CO_2 laser, the argon laser, the potassium/titanyl-phosphate (KTP) laser and the neodymium: yttrium-aluminum-garnet (Nd:YAG) laser. The mechanism by which the laser is utilized is that the endometriotic lesion is either coagulated or vaporized. The laser provides precision, control and minimal tissue damage. As a result, there is hardly any fibrosis or scarring in the surgical areas.
23. **B** (1, 2), Page 553. Approximately 15% of women with endometriosis also have coincidental anovulation. Pain is a well known symptom, but there is no correlation between pain severity or frequency with the stage of endometriosis. Although 1st trimester abortion has been reported to be associated with endometriosis, more recent data call this into question.
24. **B** (1, 2), Pages 546-547. The theory of retrograde menstruation as an etiology of en-

dometriosis is supported by clinical observations that women with menstrual flows greater than 7 days have a two times greater prevalence of endometriosis. Endometriosis is also found frequently in women with outflow obstruction of the genital tract.

25. **A** (1, 2, 3), Pages 546-548. Most authorities feel that several factors are probably involved in the etiology of endometriosis. These include retrograde menstruation, metaplasia of coelomic epithelium, and transport of endometrial cells via blood or lymphatics. A genetic predisposition has also been identified. Abnormalities of both humoral, as well as cell-mediated components of the immune system, have been implicated as well. In addition, iatrogenic dissemination of endometriosis has been reported.
26. **A** (1, 2, 3), Page 550. Endometriotic lesions have a myriad of appearances. The gross appearance of the lesion depends on the site, activity and chronicity of the endometriosis, and the day of the menstrual cycle. The predominant color depends upon the blood supply, the amount of hemorrhage, and the degree of fibrosis. New lesions are small, usually blood-filled cysts of less than 1 cm in diameter. Clinically, they are often described as a "raspberry spot" or "powder burn". Initially, they are raised above the surrounding tissue. With time they become larger and assume a light or dark brown color associated with more intense scarring. These may appear more like a blood-filled or chocolate cyst. These are usually puckered or retracted from surrounding tissue. The pattern of ovarian endometriosis is variable. Individual areas vary from 1 mm to 14 cm with associated adhesions which may be filmy or dense. Larger cysts are usually densely adherent to the pelvic sidewall or broad ligament.
27. **B** (1, 2), Page 553. The most constant pelvic findings associated with endometriosis are a fixed retroverted uterus with scarring and tenderness posterior to the uterus. Characteristic nodularity of the uterosacral ligaments and cul-de-sac of Douglas may be palpated on the rectovaginal exam. The ovaries may be enlarged, tender and often are fixed. The adnexal enlargement is rarely symmetric.
28. **C** (2, 3), Table 18-1. The staging in Table 18-1 allows for systematic follow-up of patients who have been treated for endometriosis. A separate classification by the American Fertility Society is useful for patients with infertility. (see Figure 39-27 Herbst et al.) Tubal obstruction is associated with severe disease while scattered-,scarred implants on other structures is associated with moderate disease.

TABLE 18-1. Classification of Endometriosis

Extent of Disease	Findings
Mild	1. Scattered, superficial implants on structures other than uterus, tubes, or ovaries; no scarring
	2. Rare, superficial implants on ovaries
	3. No significant adhesions
Moderate	1. Involvement of one or both ovaries with multiple implants or small endometriomas (≤2 cm)
	2. Minimal peritubular or periovarian adhesions
	3. Scattered, scarred implants on other structures
Severe	1. Large ovarian endometriomas (≥2 cm)
	2. Significant tubal or ovarian adhesions
	3. Tubal obstruction
	4. Obliteration of cul-de-sac, major uterosacral involvement
	5. Significant bowel or urinary tract disease

From Puleo JG, Hammond CB: Conservative treatment of endometriosis externa: the effects of danazol therapy. Fertil Steril 40:165, 1983. Reproduced with permission of the publisher, The American Fertility Society.

29. **A** (1, 2, 3), Page 556. Danazol has been an important medication in the treatment of endometriosis since its FDA approval in the mid 1970s. It is also useful in cases of menorrhagia, benign cystic mastitis, and hereditary angioneurotic edema.
30. **D** (1 only), Page 557. Danazol binds to androgen and progesterone receptors, and also binds to sex hormone binding globulin. It directly inhibits several steroidogenic enzymes in both the ovary and adrenal gland.
31. **E** (3 only), Page 557. The standard danazol regimen is 400-800 mg/daily for 6-9 months. The half life is 4-5 hours so that a single 200 mg tablet 4 times a day is preferable to 2 tablets twice daily. Since food does not interfere with absorption, danazol can be taken with meals. If one is certain that the patient is not pregnant, it is

better to start danazol on the first day of menstrual bleeding. By starting the hormone on the first day of the cycle rather than the 5th day as is commonly recommended, the patient will experience less breakthrough bleeding during the first 4-6 weeks.

32. **C** (2,3), Page 553. The patient described is most likely to have endometriosis. There is no history of prior infection to warrant a diagnosis of chronic PID, but this must still be included in the differential. Adenomyosis is most likely in a multiparous patient.
33. **A** (1, 2, 3), Pages 562, 567. Although the choice between medical and surgical management for endometriosis depends on many considerations, certain findings warrant surgical management. Ureteral obstruction can ultimately lead to renal failure. Large bowel involvement by endometriosis must be managed surgically to avoid extensive compromise of bowel function. A large endometrioma poses the risk of an acute accident such as torsion, rupture and hemorrhage. Furthermore, it should be remembered that an ovarian malignancy and an endometrioma can present the same clinical picture.
34. **B** (1, 2), Pages 568-569. Adenomyosis and endometriosis are different clinical entities. The glands in adenomyosis, derived from the basalis layer, are not as responsive to hormones as those in the endometrium. This may, in part, be due to the relative lack of estrogen and progesterone receptors in the glands and stroma of adenomyosis. In most cases, adenomyosis is diffusely distributed throughout the myometrium.
35. **A** (1, 2, 3), Page 564. Postoperative hormones can be given for a variety of indications. If not all the endometriosis has been removed, medroxyprogesterone is recommended for one year. To treat menopausal symptoms, cyclic estrogen and progestin can be used. Postoperative danazol or oral contraceptives may help eradicate microscopic endometriosis.
36. **E** (3 only), Page 560. GnRH agonist therapy improves symptoms in up to 90% of patients depending on the extent of the disease. The greatest effects are seen in patients whose endometriotic lesions are <1 cm in diameter. On the other hand, endometriomas and severe adhesive disease do not respond to hormonal therapy.
37. **C** (2, 3), Pages 561-562. The side effects of GnRH agonists can potentially be reduced by "adding back" low doses of estrogen or progestin. Both can diminish hot flashes and possibly produce a bone sparing effect while the patient is on GnRH agonist therapy.

CHAPTER 19 Disorders of Abdominal Wall and Pelvic Support

DIRECTIONS for questions 1 - 9: Select the one best answer or completion.

1. A 72-year-old para 3 presents with a history of a recently noticed "bulge" protruding through the vaginal introitus. Fifteen months prior to this visit, a vaginal hysterectomy was performed on this patient for uterine descensus. This "bulge" is most likely a
   A. cystocele
   B. rectocele
   C. enterocele
   D. prolapsed ovary
   E. sigmoid diverticulum
2. In performing a lower abdominal midline incision, the major anatomic landmark encountered in the abdominal wall which involves a change in the fascial investiture of the rectus muscle is
   A. Hesselback's triangle
   B. linea semilunaris
   C. linea nigra
   D. linea alba
   E. umbilicus
3. A 52-year-old para 4 woman complains of a bulging vaginal mass, constipation, and incomplete stool evacuation. The anatomic defect most likely to contribute to these is a
   A. a cystourethrocele
   B. a uterine prolapse
   C. poor anal sphincter tone
   D. a rectocele
   E. an enterocele
4. An 82-year-old woman with total vaginal vault prolapse is referred to you with a 2 month history of noticing a "bulge" between her labia. She is being treated for congestive heart failure. She had a total abdominal hysterectomy and bilateral oophorectomy 25 years prior and has been sexually inactive for more than 15 years. The best choice of a surgical procedure to correct this problem is a(n)
   A. abdominal suspension from the rectus fascia
   B. abdominal sacral colpopexy
   C. abdominal enterocele reduction
   D. vaginal colpocleisis
   E. vaginal sacrospinous ligament suspension
5. A defect in pelvic anatomy that can be correctly termed a true hernia is a(n)
   A. cystocele
   B. enterocele
   C. rectocele
   D. urethrocele
   E. ureterocele
6. The goal of an anterior colporrhaphy done to correct stress urinary incontinence in a patient who has a cystourethrocele is to
   A. foreshorten the pubovesical fascia
   B. lengthen the urethra
   C. make the bladder smaller
   D. correct the urethrovesical angle
   E. replace the bladder neck behind the pubic symphysis
7. The structure, pictured in Figure 19-1, that provides the most support in the repair of a rectocele is the
   A. levator ani muscle group
   B. perirectal connective tissue
   C. proximal fibers of the superficial transverse perinei muscle
   D. trimmed posterior vaginal mucosa
   E. anal sphincter
8. At the time of preoperative evaluation of a patient upon whom you anticipate performing a postpartum tubal sterilization, you notice a 5 cm umbilical hernia. You would now
   A. proceed with the operation as planned and repair the hernia upon completion of the sterilization
   B. proceed with the tubal sterilization and plan repair of the hernia at a later date
   C. schedule a sterilization procedure at a time when a general surgeon can assist with a herniorrhaphy
   D. proceed with the sterilization only and make a lower midline vertical incision
   E. proceed with the operation using the laparoscope
9. A 48-year-old patient with the anatomic

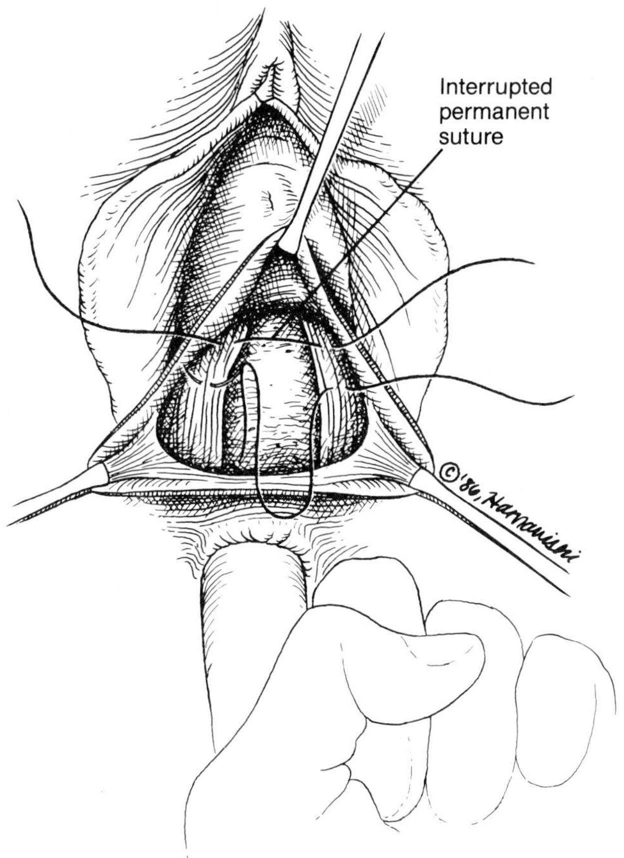

FIGURE 19-1.

(From Droegemeuller W, Herbst AL, Mishell Dr, Stenchever, MA: Comprehensive gynecology. St. Louis, The C.V. Mosby Co., 1987.)

findings illustrated in Figure 19-2 presents with symptoms of pelvic pressure, urethral irritation, and constant stress urinary incontinence with mild Valsalva. Assuming the completion of an appropriate urologic work-up that documents stress urinary incontinence, the procedure most likely to obtain good results is a(n)

A. Marshall-Marchetti-Krantz procedure
B. vaginal hysterectomy with anterior colporrhaphy
C. anterior wall colporrhaphy
D. Burch procedure
E. Pereyra operation

DIRECTIONS for questions 10 - 13: For each numbered item, select the one heading most closely associated with it. Each lettered heading may be used once, more than once, or not at all.

10-13. Choose the most appropriate surgical procedure for the patients described below

(A) Vaginal hysterectomy and anterior-posterior colporrhaphy

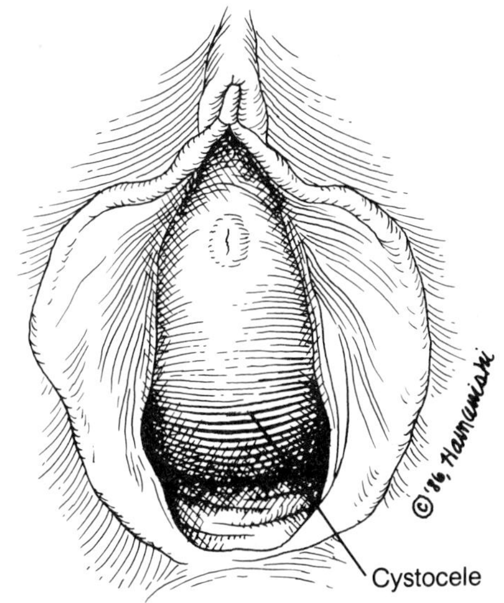

FIGURE 19-2.

(From Droegemeuller W, Herbst AL, Mishell DR, Stenchever MA: Comprehensive gynecology. St. Louis, The C.V. Mosby Co., 1987.)

(B) Manchester-Fothergill and anterior colporrhaphy
(C) Le Fort (modified)
(D) Watkins interposition
(E) Goodall-Power

10. an 85 year-old, widowed woman with congestive heart failure and total procidentia
11. a 45 year-old with an elongated cervix, a well-supported uterus, a cystourethrocele who has stress urinary incontinence. This patient has a long history of pelvic inflammatory disease.
12. a 78 year-old, sexually inactive woman with a second degree cystocele and rectocele
13. a 45 year-old woman with a second degree cystourethrocele who has stress urinary incontinence

DIRECTIONS For each numbered item 14 - 22, indicate whether it is associated with

A only (A)
B only (B)
C both (A) and (B)
D neither (A) nor (B)

14-16. Match the operative procedure with the statement

(A) vaginal colpopexy
(B) abdominal colpopexy
(C) both
(D) neither

14. correction of associated enterocele
15. sexual function preserved
16. sacrospinous ligaments used for support

17-19. Match the anatomical finding with the statement

(A) cystocele
(B) urethrocele
(C) both
(D) neither

17. considered a true hernia
18. associated with attenuation of pubovesical cervical fascia
19. contributes to urinary incontinence

20-22. Match the anatomical finding with the statement

(A) femoral canal
(B) inguinal canal
(C) both
(D) neither

20. aperture resulting from the embryonic descent of the testes from their original retroperitoneal site to the scrotum
21. herniated peritoneum into this space may occur in both sexes
22. in a woman, the round ligament courses through this aperture

DIRECTIONS for questions 23 - 29: For each of the questions below, ONE or MORE of the responses is correct. Select the best answer based on the following

A if 1, 2, and 3 are correct
B if only 1 and 2 are correct
C if only 2 and 3 are correct
D if only 1 is correct
E if only 3 is correct

23. During the performance of a vaginal hysterectomy, a postoperative enterocele is prevented by appropriate surgical disposition of the
    1. uterosacral ligaments
    2. cardinal ligaments
    3. cul-de-sac peritoneum
24. Appropriate surgical correction in cases of vaginal vault (stump) prolapse include a recognition of the
    1. normal axis of the vagina in a standing position
    2. perineal body anatomy
    3. specific vaginal wall defects
25. A cystourethrocele is more likely to develop if a woman has
    1. a wide pubic arch
    2. delivered several children
    3. prominent ischial spines
26. The characteristics of an umbilical hernia include the fact that
    1. during repair, remnants of umbilical cord are often found
    2. this fascial defect in its severe form presents as gastroschisis
    3. this fascial defect usually closes during the first 3 years of life
27. Abdominal hernias
    1. contain visceral organ structures (e.g., bowel)
    2. contain a reflection of peritoneum (sac)
    3. represent a fascial defect
28. Following a vaginal hysterectomy, surgical culdoplasty may be performed by
    1. fixing the uterosacral ligaments to the cul-de-sac peritoneum
    2. shortening the cul-de-sac (pouch of Douglas) by suturing the uterosacral ligaments in the midline and then to the edge of the proximal vagina incision
    3. suturing the round ligaments and the ovarian ligaments to the edge of the proximal vagina incision
29. Refer to Figure 19-3. Proper placement of sutures in performing a vaginal sacrospinous ligament fixation include
    1. Suture placement at label 1

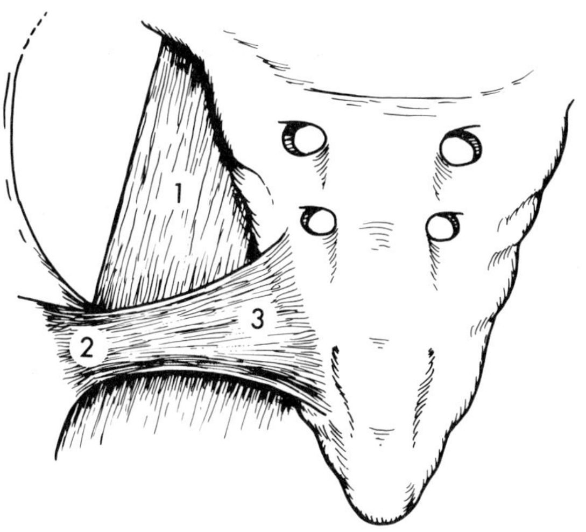

FIGURE 19-3.

2. Suture placement at label 2
3. Suture placement at label 3

ANSWERS

1. **C,** Pages 589, 591. Enteroceles frequently occur after hysterectomy and generally are due to weakened support of the pouch of Douglas. Lack of attention to the surgical repair of the supporting structures at the time of original surgery may contribute to the formation of a postoperative enterocele, especially one that presents this soon after the antecedent hysterectomy. A small preexisting herniation of peritoneum may have been overlooked during the vaginal hysterectomy. Lack of obliteration of this hernia sac and improper attention to the plication of uterosacral or cardinal ligaments may contribute to the development of an enterocele shortly after surgery. In this situation, there is often a degree of total vault prolapse perceived by the patient as a "bulge" passing through the vaginal introitus. Although a cystocele and a rectocele may be associated with an enterocele, they are usually secondary rather than primary offenders. Prolapsed adnexal structures are rare and usually are not involved in cases of vaginal vault prolapse. Likewise, prolapse of the sigmoid colon or parts of the sigmoid colon do not present in this fashion
2. **B,** Pages 578-579. Figure 19-1 (from Herbst et al.). The investing fasciae of the external oblique, internal oblique, and transversus abdominis muscles completely encase the rectus abdominis muscles cephalad to the linea semilunaris. Caudally from the semilunar line, the muscle is completely posterior to the aponeurosis of the fasciae of these muscles and lies directly on the peritoneum. In making a midline incision, this change is apparent after mobilizing the rectus muscle laterally and just prior to entry into the peritoneal cavity. In the repair of this incision, it is important to remember that this area of relative weakness contributes to a higher incidence of postoperative abdominal incisional hernias. Hesselback's triangle defines that anatomic area in which a defect in the transversalis fasciae may result in a femoral type of groin hernia. The linea alba is the midline fusion of the rectus fasciae and is not used as a superficial anatomic landmark. The linea nigra is a vertical discoloration of the skin occurring between the umbilicus and the top of the pubic symphysis.
3. **D,** Pages 586-587. In a patient with these complaints referable primarily to lower bowel dysfunction, the most likely contributing anatomic defect is a rectocele. The other anatomic defects may be associated with the presence of a rectocele but do not contribute to these symptoms. Patients may often need to "splint" the posterior vaginal wall in order to ameliorate those symptoms associated with difficulty in having bowel movements. Chronic constipation in these patients with retention of firm stool in the lower colon can be associated with degrees of discomfort during sexual intercourse. Poor anal sphincter tone may be secondary to an incompletely healed perineal laceration incurred during childbirth. Symptoms related to this defect, such as incontinence of stool or flatus, were not manifest in this patient and, when present, are not necessarily associated with other disorders of pelvic support. Operative management of a rectocele is generally performed at the time of other vaginal surgery. Likewise, perineal body reconstruction (perineorrhaphy) is also indicated in those patients where there is a marked defect in perineal support. However, this does not routinely imply reconstruction of the anal sphincter.
4. **D,** Pages 595-598. Although there are a variety of procedures to manage vaginal vault (stump) prolapse, selection of the appropriate procedure is guided by a number of factors. This includes the age of the

patient, sexual activity, the specific anatomic defects involved, and the general health of the patient. In this geriatric patient who is sexually inactive and has congestive heart failure, an extensive abdominal operation involving either suspension of the vaginal wall to the rectus fascia or any of a variety of sacral suspensions using inert gauze material is not needed. Because this patient is sexually inactive, a more extensive procedure such as vaginal sacrospinous ligament suspension is not necessary. The logical choice for this situation would be some form of vaginal closure or colpocleisis. This could be a vaginectomy or vaginal colpocleisis modified after the Le Fort procedure. When doing this procedure, it is important to identify an enterocele if it is present so that the appropriate dissection, ligation, and excision of redundant peritoneum can be performed to prevent an enterocele from forming posterior to the colpocleisis.

5. **B**, Page 589. An enterocele is a true hernia of the peritoneal cavity emanating from the pouch of Douglas between the uterosacral ligaments and into the rectovaginal septum. It may be noticed as a separate bulge above the rectocele and at times it may be large enough to prolapse through the vagina. A hernia by definition must contain a serosal sac, and it may also contain bowel or omentum. The other defects noted above are not true hernias in that they do not contain herniated peritoneum through a fascial defect. They are prolapsed distal bowel (rectocele), bladder (cystocele), or urethra (urethrocele). The latter is usually a detachment of the urethra rather than a ballooning out of this structure. A ureterocele is the most unusual of those listed above and represents sacculation of the distal ureter into the bladder as a result of stenosis of the **ureteral** meatus.
6. **E**, Pages 584-586. The overall goal of anterior colporrhaphy to correct urinary incontinence is to replace the bladder neck behind the symphysis pubis in order to increase the amount of pressure transmitted to the proximal urethra during Valsalva. The anatomic abnormality associated with urinary incontinence is discussed in Chapter 20 of Herbst et al. The other corrections noted in this question may all occur in the process of performing an adequate anterior colporrhaphy. That is, the pubovesical fascia may be drawn more closely towards the midline by appropriately placed Kelly plication sutures. Depending on the degree of urethrocele, the urethra may be somewhat lengthened, although this is not thought to lend appreciably to urinary continence. Bladder capacity may be reduced by a cystocele repair, which results in the urge to void sooner than when there is marked laxity in the vaginal wall. Finally, the urethrovesical angle may be increased in the process of anterior colporrhaphy because of appropriate elevation of the bladder neck behind the symphysis. However, the angle in and of itself is probably not important in correcting incontinence.
7. **A**, Page 587. The major contribution to the restoration of the pelvic floor anatomy when performing a posterior colporrhaphy is made by reducing the aperture of the levator hiatus. Although the levator plate is made up of a number of muscles, restoration of the anatomy of the pubococcygeus and purorectalis are probably most important. Plication of the lower margins of the bulbocavernosus and transverse perinei muscles also strengthens the support of the urogenital diaphragm. During dissection in the operating room, separation and identification of these muscles is very difficult. The superficial transverse perinei do not lend appreciably to pelvic muscle support, nor does the relatively attenuated perirectal connective tissue. The trimmed vaginal mucosa likewise does not strengthen the posterior vaginal wall. The anal sphincter is usually not involved in this repair procedure. Knowledge of the anatomy of the levator plate is important in planning the appropriate operation for patients with marked posterior vaginal wall defects.
8. **A**, Page 581. In this unexpected situation, the presence of a small umbilical hernia need not deter the surgeon in performing the original operation. A Pomeroy Tubal sterilization can be carried out with appropriate repair of the umbilical hernia after completion of the sterilization. Care should be taken to completely dissect the peritoneal sac away from the point of intraperitoneal entry. Likewise, care should be taken to find the lateral extent of the fascial defect and repair this by either direct approximation from superior to inferior using nonabsorbable sutures; close the fascia in a "vest over pants" manner. There is no point in delaying the repair of

this hernia for a later date if it can be repaired at the time of this operation. A gynecologist should have the competence to perform an umbilical herniorrhaphy without assistance from a general surgeon. There is no need to change the incision, nor is there any need to use the laparoscope. Knowledge of this anatomic defect at the time of surgery should alert the surgeon to the possibility of adherent bowel just under the peritoneal sac or the presence of a Meckel's diverticulum just beneath the peritoneal surface. Another consideration in this question has to do with the issue of informed consent. Appropriate informed consent must be obtained for all surgical procedures. With the potential alteration of the umbilicus, the surgeon should be aware that surgical alteration of this structure may carry with it the risk of patient dissatisfaction.

9. **B,** Pages 585-586, 592, 595. Although a number of options exist for surgical repair of patients with stress urinary incontinence, certain principles can be used to guide surgical decisions. The point of this question is to consider a general approach based on specific anatomic findings. Accordingly, this patient with marked anterior wall relaxation (cystourethrocele) with related pelvic pressure and irritation should have a vaginal procedure. This will best treat the anatomic defect (cystourethrocele) while at the same time offering a high degree of success in curing the incontinence. Most surgeons would agree that in a patient of this age, concomitant vaginal hysterectomy would also be indicated. Although it could be argued that a combined operation might be better, it should be appreciated that the performance of a retropubic operation such as in Marshall-Marchetti-Krantz or Burch procedure is not indicated as the sole operation. Likewise, the Pereyra operation performed without correction of the cystourethrocele will not correct the vaginal wall defect.

10-13. 10, **C**; 11, **B**; 12, **C**; 13, **A.** Pages 590-595. This series of questions deals with the choice of surgical treatment for symptomatic pelvic relaxation under different circumstances. It must be realized that there is no consensus among surgeons about the appropriate surgical treatment in every case; however, the situations described above do delineate the types of operations to be considered in certain instances. In general, eponyms should be avoided, but certain surgical procedures are named for the surgeon or surgeons who first described and popularized them. It is realized that some of these operations are rarely indicated. This series of operations underscores the need for the consultant to know a wide range of surgical options and thus assist the occasional individual patient. The Le Fort operation is usually considered the procedure of choice in elderly patients with total prolapse. This is in contrast to the Goodall-Power modification, which is used with lesser degrees of prolapse in the geriatric age group. This operation involves removing smaller triangular portions of the anterior and posterior vaginal wall mucosa instead of the traditional rectangular portions removed in the Le Fort operation. Thus, when sutured togetherafter reduction of the uterus, effective colpocleisis has been accomplished. Both operations will obliterate the vagina and should be reserved for sexually inactive women. Both operations usually are done in conjunction with a perineorrhaphy as an additional measure to assure a better long-term result. The Manchester-Fothergill operation is rarely indicated today. It is reserved for the occasional patient who has appreciable stress urinary incontinence, an elongated cervix, and excellent uterine support either by previous operation or by intercurrent inflammatory or adhesion disease. An adequate anterior colporrhaphy and plication of the vesical neck can be accomplished with this operation, which involves amputating the elongated cervix and using the cardinal ligaments to improve support. The Watkins interposition or transposition operation was used extensively for uterine prolapse in patients with a large cystocele. The operation consists of amputating the elongated cervix and suturing the fundus of the uterus beneath the large cystocele. The fundus therefore was used as an obturator to fill the defect in the anterior segment of the pelvic diaphragm. This operation is rarely used today in lieu of more popular forms of vaginal plastic procedures and because of the possibility of endometrial cancer developing in a relatively inaccessible uterus. Most instances of symptomatic vaginal relaxation associated with uterine prolapse can be surgically treated by vaginal hysterectomy and anterior and posterior colporrhaphy. This will maintain a degree of vaginal depth and caliber suitable for sexual function while at the same time correcting anatomic defects that may be associated with urinary incontinence or problems with bowel evacuation. The gynecologic surgeon should realize that although vaginal hysterectomy with colporrhaphy usually can be done, other operations are available when indicated by special circumstances to ensure the overall health of the patient.

14-16. 14, **C**; 15, **C**; 16, **A**. Pages 595-598. There are a variety of vaginal or abdominal procedures to correct vaginal stump prolapse. Within each category there are specialized surgical nuances that may be applied to individual cases. In choosing a vaginal procedure, the best results occur in those patients where vaginal length is maintained and the vagina is positioned against therectum nearly parallel to the horizontal. Similarly, when choosing an abdominal colpopexy of some variety, attention should be paid to the restoration of the anatomy so that following the procedure the anatomy is as nearly normal as possible. When performing either a vaginal or an abdominal colpopexy, an enterocele must be identified if one is present. In the case of vaginal reconstructive surgery, recognition of a dissecting enterocele sac should prompt its removal. In the abdominal operation, the deep cul-de-sac or beginning enterocele should be closed prior to the attachment of the vaginal vault to a fixed structure. If the surgical approach does not consider an existing enterocele, sac dissection may take place despite adequate support of the vaginal vault. Both abdominal and vaginal procedures may preserve sexual function. This is especially important to consider when performing an associated vaginal repair. Adequate caliber and depth can be maintained with careful attention to anatomic principles. The sacrospinous ligaments may be used for additional vaginal vault support in selected vaginal cases. This operation is technically more difficult and potentially riskier than routine vaginal colporrhaphy, but occasionally it should be chosen as a means of ensuring vaginal vault support.

17-19. 17, **D**; 18, **C**; 19, **B**. Page 584. Neither a cystocele nor a urethrocele is considered a true hernia since neither condition includes the protrusion of a peritoneal reflection or sac through a true fascial defect. Attenuation or rupture of the pubovesical cervical fascia for any reason may allow the descent of the urethra (urethrocele), bladder neck, or bladder (cystocele) into the vaginal canal. Often a cystocele is present, and in this situation the patient is generally continent of urine. When a urethrocele is also present, the woman usually suffers from stress urinary incontinence, because the urethra has rotated posteriorly. The urethra and bladder neck now lie in a position where intraabdominal pressure is not transmitted to the periurethral tissues. In other words, there is little compensatory pressure around the bladder neck and proximal urethra during times of Valsalva. In this situation, relatively more pressure is exerted on the bladder and relatively less pressure on the urethra, thereby creating urinary incontinence. Even in the presence of a cystocele, with maintenance of normal intraurethral pressures, patients generally will remain continent of urine. This observation is useful when considering surgical techniques to correct anatomically related stress urinary incontinence.

20-22. 20, **B**; 21, **C**; 22, **B**. Pages 578-579; Figure 19-2 (from Herbst). Because of embryonic descent of the testis from its original retroperitoneal site to the scrotum, the internal inguinal ring is formed at the level of the transversalis fascia. The inguinal canal runs from the internal inguinal ring obliquely medial and caudal, emerging through the external inguinal ring, opening in the external oblique aponeurosis just above the pubic tubercle, and continuing into the scrotum. In the female, the round ligament courses similarly and ends just short of the labium majus. (The femoral canal represents a potential space under the inguinal ligament medial to the femoral vessels and lateral to the lacunar ligament.) Because there is no embryonic movement of the testicle in women, their inguinal canal is less likely to be associated with herniated peritoneum. Femoral hernias are more common in women than in men. Either potential space (canal) may be involved with a hernia that includes a portion of the bowel.

23. **A** (1, 2, 3). Pages 589, 591. Enteroceles may occur after abdominal or vaginal hysterectomy and generally are due to a weakened support system around the cul-de-sac or pouch of Douglas. Inasmuch as an enterocele may form by herniation of the cul-de-sac past the uterosacral ligaments into the rectovaginal septum, ap-

propriate surgical disposition of the uterosacral ligaments, cardinal ligaments, and peritoneum overlying the cul-de-sac are imperative. Generally, if there is redundant peritoneum beginning to herniate into the rectovaginal septum, this space should be closed after the removal of the uterus to prevent further extension. Likewise, the uterosacral and cardinal ligament should be plicated in the midline or into the vaginal cuff. Each of these procedures has a number of variations, but all are termed as types of culdoplasty.

24. **A** (1, 2, 3). Pages 595-598. There is some controversy with respect to the choice of the procedure to correct a vaginal vault (stump) prolapse. Nevertheless, certain principles and facts are important. The first is that the normal position of the vagina in the standing position is against the rectum and no more than 30 degrees from the horizontal. This is important for the occasional patient in whom abdominal colpopexy is anticipated. The second principle is that pelvic relaxation is part of the problem and dictates that an existing cystocele, rectocele, or enterocele must be repaired as part of this procedure to ensure long-term success. Defects are likely to recur when appropriate recognition and repair has not taken place during the initial surgery for vaginal prolapse. The third principle acknowledges that the perineal body is almost always severely weakened in women with total vaginal vault prolapse and therefore must be reconstructed.
25. **B** (1, 2). Page 584. The factors associated with the development of a cystourethrocele are numerous and difficult to state in very specific terms, but some general associations can be noted. These include parity and a wide pelvic arch typical of the gynecoid type pelvis. Although a cystourethrocele may develop in nulliparous women, this is unusual. In such cases, the patients will often have concomitant neurologic or metabolic disease contributing to loss of pelvic support, or they may be overweight or have chronic obstructive pulmonary disease. The presence of a wide pubic arch in a gynecoid type of pelvis allows the full force of the fetal head to compress against this area during descent in the second stage of labor. Narrower arches, such as those associated with the android or anthropoid pelvis, seem to protect this region during descent of the fetal head. This may account in part for the observation that a cystourethrocele is much less common in the black race, in whom the android or anthropoid pelves are more common. Prominent ischial spines are more consistent with these latter two types of pelves than with the gynecoid type. They do not play a role in the development of a cystourethrocele.
26. **E** (3 only). Page 581. An umbilical hernia is an example of a congenital malformation. Before 10 weeks of gestation, the abdominal contents are partially herniated through the umbilicus into the extra embryonic coelomic cavity. Shortly thereafter, the visceral contents return to the abdominal cavity and the defect in the abdominal wall closes during subsequent fetal growth. Generally, at birth this space contains only the umbilical cord. Following the cutting of the cord the area heals so that the skin in the area of the umbilicus fuses over the closed fascial layer. Small umbilical hernias at birth usually close in the first three years of life. In rare cases, with a less complete closure of the abdominal wall, an omphalocele forms, which is a hernia sac in the umbilicus covered only by peritoneum and including bowel and sometimes other abdominal contents. This is in contrast to gastroschisis, which is a failure of fusion to the right of the midline. In the repair of an umbilical hernia, usually all that is encountered is an empty hernia sac protruding through the small fascial defect.
27. **A** (1, 2, 3). Pages 578-581. Characteristics of abdominal hernias by definition include a reflection of peritoneum through a fascial defect. When intraperitoneal organ structures are part of the hernia, they are called sliding hernias. Although most hernias occur at anatomic weak spots, they generally are not considered congenital anomalies. The only exception is an omphalocele. When considering surgical repair of abdominal hernias, it is important to remember that there is almost always a peritoneal reflection to dissect and close, in addition to closing the original fascial defect.
28. **B** (1, 2). Pages 589, 591. If a significant redundancy exists in the cul-de-sac peritoneum following vaginal hysterectomy, it is important to obliterate this space to prevent a future enterocele. If uterosacral ligaments can be identified, they should be used in the repair. This can be accomplished by fixing the uterosacral ligaments

to the peritoneum of the sac and the vaginal vault. The peritoneum of the sac, and the uterosacral ligaments and vagina of the opposite side are similarly used closing this potential space with multiple sutures if necessary. This effectively shortens the cul-de-sac and also supports the attendant enterocele neck. Suturing the round ligaments and the ovarian ligaments will not prevent either an enterocele or vaginal prolapse. Suturing the ovaries can be a cause of dyspareunia.

29. **E** (3 only). Pages 596-597. In performing a sacrospinous ligament fixation the proper placement of the supporting suture is critical. Usually only one suture is used and placed approximately 2 finger-breadths or 3 cm medial to the ischial spine. This can be done with either a suture ligature carrier or an aneurysm needle. It is important not to place the suture around or adjacent to the ischial spine because of danger to the underlying pudendal vessels and nerve. The sacrotuberous ligament will not offer proper support since an aneurysm needle or suture ligature carrier will not surround this structure.

CHAPTER

20 Gynecologic Urology

DIRECTIONS for questions 1 - 16: Select the one best answer or completion.

1. A 24-year-old, healthy appearing woman complains of the recent onset of urgency with loss of urine. She has never had such symptoms before. The best single test to make a diagnosis in this case is
   A. residual urine
   B. cystometrics
   C. urinalysis
   D. Bonney test
   E. urethroscopy
2. The major action of urethral support operations is to
   A. decrease bladder activity
   B. increase urethral sphincter tone
   C. decrease the parasympathetic nerve supply to the urethra
   D. decrease the caliber of the urethral lumen
   E. increase the transmission of abdominal pressure to the urethra
3. The major risk for a patient who has had a Mersilene sling procedure for urethral suspension is
   A. intraoperative hemorrhage
   B. infection
   C. transection of the urethra by the Mersilene
   D. reabsorption of the Mersilene sling
   E. loss of bladder innervation
4. A 72-year-old diabetic female has been sent to you from a nursing home for evaluation because she is always incontinent. She has no complaints other than the wetness. The test most likely to demonstrate the etiology is
   A. urinalysis
   B. urethroscopy
   C. determination of residual urine
   D. Bonney test
   E. transurethral injection of methylene blue
5. A woman complains that a large volume of urine is lost shortly after coughing or jumping. She occasionally has a loss of urine while in bed at night if she happens to cough vigorously. She is unable to stop the urinary stream once it has begun. Given this history the most likely diagnosis is
   A. genuine stress incontinence
   B. a urethrovaginal fistula
   C. detrusor dyssynergia
   D. a urinary tract infection
   E. an ectopic ureter
6. A 24-year-old woman complains of frequency, urgency, and dysuria of 2 days duration. The most likely etiologic agent causing these symptoms is
   A. *Enterobacter aerogenes*
   B. *Streptococcus faecalis*
   C. *Chlamydia trachomatis*
   D. *Klebsiella aerogenes*
   E. *Escherichia coli*
7. Four weeks after a MMK (Marshall-Marchetti-Krantz) repair for stress incontinence, a patient complains of increased pain in the suprapubic area that is aggravated by walking. She is continent, afebrile, and has a white blood count of 11,000. Her urinalysis is normal. On examination, she has tenderness over the mons pubis. The pelvic exam is unremarkable. The mostly likely diagnosis is
   A. a urinary tract infection
   B. a retropubic abscess
   C. osteitis pubis
   D. osteomyelitis
   E. a hematoma in the space of Retzius
8. A 44-year-old woman complains of copious (approximately one-half cup) urine loss that she is unable to stop once it begins to flow. She states that the loss begins shortly after a cough or sneeze and that she frequently feels she has to void. If she doesn't void within a few minutes after this sensation, she will also lose urine. The most likely diagnosis is
   A. urge incontinence
   B. stress incontinence

C. a urethrovaginal fistula
D. a urethral diverticula
E. overflow incontinence

9. A premenopausal woman who has completed her family and has mild genuine stress incontinence requests treatment. Initially, this would include
A. estrogen
B. Kegel exercises
C. an alpha adrenergic agent
D. a Kelly plication
E. a Marshall-Marchetti-Krantz procedure

10. A 50-year-old woman has a history of recurrent dysuria and frequency as well as dyspareunia and postvoid dribbling. On examination she has a tender nodule palpable through the anterior vaginal wall. The most likely diagnosis is a(n)
A. ectopic ureter
B. Bartholin duct abscess
C. urethral diverticulum
D. urethrocele
E. Gartner's duct cyst

11. A cystourethrocele is a herniation of
A. the bladder
B. the urethra
C. both the urethra and the bladder
D. the bladder and a detachment of the urethra
E. the bladder and a diverticulum of the urethra

12. A patient with genuine stress incontinence is most apt to have
A. a short urethra
B. an abnormal bead chain cystourethrogram
C. loss of the pubourethral vesical angle
D. a positive Q-tip test
E. lack of transmission of intraabdominal pressure to the urethra

13. Instructions for Kegel exercises include contraction of the pubococcygeal muscles and which of the following?

	Repetitions during one sitting	Repetitions during one day	Breathing	Position
A.	5	2-4	panting	sitting
B.	5	2-4	deep breathing	sitting
C.	10	4-6	doesn't matter	doesn't matter
D.	10	6-8	deep breathing	supine
E.	10	6-8	hold breath	doesn't matter

14. A woman has genuine stress incontinence and symptoms and signs of anterior vaginal wall excoriation from a fourth degree cystourethrocele. Her stress incontinence has improved minimally with adequately performed Kegel exercises. She wishes to remain fertile, but she wants to have a surgical procedure to relieve her symptoms. The appropriate recommendation is a(n)
A. vaginal hysterectomy and anterior and posterior repair
B. retropubic urethropexy such a Marshall-Marchetti-Krantz procedure
C. trial on an anticholinergic drug
D. anterior colporrhaphy with a Kelly plication
E. fascial Sling procedure

15. A patient complains of leakage of urine. Of the following information uncovered in taking a history, the one most helpful in solving the problem is that she
A. is 45 years old and stopped menstruating 9 months ago
B. is not on estrogen replacement therapy
C. drinks 20 - 30 cups of coffee a day
D. takes terbutaline for her asthma
E. jogs 2 miles every morning

16. A patient whose history and assessment suggests detrusor dyssynergia is likely to benefit from
A. digitalis
B. haloperidol
C. imipramine
D. reserpine
E. hydralazine

DIRECTIONS for questions 17 - 20: For each numbered item, select the one heading most closely associated with it. Each lettered heading may be used once, more than once, or not at all.

17-20. Match the procedure with the technique.
(A) Passing a needle with a suture from the rectus fascia through the space of Retzius to the paravaginal tissue

(B) Suturing lateral paravaginal fascia together beneath the urethra to support the bladder neck
(C) Suturing the paravaginal fascia to the symphysis pubis
(D) Suturing the rectus fascia beneath the urethra
(E) Suturing the paravaginal fascia to Cooper's ligament

17. Burch
18. Kelly
19. Marshall-Marchetti-Krantz
20. Pereyra

DIRECTIONS For each numbered item 21 - 27, indicate whether it is associated with
A only (A)
B only (B)
C both (A) and (B)
D neither (A) nor (B)

21-24. Match the type of incontinence with the description or pathophysiology.
(A) Urge incontinence
(B) Genuine stress incontinence
(C) Both
(D) Neither

21. An objectively demonstrated involuntary loss of urine that is a social or hygienic problem
22. Involuntary loss of urine associated with bladder pressure greater than urethral pressure in the absence of detrusor contractions
23. Involuntary loss of urine associated with uninhibited detrusor contractions
24. Involuntary loss of urine due to a bladder pressure greater than the urethral pressure because of bladder distension without detrusor activity

25-27. Match the innervation with the action.
(A) Inhibits bladder contraction
(B) Stimulates urethral contraction
(C) Both
(D) Neither

25. The micturition feedback nerve circuit from the cortex to the brain stem (loop I)
26. Parasympathetic stimulation
27. Stimulation of adrenergic receptors

DIRECTIONS for questions 28 - 30: For each of the questions below, ONE or MORE of the responses is correct. Select the best answer based on the following
A if 1, 2, and 3 are correct
B if only 1 and 2 are correct
C if only 2 and 3 are correct
D if only 1 is correct
E if only 3 is correct

28. A patient has had the diagnosis of genuine stress incontinence made. It is recommended that she have corrective surgery. Risk factors that should be discussed with her at this time encompass
    1. increased incontinence
    2. failure to achieve correction
    3. difficulty in urinating after the procedure
29. Urinary continence is achieved by maintaining urethral pressures greater than the intravesical pressures. Factors that contribute to the maintenance of intraurethral pressure include
    1. smooth and striated muscle in the urethral wall
    2. vascularity of the urethral submucosa
    3. the distal 1 cm of the urethra
30. Urethral diverticula are thought to arise as a result of
    1. a congenital defect
    2. a gonococcal infection
    3. childbirth

ANSWERS

1. **C,** Pages 608-609. In an otherwise healthy woman who has had the recent onset of urinary urgency and loss of urine, the differential diagnosis should include urethritis, trigonitis, or cystitis. If the clean void urinalysis has WBCs and bacteria, cystitis is likely. If only WBCs are found, urethritis with an organism such as chlamydia is likely. In such a case, treatment of the infection is the first priority and other tests (with the exception of urine culture to determine the type of organism) are not indicated unless symptoms persist later in the absence of an infection.
2. **E,** Page 622. The basic defect in genuine stress incontinence is lack of transmission of abdominal pressure to the urethra. The urethral support procedures all attempt to accomplish the same goal. This goal is to ensure adequate intraabdominal pressure transmission so that it, together with the sphincter muscles of the urethra and the epithelium of the urethra, combine to make the intraurethral pressure greater than the intravesical pressure, thereby insuring continence.
3. **B,** Page 622. A foreign body left in place always creates a risk of infection. This is a major complication of a urethral sling, which utilizes synthetic materials. The Mersilene will not absorb, but it has been known to work its way into, or through, the urethra with a resulting fistula. The

patient is at no greater risk of hemorrhage or loss of bladder innervation than with any other suspension procedure.

4. **C,** Pages 608-610. This patient is quite likely to have overflow incontinence secondary to a neurogenic bladder with incomplete emptying. Her age, history of diabetes, and the history of constant wetting are significant clues to this etiology. If this is the case, large amounts of urine will remain in the bladder after voiding and may easily be detected by simple catheterization after an attempt to void. If the diagnosis of a neurogenic bladder is established, treatment of the underlying disease may be helpful to decrease incontinence, but usually it is not. Voiding frequently at specific times or using intermittent catheterization may be the best management. Catherization does carry a risk of infection.
5. **C,** Pages 623-624. Detrusor dyssynergia, which has also been known as detrusor instability, detrusor irritability or an unstable bladder, is associated with uninhibited bladder contractions. These are often triggered by an intraabdominal stress, such as coughing. Therefore it is easily confused with genuine stress incontinence. However, a careful history usually will reveal that a few seconds elapse between the stress and the onset of the urine flow. The bladder hyperactivity should be demonstrated by a cystometrogram. Treatment with bladder drills, such as voiding at specific time intervals, and anticholinergic or beta-adrenergic drugs are often helpful. A patient with a urethrovaginal fistula is likely to have a less predictable urinary stream during micturition and will complain of a watery vaginal discharge or that she loses urine upon standing or at unpredictable times. A patient with a bladder infection is apt to have detrusor dyssynergia. In addition she usually experiences frequency, dysuria, and pyuria. The symptoms associated with an ectopic ureter include constant leaking of urine.
6. **E,** Page 611. *Escherichia coli* is the most frequently found bacterium in uncomplicated urinary tract infections. The causative bacteria are usually present in accumulations of more than 100,000 organisms per ml. In cases of urethritis and trigonitis the presence of as few as 100 organisms per ml may indicate an infection because of the dilution factor of bladder urine. At least 20% of all women will develop urinary tract infections at some time in their life.
7. **C,** Pages 620-621. It is possible that this patient, who has suprapubic pain 4 weeks after an Marshall-Marchetti-Krantz repair, could have a urinary tract infection, an abscess, or a hematoma. However, the lack of WBCs in the urine, a normal white count, absence of fever, and no mass on exam make these all unlikely. Osteitis pubis is rare, but with this presentation of pain over the symphysis without fever or mass, it is the most likely diagnosis. Osteomyelitis is another possibility, and clinical differentiation between osteomyelitis and osteitis pubis may be difficult. Diagnosing osteomyelitis requires X-ray changes of cortical bone, marrow biopsy demonstrating infection, and recovery of microorganisms. Osteomyelitis pubis may be the eventual end to the continuum of an inflammatory process involving the pubic bone. Osteitis pubis is an inflammation of the periosteum of the pubis and represents an early stage in this process.
8. **A,** Page 623. With a history of short delay after the cough, the copious uncontrollable urine loss, and the urgency she often feels, urge incontinence is likely. Stress incontinence is usually described as loss of a small amount of urine and occurs immediately after or during the cough or valsalva. A urethrovaginal fistula causes an unpredictable urinary stream and/or loss of urine from the vagina. Typically a patient with overflow incontinence complains of voiding small amounts and still having the feeling that there is urine in the bladder. These women almost constantly lose small amounts of urine without any control. A urethral diverticulum tends to leak after voiding. This patient should be evaluated for infection and detrusor contractility prior to any surgery.
9. **B,** Pages 617-622. As this woman is premenopausal, estrogen is probably not indicated, although it is helpful in treating postmenopausal women. Kegel pubococcygeal muscle exercises often yield good results if done correctly. While the severity of the symptoms before therapy and the patient's age had no effect on outcome in one study evaluating the efficacy of Kegel exercises, the treatment was noted to be more effective when the symptoms were present for less than a year. Alpha adrenergic drugs are mildly effective in increasing urethral pressure, but usually are

not the best choice for the initial treatment of patients with mild symptoms of stress incontinence although this might be tried in conjunction with Kegel exercise. Surgical treatment, whether by the vaginal or abdominal route, should be reserved until the effect of Kegel exercises can be evaluated.

10. **C**, Page 613. With a history of dysuria, frequency, urinary dribbling, and dyspareunia, coupled with a palpable tender nodule, a urethral diverticulum is highly suspect. An ectopic ureter causes constant incontinence. The anatomic location is wrong for both Bartholin and Gartner's duct pathology. A urethrocele is not detected as a tender nodule, whereas a urethral diverticulum often presents as a tender suburethral mass. Urethral diverticula are relatively uncommon occurring in only 3% to 4% of all women sometime during their lifetime. They should be considered when these signs and symptoms occur however.
11. **D**, Pages 616-617. A urethrocele is somewhat of a misnomer, as the urethra most often does not balloon out or herniate. The urethra instead becomes detached. Then both the urethra and bladder rotate caudally out of the space beneath the symphysis pubis so that pressure from the intraabdominal cavity can no longer be transmitted to the urethra. Loss of this pressure transmission often results in genuine stress incontinence as the pressure transmission to the bladder continues increasing the intravesical pressure above that of the urethra.20
12. **E**, Pages 615-617. Genuine stress incontinence is due mainly to a lack of transmission of intraabdominal pressure to the urethra. The length of the urethra or its angle, as measured by the Q-tip test, or the amount of funnelling of the bladder neck, as determined by the bead chain cystourethrogram, do not correlate well with the presence or absence of genuine stress incontinence. However, in all cases of genuine stress incontinence the intravesical pressure exceeds the the maximum urethral pressure in the absence of detrusor activity.
13. **C**, Page 617. Patients are frequently told to do Kegel exercises, but they are not told how often to perform them. If they are not done frequently, they are ineffective. Kegel reported excellent results when the pelvic floor muscles were intermittently contracted and relaxed 5 times on waking, 5 times on rising, and 5 times every half hour through-out the day. Adequate pelvic floor musculature must exist in order for the exercises to cause hypertrophy and yield a beneficial result. If the pelvic floor muscles have been attenuated or are in any way obliterated, the exercise regime is less helpful as muscles cannot be developed if they are not present. Five to 10 repetitions should be performed at any one time. These sets should be repeated several times a day. The critical point in this question is that this is an isometric exercise. It is not possible to deep breathe or pant and adequately contract the pelvic floor muscles.
14. **D**, Pages 618-619. In this patient, who wishes to remain fertile, removal of the uterus is contraindicated. An anterior repair with a Kelly plication will support the bladder and urethra, thereby relieving her symptoms. There is no need for posterior repair if there are no symptoms of posterior relaxation. A retropubic urethropexy such as a Marshall-Marchetti-Krantz procedure will relieve her stress incontinence, but it will not replace the cystocele; therefore, her anterior vaginal wall will still be excoriated from extrusion. Modifications of the Marshall-Marchetti-Krantz, such as the Burch procedure, also would be of little benefit in this case. Anticholinergics are of some value in the treatment of detrusor dyssynergia not genuine stress incontinence. A fascial sling procedure is usually reserved for patients with previous operative failures. It too would not correct the cystocele. An anterior colporrhaphy with a Kelly plication should correct this patient's problems.
15. **C**, Pages 618, 623, (Office Practice and Practice Management: Initial Evaluation of Urinary Symptoms. The American College of Obstetricians and Gynecologists. Precis III: An Update in Obstetrics and Gynecology. Washington, D.C.: The American College of Obstetricians and Gynecologists 1986; Chapter 8). It is important to take a complete history from patients complaining of leakage of urine. Obviously, all answers are important. In this case the fact that the patient is menopausal and not on estrogen is probably not related to her incontinence. It is too soon for her to have developed atrophy. The fact that she jogs 2 miles every day would indicate that she is in good physical condi-

tion, but does not tell us anything about her pelvic floor musculature. Terbutaline can cause urinary retention and should have a beneficial effect. Caffeine on the other hand can decrease the urethral closing pressure. This patient drinks an excessive amount of fluid. It would be important to know the specific gravity of her urine. Does she have diabetes insipidus? Does she have polyuria? It would be more common to find that she is a nervous person and that this is a learned habit. Such a patient will benefit from bladder training if the remainder of her history and physical are normal. This patient should keep a diary and attempt to decrease the amount of fluid she drinks and the number of times she voids.

16. **C**, Page 624. All are medications not usually associated with the urinary tract. Digitalis is a cholinergic agonist. It will increase bladder wall tension. Haloperidol is a neuroleptic. It will block dopamine receptors leading to internal sphincter relaxation. Imipramine is a tricyclic antidepressant with alpha-adrenergic enhancement characteristics which have been found to be beneficial in patients with detrusor dyssynergia. Both reserpine andhydralazine are antihypertensives. They block adrenergic activity.

17-20. 17, **E**; 18, **B**; 19, **C**; 20, **A**. Pages 617-620. In the Marshall-Marchetti-Krantz procedure, the paravaginal fascia is sutured to the symphysis pubis in the space of Retzius. The Burch procedure is a modification of the Marshall-Marchetti-Krantz procedure and requires suturing the paravaginal fascia to Cooper's ligament. The Kelly plication sutures lateral paravaginal fascia in the midline beneath the urethra. The Pereyra procedure involves passing a needle with a suture attached through the space of Retzius from the rectus fascia to the paravaginal fascia on either side of the urethra. Each procedure is designed to place the proximal third of the urethra in an area where the intraabdominal pressure can be transmitted to it, while maintaining support of the urethra that will not allow it to move out of that pressure zone. This results in an increase in intraurethral pressure which, together with the urethral sphincters and mucous membrane, creates an intraurethral pressure greater than the intravesical pressure resulting in urinary continence.

21-24. 21, **C**; 22, **B**; 23, **A**; 24, **D**; Page 601. Incontinence is the involuntary loss of urine and if in a significant amount is both a social and a hygienic problem. Genuine stress incontinence is by definition the involuntary loss of urine associated with a bladder pressure greater than urethral pressure in the absence of detrusor contractions. Motor urge incontinence is the desire to void along with the involuntary loss of urine associated with uninhibited detrusor contractions. Overflow incontinence is the involuntary loss of urine due to a bladder pressure greater than the urethral pressure because of bladder distension without detrusor activity. The various types of incontinence are defined according to the cause of the pressure gradient. Successful treatment is based on correcting the specific reason for the higher bladder pressure, the lower urethral pressure, or both. Therefore, diagnostically it is important to determine the reason for the pressure differential as the treatment differs depending on the underlying cause.

25-27. 25, **A**; 26, **D**; 27, **C**; Pages 602-604, Figure 20-1.

Loop I of the micturition feedback nervous system circuit runs from the cortex to the brain stem to inhibit urination by modifying sensory stimuli from loop II, thereby inhibiting the bladder. The parasympathetic system generally initiates voiding with detrusor muscle stimulation and relaxation of urethral sphincters. Activating the beta adrenergic receptors of the sympathetic system inhibits the detrusor muscle through beta receptors within the bladder while activation of the alpha adrenergic receptors cause urethral muscle constriction. Knowing these facts allows one to plan rational therapy for urge incontinence, which is due to uninhibited bladder muscle spasms.

28. **A** (1, 2, 3), Page 622. Any surgical candidate should be informed of several basic surgical risks—infection, hemorrhage, damage to other structures, failure to achieve cure, and the risks of anesthesia. These general risks should all be documented on the patient's record. Specific procedures carry specific complications and these should also be outlined. In the case of urethral suspension, failure to spontaneously void may be a major factor. The patient should recognize the possible need for long-term urinary catheterization. Eventually nearly all patients with these repairs will void spontaneously.

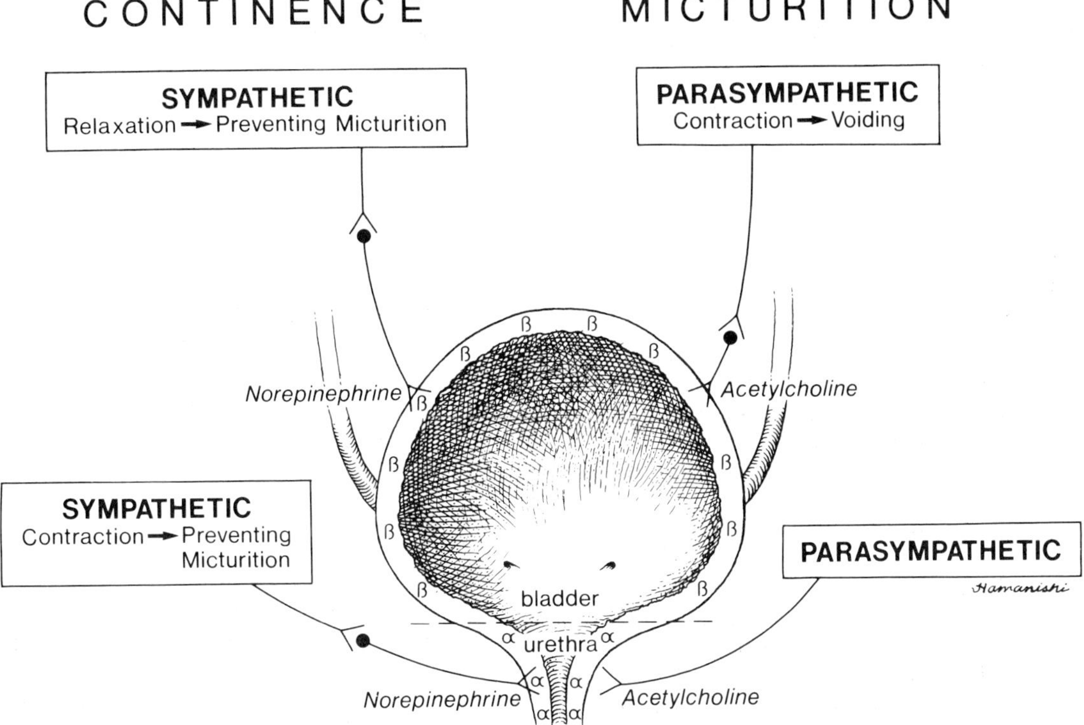

FIGURE 20-1.
The innervation of the bladder and urethra. Parasympathetic fibers arising in S2 through S4 have long preganglionic fibers and pelvic ganglia close to the bladder and urethra. These parasympathetic fibers excrete acetylcholine. Sympathetic fibers that have long postganglionic fibers discharge norepinephrine to beta receptors, primarily in the bladder, and alpha receptors, primarily in the urethra.
(Redrawn and modified from Raz S: Urol Clin North Am 5:323, 1978).

Some patients—particularly those who have minimal stress incontinence or have urge incontinence rather than stress incontinence, will actually have more incontinence postoperatively. Patients who preoperatively have only genuine stress incontinence sometimes develop detrusor instability after surgery and may require further medical therapy.

29. **B** (1, 2,), Page 605. The muscles, the vascularity, and the transmission of increased intraabdominal pressure are all important factors in maintaining a high urethral pressure with resultant continence. The vascularity and mucosal thickness of the urethra increase in response to estrogen. This may be the reason that estrogen helps in the treatment of incontinence in some estrogen-deficient women. The distal urethra is usually not important in maintaining continence as it is beyond the sphincter action of the striated muscle and beyond the area of intraabdominal pressure transmission.
30. **A** (1, 2, 3), Page 613. There are several ways in which a urethral diverticulum may develop. These include a congenital defect, acute and chronic inflammation and trauma. The congenital theory stems from the fact that cases have been reported in children and neonates. Infection of the periurethral glands with such organisms as the gonococcus or *E. coli* can result in the formation of retention cysts that when repeatedly infected may rupture into the lumen of the urethra, giving rise to a diverticulum. Urethral trauma from multiple catheterizations or via childbirth has been mentioned as an etiologic factor.

CHAPTER 21

Infections of the Lower Genital Tract

DIRECTIONS for questions 1 - 15: Select the one best answer or completion.

1. A 22-year-old woman complains of urgency, frequency, and dysuria. Urinalysis reveals more than 20 WBCs per high power field, and culture reveals 10 colonies per ml. The most likely diagnosis is
   A. pyelonephritis
   B. vulvovaginitis
   C. cystitis
   D. cervicitis
   E. acute urethral syndrome
2. A 19-year-old woman complains of headache, myalgia, dizziness, and low grade fever with each menstrual period for the past 6 months. She feels well at other times and denies depression or dysmenorrhea. She takes birth control pills and uses tampons. Of the following the most likely diagnosis is
   A. Weil's disease
   B. premenstrual syndrome
   C. flu
   D. Lyme disease
   E. forme fruste of toxic shock syndrome
3. A 22-year-old woman complains of severe itching of her perineum, wrists, and breasts. The symptoms are worse at night. Exam reveals excoriation in all the above areas. No hives are seen. The most likely diagnosis is
   A. allergy
   B. scabies
   C. molluscum contagiosum
   D. lice
   E. pityriasis rosea
4. A 26-year-old woman from the British Virgin Islands is found to have several painless, beefy red ulcers on the vulva. A biopsy is taken and depicted in Figure 21-1. The diagnosis is
   A. syphilis
   B. chancroid
   C. herpes simplex
   D. lymphogranuloma venereum
   E. granuloma inguinale
5. After injecting Xylocaine anesthesia for suturing a wound, the correct needle handling procedure is
   A. break or bend needle so it cannot be reused
   B. dispose of the needle and syringe separately
   C. recap the needle before disposal
   D. drop the needle in a bleach solution
   E. place the needle and syringe in a puncture proof container
6. A patient with severe toxic shock syndrome is most likely to have
   A. total lymphocytes greater than 1000 per cc
   B. polymorphonuclear cells less than 80%
   C. SGOT less than 30 units per liter
   D. BUN greater than 20 milligrams per deciliter
   E. platelets greater than 300,000
7. The basic underlying pathophysiologic disturbance in a patient with AIDS is
   A. infection with opportunistic organisms such as pneumocystis carinii
   B. a cancer that affects the cell-mediated immune system
   C. a decrease in number and function of T-4 lymphocytes
   D. decrease in serum immunoglobulins, IgG and IgA
   E. thrombocytopenia
8. How many different species of bacteria are found in the vaginas of normal asymptomatic women when careful culturing is done?
   A. 2-3
   B. 6-10
   C. 12-15
   D. 17-20
   E. more than 30
9. The most specific test commonly used to detect AIDS is
   A. enzyme-linked immunosorbent assay (ELISA)
   B. Southern blot
   C. Polymerase Chain Reaction (PCR)
   D. Northern blot
   E. Western blot
10. A young woman complains of a bad odor

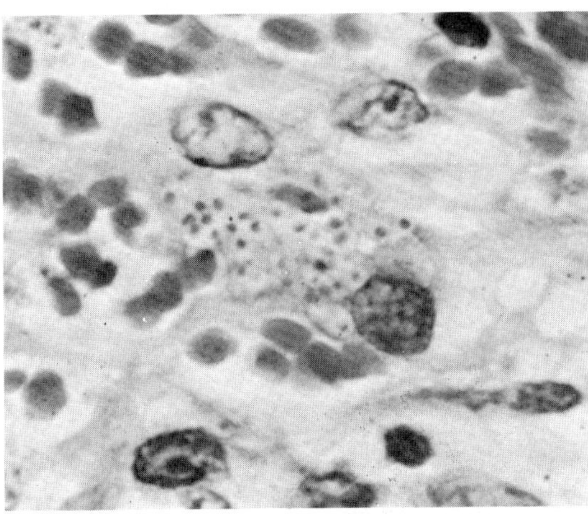

FIGURE 21-1.

(From Hart G. In Holmes KK, Mårdh PA, Sparling PF, et al, eds: Sexually transmitted diseases. New York, McGraw-Hill, 1984, p. 394.)

from the vaginal area after intercourse and during menses. She has very little discharge but it is irritating. The direct reason for the odor is most likely

A. breakdown of blood or protein in semen
B. increased numbers of anaerobes
C. *E. coli*
D. normal vaginal secretions
E. release of amines in an alkaline milieu

11. A 26-year-old woman complains of a vaginal discharge associated with itching and burning. The pH of the discharge is 5.5. Which of the following is the **LEAST** likely diagnosis?
    A. chlamydia cervicitis
    B. gonorrhea cervicitis
    C. yeast vaginitis
    D. *Trichomonas vaginitis*
    E. bacterial vaginosis
12. A young woman whose partner is an IV drug abuser feels well but wishes to be tested for HIV antibodies. Both the enzyme-linked immunosorbent assay (ELISA) and Western Blot tests are positive. Into which CDC group of HIV infections should she be classified?
    A. not infected
    B. group I
    C. group II
    D. group III
    E. group IV
13. Clue cells are often seen in the wet mount of the vaginal secretions of a patient with bacterial vaginosis. A clue cell is a(n)
    A. WBC with phagocytized bacteria
    B. epithelial squamous cell covered with bacteria
    C. epithelial columnar cell covered with bacteria
    D. WBC containing gram-negative paired cocci
    E. squamous epithelium containing macrophages
14. After candida albicans, the yeast most often found in the vagina is
    A. *tricophyton rubrum*
    B. *candida glabrata*
    C. microsporum canis
    D. *candida tropicalis*
    E. pityrosporum orbiculare
15. A 21-year-old woman is seen in the Emergency Room with hypotension, fever, diarrhea, headache, myalgia, red eyes, and a skin rash. She states she has felt ill for 2 days and the symptoms are worse. She is sexually active and uses barrier contraception. She denies abdominal pain, vaginal discharge, or any drug ingestion except aspirin. Her periods are regular. Her last normal period began 4 days ago. The most likely diagnosis is
    A. Rocky Mountain spotted fever
    B. scarlet fever
    C. toxic shock syndrome
    D. meningococcemia
    E. leptospirosis

DIRECTIONS for questions 16 - 23: For each numbered item, select the one heading most closely associated with it. Each lettered heading may be used once, more than once, or not at all.

16-19. Match the causative organism with the disease or lesion

(A) *Calymmatobacterium*
(B) *Chlamydia trachomatis*
(C) Spirochete
(D) Mycobacterium
(E) *Hemophilus ducreyi*

16. Gumma
17. Granuloma inguinale
18. Chancroid
19. Condyloma lata

20-23. Match the disease with the Figure

(A) primary herpes
(B) Molluscum contagiosum
(C) Condyloma acuminatum
(D) Lymphogranuloma venereum
(E) invasive cancer

20. Figure 21-2
21. Figure 21-3
22. Figure 21-4
23. Figure 21-5

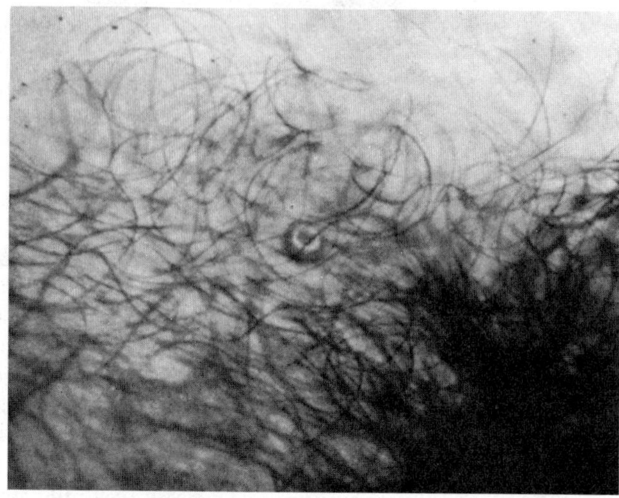

FIGURE 21-2.
(From Brown ST. In Holmes KK, Mårdh PA, Sparling PF, et al, eds: Sexually transmitted diseases. New York, McGraw-Hill, 1984, p. 394.)

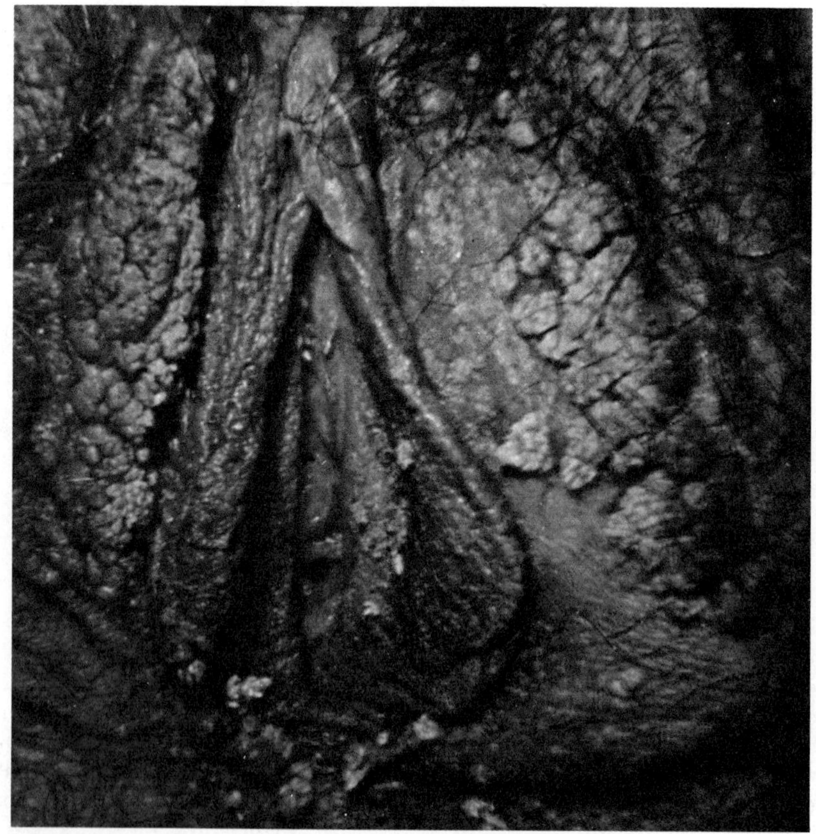

FIGURE 21-3.
(From Friedrich EG: Vulvar disease, 2nd ed. Philadelphia, W.B. Saunders Co., 1983, p. 25.)

DIRECTIONS: For each numbered item 24 - 26, indicate whether it is associated with
A only (A)
B only (B)
C both (A) and (B)
D neither (A) nor (B)

24-26. Match the organism
(A) *Chlamydia trachomatis*
(B) *Neisseria gonorrhoeae*
(C) both
(D) neither

24. causes a mucopurulent cervicitis
25. cultured on agar media
26. treated with tetracycline

DIRECTIONS for questions 27 - 32: For each of the questions below, ONE or MORE of the responses is correct. Select the best answer based on the following
A if 1, 2, and 3 are correct
B if only 1 and 2 are correct
C if only 2 and 3 are correct
D if only 1 is correct
E if only 3 is correct

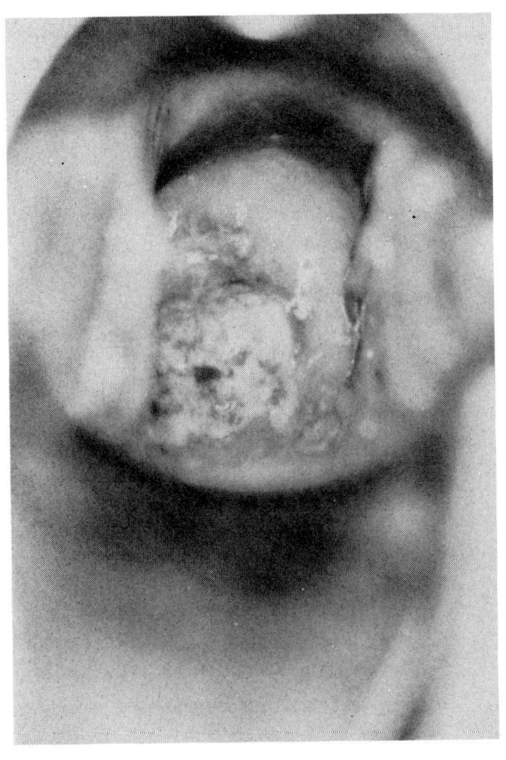

FIGURE 21-4.
(From Kaufman RH, Faro S: Clin Obstet Gynecol 28:154,1985.)

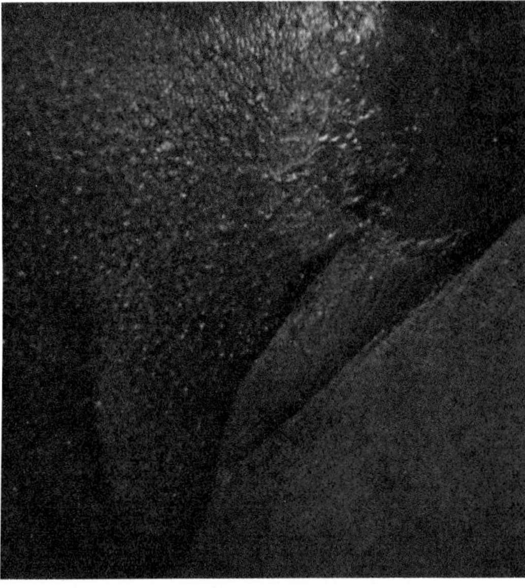

FIGURE 21-5.
(From Friedrich EG: Vulvar disease, 2nd ed. Philadelphia, W.B. Saunders Co., 1983, p. 229.)

27. A 16-year-old patient presents during a menstrual period with hypotension, skin rash, fever, and myalgia. She is found to have staphylococci in her vaginal culture. Her mother asks you to explain her daughter's illness and wants to know the proposed treatment plan. You should tell her
    1. symptoms are due to staphylococcus aureus bacteremia
    2. almost all cases are sexually transmitted
    3. antibiotic treatment is helpful
28. A 24-year-old woman has had several sexual contacts in the last 20 days, but no sexual contact for several months prior to this time. She presents with a small tender ulcer on her vulva of 3 days' duration. She also has enlarged, slightly tender inguinal nodes. She has no other signs or symp-

toms. At this visit you should culture for herpes simplex virus and
1. obtain a serologic test for syphilis
2. perform a dark field study
3. biopsy for cancer

29. Clinical AIDs (Group IV) from HIV infection includes
1. low CD4 lymphocyte count
2. monocytes infected with HIV
3. lymphomas

30. In which of the following situations would one regularly expect to find >10 WBCs (per hpf) in a specimen of cervical mucus?
1. when sperm is present in cervical mucus
2. with a positive gonorrhea culture
3. *Chlamydia* cervicitis

31. A woman with florid condyloma acuminata on the vulva desires their removal. Her PAP smears are negative. Methods of treatment include
1. interferon
2. trichloracetic acid
3. cryocautery

32. A 26-year-old woman complains of burning of the vulva, which has been present for 6 days and is increasing in severity. The differential diagnosis should include a
1. primary vaginal infection
2. primary skin irritant
3. contact dermatitis

ANSWERS

1. **E,** Page 634. Fever and chills are usually a major feature in pyelonephritis, which also presents with increased bacteria and WBCs in the urine. Vulvovaginitis may be associated with dysuria, but a careful history reveals that the pain is external, away from the urethra, and due to urine contact on the tender vulva. Physical exam reveals vaginal discharge. Patients with cystitis may have symptoms similar to the urethral syndrome, but have greater than 100 bacteria per ml cultured from the urine. Cervicitis usually does not cause urinary symptoms unless there is a concomitant infection of the urethra, which is often true with organisms such as gonorrhea or chlamydia. The acute urethral syndrome is defined by symptoms of dysuria and frequency and pyuria without significant numbers of bacteria in the urine.
2. **E,** Page 669. The repetitive and cyclic nature of the symptoms makes flu and Lyme disease unlikely. Lyme disease is due to a spirochete carried by a tick and may cause similar early symptoms. Later it often causes a significant arthritis. It is not repetitive and has a classic skin lesion erythema migrans. Weil's disease is the sequel of a severe infection with leptospirosis, which is a rare condition and much more severe than the symptoms outlined. However, it is one of the differential diagnoses in cases of severe toxic shock syndrome (TSS). The premenstrual syndrome occurs prior to the menses. A mild form, or "forme fruste," of toxic shock syndrome is likely with the use of tampons. Vaginal cultures for staphylococcus aureus should be done and the use of tampons discontinued until the bacteria are eradicated. Then tampons should be worn for no longer than 6 hours.
3. **B,** Page 639. The distribution, with increased itching at night, makes scabies the most likely diagnosis. This diagnosis can be proven by an Indian ink test to identify the burrows, or by making a slide of the scrapings from the affected skin and using mineral oil to prevent loss of specimen. Allergies are unlikely to have a concomitant genital, wrist, and breast distribution and are often associated with hives. Molluscum contagiosum has classic umbilicated papules, and lice tend to be located in hair-bearing areas. Pityriasis rosea has a truncal and upper extremity distribution, often with a history of a herald patch.
4. **E,** Page 649 and Table 21-1

   Granuloma inguinale is due to a gram negative, nonmotile, encapsulated rod, calymmatobacterium granulomatis. The pathognomonic Donovan bodies are clusters of dark-staining, bipolar-appearing (safety pin) bacteria in large mononuclear cells. The disease is found in subtropical areas and is rare in the United States. Treatment is with tetracycline. The differential diagnoses are discussed under questions 16-19.
5. **E,** Page 675. Because of the danger of hepatitis and HIV infection from a needle stick exposure, the safest technique is to dispose of both needle and syringe in a puncture resistant disposable container. Any manipulation of the needle including capping, breaking, or removal, increases the risk of inadvertent skin puncture and contamination.
6. **D,** Page 670 and Table 21-3. A patient with severe toxic shock syndrome usually has less than 860 lymphocytes per ml, polymorphonuclear cells greater than 90%, platelets less than 150,000, a SGOT

TABLE 21-1. Characteristic Features Which Differ in the Three Major Causes of Dysuria in Women

	Acuate Bacterial Cystitis	Urethritis	Vulvitis
Predisposing factors	Previous cystitis Diaphragm use Onset of symptoms within 24 hours after intercourse	New sex partner	History of genital herpes Partner with genital herpes Antibiotic use History of recurrent vulvovaginal candidiasis
Symptoms	Internal dysuria Duration of symptoms ≤4 days Frequency and urgency Gross hematuria	Internal dysuria Duration of symptoms often ≥7 days with chlamydial urethritis	External dysuria Vaginal discharge Vulvar irritation, burning, pruritus, or lesions
Signs	Suprapubic tenderness	Mucoprurulent cervicitis Vulvar lesions	Vulvar lesions Vulvitis Curdlike vaginal exudate
Laboratory	Pyuria Microscopic hematuria Rapid nitrite test Urine Gram stain Urine culture	Pyuria Urethral discharge or bartholinitis Endocervical exudate Cervical and urethral tests for *C. trachomatis* and *N. gonorrhoeae* Test lesion for HSV	No pyuria Test lesion for HSV Test vaginal discharge for *C. albicans*

From Holmes KK, Mårdh PH, Sparling PF, et al, editors: Sexually transmitted diseases, ed 2, New York, 1990, McGraw-Hill Book Co.

greater than 40 units per deciliter, and a BUN greater than 20 milligrams per deciliter. The last two indicate liver and kidney involvement, which occurs in severe disease. An elevated creatine phosphokinase is also frequently found due to muscle damage.

7. **C,** Page 671. AIDS victims often acquire the disease from contact with homosexuals or shared IV drug needles. They may suffer infection with opportunistic bacteria, viruses, or parasites, develop thrombocytopenia, Kaposi's sarcoma, or have increased immunoglobulins. The basic problem is infection of the T lymphocytes with RNA human immunodeficiency virus. This causes a decrease in function of the T-4 lymphocytes, resulting in breakdown of cell-mediated immune responses that allow the secondary infections or Kaposi's sarcoma to occur.
8. **D,** Page 658. The most common bacteria in the vagina are the lactobacillus found in 60-80% of normal women. Other facultative aerobes include Diphtheroids, *Streptococcus*, *Staphylococcus*, *Gardnerella vaginalis*, and *E. coli*. Anaerobes can be cultured in the vaginas of approximately 80% of normal women. These include *Peptostreptococcus*, *Peptococcus*, and *Bacteroides*. Normal asymptomatic women harbor 17-29 species of bacteria. Candida is also commonly found. The quantity of the different species varies. Both anaerobes and aerobes are found in significantly increased amounts in patients with bacterial vaginosis.
9. **C,** Page 674. Enzyme-linked immunosorbent assay (ELISA) is a screening test for antibodies against the HIV that has a significant number of false positives and negatives. Western blot is another method of detecting specific antibodies to proteins of the human immunodeficiency virus (HIV). Southern blot and Northern blot use the same methodology to detect DNA and RNA, respectively. PCR (Polymerase Chain Reaction) is an extremely sensitive and specific method for testing specific types of DNA. It can be used as a test for

HIV viral DNA, which if present, documents infection with HIV.

10. **E,** Page 661. Volatile amines are released in an alkaline media. The normal pH of the vagina is less than 4.5, but both blood and semen have a high pH (around 7.2-7.4). The amines are formed by anaerobic bacteria and become volatile, and therefore noticeable, when the pH rises above the normal vaginal pH of 4.5. Addition of KOH to vaginal secretion volatilizes the amines. This forms the basis for the "sniff test," the fishy smell associated with bacterial vaginosis.
11. **C,** Page 657. The normal pH of the healthy vagina is 3.8 to 4.2. If the pH is greater than 5.0, bacterial vaginosis, trichomonas, or some other bacteria infection is likely. A yeast infection or physiologic discharges are more likely if the pH is normal. Testing the pH is quick and easy, and it divides symptomatic vaginal discharges into bacterial infections versus yeast and physiologic discharge quite well. It should be measured routinely in patients with complaints of vaginal discharge and can be easily done by using Nitrazine or pH paper.
12. **C,** Pages 671-672. HIV infection has be categorized by symptomatology and laboratory tests into 4 groups. Group I patients are those with initial viremia who may have symptoms ranging from nothing to a mononucleosis type illness. Antibodies to HIV may be absent or low. Group II patients are those who are in a latent phase and is by far the most common situation. HIV antibodies are present and in a few individuals each year the infection will progress to Group III or IV. Group III includes those patients with generalized lymphadenopathy. Group IV patients have clinical AIDs that is manifest by malignancy (most commonly lymphomas or Kaposi's sarcoma), weight loss, diarrhea, CNS symptoms and repeated opportunistic infection.
13. **B,** Page 660 and Figure 21-19 (from Herbst). A clue cell is a squamous epithelial cell so heavily covered with numerous bacteria that its outline is obscured. These cells are found in high numbers in patients with bacterial vaginosis. Columnar cells are rarely seen in wet mounts. WBCs with intracellular gram-negative diplococci are indicative of gonococcal infection. Macrophages in the epithelium are seen on histologic specimens, not on wet mounts.
14. **B,** Page 665. Candida are found normally in 25% of women. They are an opportunistic pathogen and grow in the G.I. tract from the mouth to the anus, even more readily than in the vagina. *Candida glabrata* is occasionally found in the vagina and is said to cause burning rather than itching. It does not produce filaments. Therefore, spores only are found. It does not respond well to the imidazoles but may be treated with gentian violet. *Trichophyton rubrum* is the fungus that usually causes *tinea cruris* (jock itch) or *tinea corporis*. Microsporum canis causes *tinea capitis* and pityrosporum orbiculare causes *tinea versicolor*.
15. **C,** Page 669. The onset with the period and symptoms make toxic shock syndrome the most likely of the diagnoses mentioned. She has hypotension, rash, fever and three organ symptom manifestations, thereby meeting the criteria for the diagnosis of toxic shock syndrome. However, one must not forget other diseases that cause similar symptoms, such as Rocky Mountain spotted fever, scarlet fever, meningococcemia, leptospirosis, measles, Kawasaki's disease, and Lyme disease.

16-19. 16, **C**; 17, **A**; 18, **E**; 19, **C**; Pages 649, 651, and 655. *Chlamydia* is well known to cause cervicitis, nonspecific urethritis, PID, and trachoma. It also causes lymphogranuloma venereum, which is not as common. Gummas and condyloma lata are lesions of secondary syphilis, which are not often seen, and not as well known as the chancre of primary syphilis. Chancroid is a rare disease caused by *Hemophilus ducreyi*, which may form the classic "school of fish" appearance of extracellular streptobacillary chains on a gram smear. It is hard to remember the signs, symptoms, causative agents, diagnostic methods, and treatment of rare diseases; yet these rare manifestations should be reviewed regularly, as they are all in the differential diagnosis for genital lesions that are frequently seen, such as condyloma acuminata, herpes, or the less common, but serious, vulvar carcinoma. Granuloma inguinale is caused by *calymmatobacterium granulomatis* and is very rare in the United States. It generally starts as an asymptomatic nodule, which then develops into a painless ulcer.

20-23. 20, **B**; 21, **C**; 22, **A**; 23, **D**; Pages 641, 643, 647, and 651. Visual identification of some vulvar lesions is easy, but confirmation by culture or biopsy is usually indicated.

Molluscum contagiosum lesions appear umbilicated and have a central core of hyperkeratotic epidermis, which is easily expelled. Microscopically, it contains intracytoplasmic inclusions. Treatment is by curettage. Lymphogranuloma venereum is caused by chlamydia trachomatis, and in its secondary stage has enlarged lymph nodes, which coalesce forming skin depressions between groups of the inflamed nodes, yielding the groove sign. Fluctuant nodes may be aspirated for diagnosis. Treatment is 3 to 6 weeks of tetracycline or erythromycin. Herpes simplex may form a necrotic ulcer of the cervix with remarkably few systemic symptoms. One must remember that the herpes simplex virus is likely in a young woman and obtain cultures for the herpes virus. In such cases, if culture does not confirm the diagnosis, and the ulcer persists, biopsy should be done to rule out cancer. A course of Acyclovir should be given for treatment of a significant herpes infection. Treatment will decrease the time and severity of symptoms, but does not affect the frequency of recurrences. In the majority of women, the diagnosis of condyloma acuminatum can be made by direct inspection. The warts tend to occur on moist skin. Initial infections usually begin in the vestibule and adjacent areas of the labia. However, all adjacent, moist epithelium may be involved with condyloma. Initial lesions are pedunculated, soft papules approximately 2 to 3 mm in diameter and 10 to 20 mm long. They may occur as a single papule or in clusters. The management of the individual case depends on the location, size, and extent of the condyloma and whether the woman is pregnant. There is a wide range of therapeutic choices, including chemical, cautery, and immunologic therapy. All of these lesions can be confused with cancer, and one should not be hesitant to biopsy a lesion if there is doubt. Perhaps the onlyexception to biopsy is the fluctuant nodes of lymphogranuloma venereum, which tend to form draining sinuses after incision.

24-26. 24, **A**; 25, **B**; 26, **C**; Pages 635-636. *Chlamydia trachomatis*, *Neisseria gonorrhoeae*, and the herpes simplex virus can all produce cervical mucopus. However, neither herpes simplex virus nor *Neisseria gonorrhoeae*-positive cultures correlated significantly with mucopus when mucopus was defined as purulent endocervical discharge from which a gram stain shows equal to or greater than 10 WBCs per high power field. Gonorrhea grows well on modified Thayer-Martin agar, while *chlamydia*, being an obligate, intracellular organism, requires cell cultures. *Chlamydia* is treated with doxycycline, erythromycin, or trimethoprim-sulfamethoxizole, in both males and females. Gonorrhea is somewhat sensitive to doxycycline or tetracycline, but the third generation cephalosporins are the first line drugs for therapy.

27. **E** (3), Page 669. The symptoms are due to absorption of an exotoxin produced by the staphylococcus aureus. Blood cultures are rarely positive. The use of tampons allows the staphylococcus to grow and excrete the exotoxin, which is then absorbed through the vaginal mucosa. Sexual transmission is not a common factor, as the staphylococcus can commonly be cultured from the vaginas of many sexually inactive women. Treatment with an anti-staphylococcal antibiotic will prevent recurrent episodes, which occur in approximately 1/3 of untreated women even if they stop using tampons. The 16-year-old should be encouraged to stop using tampons or at least change them every 6 hours during the day and use sanitary napkins at night.

28. **B** (1, 2), Pages 644-646. In a woman with this history, the primary possibility is herpes simplex virus, though the differential must include syphilis along with several less common possibilities such as chancroid, granuloma inguinale, and cancer. A herpes simplex virus culture would be indicated, as would a dark field study. A serologic test for syphilis should be obtained in case she had prior syphilis, but it is too soon to have developed a positive test from her recent exposure. It takes 4 to 6 weeks for a positive serologic test for syphilis to develop. Cancer is unlikely in this age group, but could be ruled out by biopsy if the lesion is not healed or markedly improved within two weeks.

29. **A** (1, 2, 3), Pages 672-673. The decrease in number and quality of CD4 lymphocytes (T4 lymphocytes with CD4 receptors) allows opportunistic infections as those lymphocytes modulate many of the human immune system functions. Without the protection offered, organisms that normally would not cause a problem result in serious disease (e.g., pneumocystis). HIV infected monocytes migrate into the CNS causing CNS symptoms, which are the presenting complaints in 1/3 of AIDs pa-

tients and occur in over 80% at some time during the illness. Karposi's sarcoma is the most well known associated malignancy, but lymphomas are also commonly found.

30. **E** (3 only), Page 677. *Chlamydia* infection of the cervix causes mucopus, which can be seen on a white Q-tip if there is sufficient cervical mucus. A gram stain will reveal 10 WBCs per high power field. Both gonorrhea and sperm will result in increased WBCs in the cervical mucus but usually in smaller numbers.
31. **A** (1, 2, 3), Pages 641 and 644. Several therapeutic modalities for visible warts are available. For recently developed florid condyloma acuminata, podophyllin and trichloracetic acid work quite well. If the warts are more mature, surgical excision, cryocautery, and laser are more effective. Interferon has been used both systemically and locally with some improvement in resolution of visible warts. However, none of these modalities destroy the viable viral DNA in the basal cells, or virons in the epithelium, which are located at a distance from the florid wart. Therefore, close observation and follow-up are required. Frequent recurrence is common.
32. **A** (1, 2, 3), Page 634. The vulva is often irritated by primary vaginal infections, which are the most common cause of the above symptoms. However, allergens such as soap and perfumes, contact toxins (such as poison oak and ivy, which are primary skin irritants), as well as secondary skin infections, which occur after a primary insult should be remembered as causes of this frequent complaint.

CHAPTER

22 Upper Genital Tract Infections

DIRECTIONS for questions 1 - 11: Select the one best answer or completion.

1. In a tubo-ovarian complex associated with acute pelvic inflammatory disease, the flora is predominantly
   A. Group D enterococcus
   B. mixed anaerobes
   C. *Chlamydia trachomatis*
   D. *Neisseria gonorrhoea*
   E. *Escherichia coli*
2. A 16-year-old nullipara has bilateral lower abdominal pain, a fever of 38°C, and a tender left adnexal thickening. A cervical culture is positive for *Chlamydia trachomatis*. Assuming a correct diagnosis of acute pelvic inflammatory disease (PID), the best treatment would be
   A. outpatient treatment with I.M. cefoxitin and oral doxycycline
   B. oral doxycycline alone
   C. I.M. procaine penicillin
   D. hospitalization with parenteral doxycycline and cefoxitin
   E. hospitalization with parenteral cefoxitin alone
3. Empiric antibiotic protocols used to treat acute pelvic inflammatory disease should cover a wide range of bacteria which includes all the following **EXCEPT**
   A. *Neisseria gonorrhoeae*
   B. *Chlamydia trachomatis*
   C. *Bacteroides* species
   D. *Peptococcus* species
   E. *Clostridium* species
4. The most accurate method of diagnosing acute pelvic inflammatory disease is
   A. history
   B. pelvic examination
   C. ultrasound
   D. leukocytosis
   E. diagnostic laparoscopy
5. Of the following contraceptive methods, the one that does not lower the relative risk of incurring a sexually transmitted disease is
   A. Nonoxynol 9 (spermicidal jelly or cream)
   B. an intrauterine device
   C. condoms
   D. oral contraceptives
   E. a diaphragm
6. When using clinical criteria alone to diagnose acute pelvic inflammatory disease, the percent of false positives is approximately
   A. 15%
   B. 25%
   C. 35%
   D. 45%
   E. 55%
7. Bacteriologic and immunologic studies suggest the most prevalent sexually transmitted organism causing upper tract disease in the United States is
   A. the human immunodeficiency virus (HIV)
   B. Herpes simplex virus
   C. *Neisseria gonorrhoea*
   D. *Chlamydia trachomatis*
   E. *Mycoplasma hominis*
8. A 27 year-old patient who is hospitalized for treatment of acute salpingitis has a cervical culture that is positive for *Neisseria gonorrhoeae*. The likelihood of her having a fallopian tube culture positive for the same organism is
   A. 5%
   B. 10%
   C. 25%
   D. 50%
   E. 75%
9. The most frequent symptom of acute pelvic inflammatory disease is
   A. vaginal discharge
   B. abnormal bleeding
   C. nausea and vomiting
   D. lower abdominal pain
   E. urinary frequency
10. A 32 year-old multipara with an intrauterine device (IUD) in place is hospitalized for treatment of acute pelvic inflammatory disease. The IUD should be removed
    A. as soon as the diagnosis has been made

B. as soon as antibiotics have been started
C. as soon as adequate levels of antibiotics have been achieved
D. 24 hours after antibiotics have been initiated
E. at the conclusion of parenteral antibiotic therapy

11. A 24-year-old nullipara is being treated for bilateral tubo-ovarian abscesses noted on ultrasound. Triple antibiotics, including clindamycin, gentamicin and ampicillin, have been given for 72 hours. Pain and fever persist. The abscess is **not** pointing into the cul-de-sac. The recommended surgical procedure is
A. total abdominal hysterectomy with bilateral salpingo-oophorectomy
B. total abdominal hysterectomy
C. bilateral salpingo-oophorectomy
D. colpotomy drainage of abscess
E. percutaneous aspiration of abscess under ultrasound guidance

DIRECTIONS for questions 12 - 17: For each numbered item, select the one heading most closely associated with it. Each lettered heading may be used once, more than once, or not at all.

12-14. Percent affected
(A) 1-4%
(B) 5-10%
(C) 20-25%
(D) 40-50%
(E) >51%

12. mortality rate associated with ruptured tubo-ovarian abscess
13. recurrence rate of pelvic inflammatory disease
14. percentage of ectopic pregnancies occurring in tubes damaged by previous salpingitis

15-17. Match the findings with the preferred therapy
(A) intravenous doxycycline and cefoxitin
(B) intravenous clindamycin and gentamicin
(C) intramuscular cefoxitin plus oral probenecid
(D) intramuscular ceftriaxone plus 10 days of tetracycline
(E) intramuscular ceftriaxone plus 10 days of erythromycin

15. positive *Neisseria gonorrhoeae* culture from cervix, no fever, no tenderness
16. 7 cm abscess, fever, negative cervical culture
17. bilateral adnexal tenderness, low grade temperature

DIRECTIONS: For each numbered item 18 - 26, indicate whether it is associated with
A only (A)
B only (B)
C both (A) and (B)
D neither (A) nor (B)

18-19. Match the statements about acute pelvic inflammatory disease with the causative organism
(A) *Chlamydia trachomatis*
(B) *Neisseria gonorrhoeae*
(C) both
(D) neither

18. 5-10% are associated with Fitz-Hugh-Curtis syndrome (perihepatic inflammation)
19. more than two thirds of patients will have temperature elevation of greater than 38° C

20-21. Match the appropriate antibiotic or antibiotics with the situation
(A) ceftriaxone 250 mg
(B) doxycycline 100 mg b.i.d.
(C) both
(D) neither

20. acute PID without fever, nausea, or vomiting
21. a pharyngeal culture positive *Neisseria gonorrhoeae*

22-23. Relationship with upper tract infection or colonization
(A) ectopic pregnancy
(B) chronic pelvic pain
(C) both
(D) neither

22. at least a fourfold increase in patients with acute PID
23. related to colonization of endosalpinx by anaerobic bacteria

24-26. Frequency, cause, and effect of two of the more uncommon organisms associated with pelvic infections
(A) *Actinomyces* infection
(B) Tuberculosis infection
(C) both
(D) neither

24. rare cause of upper genital tract infection in United States
25. associated with intrauterine device (IUD) use
26. a cause of infertility

DIRECTIONS for questions 27 - 32: For each of the questions below, ONE or MORE of the responses is correct. Select the best answer based on the following
A if 1, 2, and 3 are correct
B if only 1 and 2 are correct
C if only 2 and 3 are correct

D if only 1 is correct
E if only 3 is correct

27. Acute pelvic inflammatory disease caused by *Neisseria gonorrhoeae* can resist therapy by
    1. suppressing the antibody response in patients
    2. causing necrotic destruction of tubal epithelium
    3. producing penicillinase
28. Organisms associated with **non-puerperal** endometritis include
    1. the cytomegalovirus
    2. *Neisseria gonorrhoeae*
    3. *Chlamydia trachomatis*
29. Oral contraceptives protect against the development of sexually transmitted diseases by
    1. altering bacterial flora of the vagina
    2. altering the cervical mucus
    3. decreasing the duration of menstruation
30. True statements regarding the pathogenesis of acute pelvic inflammatory disease (PID) include that it is
    1. associated with menstruating women
    2. an ascending infection from the flora of the cervix and vagina
    3. polymicrobial
31. A 62-year-old patient is being treated for pelvic inflammatory disease. The differential should include
    1. diabetes
    2. genital tract malignancy
    3. intestinal disease
32. Risk factors for acute pelvic inflammatory disease include
    1. vaginal douching
    2. intrauterine device (IUD) use
    3. a history of a tubal ligation

ANSWERS

1. **B,** Page 697. Abscesses caused by acute pelvic inflammatory disease contain a mixture of anaerobes and facultative or aerobic organisms. The environment of an abscess cavity results in a low level of oxygen tension. Therefore, anaerobic organisms predominate and have been reported to be present in between 60% and 100% of cases.
2. **D,** Pages 706-707. This question addresses optimal treatment of acute pelvic inflammatory disease. Especially important in this patient are her young age, nulliparity, demonstrable fever and the presence of a palpable inflammatory thickening. Outpatient therapy does not provide high enough levels of appropriate antibiotics to penetrate successfully a developing tubo-ovarian complex. The presence of the *Chlamydia trachomatis* mandates treatment with Doxycycline and the presence of a palpable inflammatory thickening implicates other opportunistic organisms as pathogens. Cefoxitin is an excellent antibiotic for *Peptococcus* and *Peptostreptococcus* as well as *E coli.* An alternative to this regimen would include parenteral Clindamycin and an aminoglycoside. This combination has an advantage of providing better coverage for anaerobic infections and facilitative gram negative rods.
3. **E,** Page 707, Table 22-16. Empiric antibiotic protocols should cover a wide range of bacteria, including *Neisseria gonorrhoeae, Chlamydia trachomatis,* anaerobic rods and cocci, gram negative aerobic rods, gram positive aerobes, and *Mycoplasma* species. *Clostridium* species are rarely implicated in acute tubo-ovarian disease, and therefore, treatment for this group of organisms is not indicated initially. Selection of one antibiotic protocol over another will often depend on the clinical history and combinations of findings such as those shown in Table 22-16 (from Herbst et al.). Unfortunately, recent epidemiologic studies have shown that most women with acute pelvic inflammatory disease are treated as outpatients and have received only a single antibiotic regimen. Of these, less than one-third of the patients received tetracycline to treat possible chlamydial infection. This underscores the need for thorough knowledge of the bacteriology of acute pelvic inflammatory disease as a polymicrobial infection.
4. **E,** Page 705. Direct visualization of the pelvic organs is the most accurate method of diagnosing acute pelvic inflammatory disease. Therefore, laparoscopy is the gold standard. The pelvic organs may appear red, with an indurated, edematous oviduct, or there may be obvious purulent material. Laparoscopy should be used for patients who are not responding to antimicrobial therapy, or for those patients in whom cultures of purulent material need to be obtained.
5. **B,** Pages 698-700, Table 22-7. Using arbitrary risk rating scales in which the risk of developing acute pelvic inflammatory disease in sexually active women not using

contraception is assigned a score of 1, the following observations have been calculated. The corresponding risk of women wearing an intrauterine device is 2 to 4 among women using oral contraceptives 0.3, and among women using a barrier method including spermicidal preparations 0.4. Nonoxynol 9, the material found in spermicidal preparations, is both bactericidal and viricidal and laboratory tests have demonstrated its effectiveness among all sexually transmitted diseases including the human immunodeficiency virus (HIV).

6. **C,** Page 701. Patients with acute pelvic inflammatory disease present with a wide range of nonspecific clinical symptoms. Since the diagnosis is usually based on clinical criteria, there is both a high false positive rate and a high false negative rate. Laparoscopic studies of women with a clinical diagnosis of acute pelvic inflammatory disease suggest that this diagnosis is in error in over one-third of patients. Of this approximately 35%, 20% have no identifiable intra-abdominal or pelvic disease and approximately 15% have other entities such as ectopic pregnancy, acute appendicitis or torsion of an adnexa.
7. **D,** Page 694. *Chlamydia trachomatis* is an intracellular, sexually transmitted bacterial pathogen. This organism has recently become more prevalent than gonorrhea. From 20% to 40% of sexually active women have antibodies against *Chlamydia trachomatis*. From 10% to 30% of women with acute pelvic inflammatory disease who do not have cultures positive for *Chlamydia* have evidence of acute chlamydial infection by serial antibody testing. Although considered sexually transmitted organisms, herpes is generally not associated with acute upper tract infection and human immunodeficiency virus is considered a systemic illness rather than an infection limited to the upper gynecologic tract. *Mycoplasma hominis* appears in direct tubal cultures in approximately 15% of women with acute inflammatory disease while the gonococcus is cultured less than 15% of the time in women with upper tract disease.
8. D, Page 694. Approximately 15% of women with cervical infection caused by *Neisseria gonorrhoeae* subsequently develop acute salpingitis. Fifty percent of women with endocervical cultures which are positive for this organism at the time of treatment for acute salpingitis will have the same organisms cultured from the fallopian tubes. If *Neisseria gonorrhoeae* is the only organism cultured from the tubes, a patient should respond rapidly to antimicrobial therapy.
9. **D,** Page 703. By far, the most frequent symptom of acute pelvic inflammatory disease is pain in the lower abdomen. Over 90% of women present with diffuse bilateral lower abdominal pain, usually described as constant and dull. It is usually of short duration; if the pain has been present for longer than three weeks, it is unlikely that the patient has acute pelvic inflammatory disease. Approximately 75% of patients have an associated endocervical infection with vaginal discharge. Abnormal vaginal bleeding is noted in approximately 40% of patients. Nausea and vomiting are late symptoms in the course of this disease.
10. **C,** Page 708. Acute pelvic inflammatory disease associated with the presence of an intrauterine device (IUD) is usually more advanced at the time diagnosis is made. This is due to both physician and patient delays in the diagnosis. The patient misinterprets early signs and symptoms of pelvic inflammation as being related to the presence of the IUD. Patients with an IUD should be hospitalized and given parenteral antibiotics. The IUD should be removed as soon as therapeutic levels of intravenous antibiotics have been obtained.
11. **E,** Page 710. Management of a tubo-ovarian abscess should be medical with operative intervention only undertaken if medical treatment fails. In women who have not completed their families, every effort should be made to conserve reproductive potential. Consideration might be given to unilateral removal of the tubo-ovarian complex or abscess if the disease is unilateral. Similarly, colpotomy would be appropriate if the abscess were pointing posteriorly. In a young patient as described, given the clinical circumstances, a new approach that would retain as much reproductive potential as possible would be percutaneous aspiration under ultrasound guidance. Laparoscopic aspiration has also been used, but does not appear to have any greater benefit than ultrasound-guided aspiration.

12-14. 12, **B;** 13, **C;** 14, **D;** Page 711. Before antibiotic therapy, the mortality associated with acute pelvic inflammatory disease was 1% of all patients. Although the death rate has improved with modern treatment, it has been estimated that there still is one death every other day in the United States directly related to pelvic inflammatory disease. Most of these deaths result from rupture of a tubo-ovarian complex which carries with it a mortality rate of between 5 and 10%. Recurrent pelvic inflammatory disease is experienced by approximately 25% of patients. Younger women become reinfected twice as often as older women. The number of ectopic pregnancies has doubled over the past ten years and is directly related and proportional to the increase in sexually transmitted diseases. Pathologic studies estimate that approximately one half of ectopic pregnancies occur in oviducts damaged by previous salpingitis.

15-17. 15, **D**; 16, **B**; 17, **A**; Pages 708-709. Patients without evidence of upper tract disease who have positive screening cultures only may be treated with outpatient antibiotics such as intramuscular ceftriaxone plus 10 days of tetracycline. Treatment with intramuscular cefoxitin plus oral probenecid without a tetracycline does not take into consideration the likelihood of a co-existent *Chlamydia* infection. Erythromycin has been substituted for tetracycline in patients who are allergic to the latter. This regimen is based on limited data and the question made no mention of a tetracycline allergy. In the presence of an abscess or tubo-ovarian complex, one assumes the presence of anaerobic organisms and facultative gram negative rods. Therefore, a regimen of treatment including parenteral clindamycin and an aminoglycoside is preferable. Cervical cultures are often times negative in the presence of a pyosalpinx. In cases of acute salpingitis without a palpable abscess, doxycycline accompanied by broad spectrum agents such as cefoxitin is adequate since there is no need to penetrate an abscess cavity.

18-19. 18, **C**; 19, **D**; Pages 704-705. Five to 10% of women with acute pelvic inflammatory disease caused by either *Chlamydia trachomatis* or *Neisseria gonorrhoeae* develop symptoms of perihepatic inflammation—the Fitz-Hugh-Curtis syndrome. This condition is often mistakenly diagnosed as either pneumonia or acute cholecystitis. The symptoms include right upper quadrant pain, pleuritic pain, and tenderness in the right upper quadrant when the liver is palpated. It develops from the transperitoneal or vascular dissemination of the organisms causing the acute pelvic inflammatory disease. Only one out of three women with acute pelvic inflammatory disease presents with a temperature greater than 38°C as borne out in laparoscopically confirmed cases of acute pelvic inflammatory disease. Whereas the gonococcus survives no more than a few days in the endosalpinx of untreated patients, chlamydia may remain in the fallopian tubes for months following initial colonization of the upper genital tract.

20-21. 20, **C**; 21, **C**; Page 707. Recommended therapy for the ambulatory management of pelvic inflammatory disease includes ceftriaxone 250 mg intramuscularly plus doxycycline 100 mg orally two times per day for ten to 14 days. Both rectal and pharyngeal gonorrheal infections are difficult to treat. The Centers for Disease Control advises the use of ceftriaxone 250 mg in a single intramuscular dose along with doxycycline 100 mg orally twice per day for seven days for either pharyngeal or rectal gonorrheal infections.

22-23. 22, **C**; 23, **D**; Pages 712-713. Acute pelvic inflammatory disease can be directly related to medical sequelae in 25% of patients. Following acute pelvic inflammatory disease the rate of ectopic pregnancy climbs six to tenfold, and the chance of developing chronic pelvic pain increases fourfold. In the United States each year, 26,000 ectopic pregnancies and 90,000 new cases of chronic abdominal pelvic pain are directly related to pelvic inflammatory disease. Neither entity is directly related to species-specific anaerobic colonization of the endosalpinx. The term chronic pelvic inflammatory disease should not be used since the majority of cases with sequelae of chronic pelvic infection are bacteriologically sterile, including a hydrosalpinx. Chronic pelvic pain may exist with minimal visual anatomic changes and in the absence of positive endosalpingeal cultures.

24-26. 24, **C**; 25, **A**; 26, **B**; Page 714. Both *Actinomyces* and tuberculosis are rare causes of upper genital tract infection. Tuberculosis is, however, a frequent cause of chronic pelvic inflammatory disease and infertility in parts of the world other than the United States. Most cases of *Actinomyces* infection have occurred in women wearing an intrauterine device (IUD). It is, in fact, controversial as to whether or not a woman with an IUD in place who has *Actinomyces* found on pap smear should have the IUD removed or not. Some clinicians will remove the IUD and treat with penicillin. If *Actinomyces* is part of a polymicrobial infection, histologic evidence for this organism is the presence of "sulfur granules." The primary site of infection for tuberculosis is usually the lung. The bacteria is spread hematogenously and the infection becomes located in the fallopian tube. From there, it spreads to the endometrium and to the ovaries. Primary symptoms are infertility and abnormal bleeding.

27. **E** (3 only), Page 696. Acute pelvic inflammatory disease caused by *Neisseria gonorrhoeae* can resist therapy by producing penicillinase. These strains of gonorrhea become resistant to penicillin by acquiring a resistance factor plasmid. By 1989, 6% of gonorrhea strains were resistant to penicillin. Resistance is not caused by suppressing the antibody response as 70% of women with severe pelvic infection develop antibodies against the outer membrane of the gonococcus. By its natural course, the gonococcus produces an intense inflammatory reaction in the tubes, which causes the tubal lumen to swell with necrotic debris and purulent material.
28. **A** (1, 2, 3), Page 692. Non-puerperal endometritis is an obscure chronic infection of the lining of the uterus. Although research about this entity is scant, it probably represents an intermediate state of ascending infection which is spreading through the canaliculi, which connect the lower genital tract to the upper genital tract. There is a correlation between serum antibody levels against both *Mycoplasma hominis* and *Chlamydia trachomatis* with the prevalence of non-puerperal endometritis. Organisms commonly found associated with non-puerperal endometritis include *Chlamydia trachomatis*, *Neisseria gonorrhoeae*, *Streptococcus agalactiae*, the cytomegalovirus, and the herpes simplex virus.
29. **C** (2, 3), Page 700. Oral contraceptive use is associated with a lower incidence of acute pelvic inflammatory disease and a milder form of upper tract genital infection when it does occur. The decrease in incidence of upper tract disease is believed to be secondary to a thicker cervical mucus which is caused by the progestin component of oral contraceptives. The decrease in duration of menstrual flow theoretically creates a shorter interval for bacterial colonization of the upper tract.
30. **A** (1, 2, 3), Page 693. Factors associated with the pathogenesis of acute pelvic inflammatory disease include that it represents an ascending infection from bacteria in the vagina or cervix in 99% of the cases; that it is rare in women without menstrual periods; and that it involves a mixture of aerobic and anaerobic bacteria which appear clinically as a single complex infection. More than 20 species of microorganisms have been cultured from direct aspiration of purulent material from infected fallopian tubes. Usually the inciting organism is one of the more common sexually transmitted diseases such as *Chlamydia* or *N. gonorrhoeae* with subsequent upper tract disease associated often with coliform organisms and anaerobic organisms which become involved in an opportunistic fashion.
31. **A** (1, 2, 3), Page 693. Spontaneous pelvic inflammatory disease is extremely unusual in women who are not sexually active or who are amenorrheic. If pelvic inflammatory disease is found in a postmenopausal women, genital malignancies, diabetes or a concurrent intestinal disease are also usually present.
32. **B** (1, 2), Page 700. Frequent vaginal douching increases the risk of pelvic inflammatory disease 3.6 fold over women who douche less than once a month. In addition, despite criticism of the epidemiologic studies, the risk of acute pelvic inflammation in women who wear an IUD appears to be two to three times greater during the first four months after the IUD is inserted over those women who do not use any contraception. Salpingitis does occur after tubal ligation, but does so infrequently. In one series, salpingitis of the proximal stump of previously ligated fallopian tubes was one in 450.

CHAPTER

23 Preoperative Management

DIRECTIONS for questions 1 - 16: Select the one best answer or completion.

1. The parts of the preoperative evaluation most likely to reveal medically important information are the
   A. medical history and physical exam
   B. medical history and laboratory evaluation
   C. physical examination and laboratory evaluation
   D. history and nursing evaluation
   E. physical and nursing evaluation
2. Of the following, the cephalosporin with the longest half-life is
   A. cephalothin
   B. cephazolin
   C. cefoxitin
   D. cefotaxime
   E. moxalactam
3. The overall mortality rate from a nonradical hysterectomy is
   A. 1 in 10,000
   B. 6 in 10,000
   C. 12 in 10,000
   D. 18 in 10,000
   E. 24 in 10,000
4. An intravenous pyelogram is ordered for a 48-year-old woman scheduled to have a hysterectomy for large uterine myomata. The risk of mortality is
   A. 1 per 1000
   B. 1 per 10,000
   C. 1 per 100,000
   D. 1 per 1,000,000
   E. nonexistent in nonallergic people
5. A 35-year-old woman with heart disease, who has difficulty walking one block without becoming short of breath, is in need of an emergency laparotomy for a suspected ectopic. According to the DRIPPS American Society of Anesthesiology risk classification, she is class
   A. 1
   B. 2
   C. 3
   D. 4
   E. 5
6. Which of the following antihypertensive medications should be discontinued prior to a surgical procedure?
   A. beta blockers
   B. diuretics
   C. clonidine
   D. calcium channel blockers
   E. MAO inhibitors (Monoamine oxidase inhibitors)
7. The usual dose for heparin as prophylaxis against postsurgical thromboembolism is
   A. 5,000 U IM every 12 hours
   B. 10,000 U IM every 12 hours
   C. 5,000 U IM every 8 hours
   D. 10,000 U SQ every 8 hours
   E. 5,000 U SQ every 12 hours
8. A 37-year-old obese female with stage 1B carcinoma of the cervix is scheduled for a radical hysterectomy and node dissection. She has been on birth control pills for contraception, and has a history of varicose veins. Which of the following factors place her at the greatest risk for postoperative thromboembolism?
   A. obesity
   B. carcinoma of the cervix
   C. varicose veins
   D. age
   E. estrogen use
9. A 42-year-old diabetic woman is on 28 units of insulin each day and has fasting blood sugars between 105 and 180 milligrams per deciliter. She also has stress urinary incontinence amenable to surgical repair. The next appropriate step is to
   A. schedule the surgery as usual for next week
   B. refuse to operate
   C. set up appointments to evaluate and control her diabetes better
   D. admit her to the hospital for diabetic control
   E. increase her insulin 5 units a day and schedule the surgery
10. An otherwise healthy 29-year-old woman with a tender pelvic mass is scheduled for exploratory laparotomy. She has no urinary or bowel symptoms. Each of the following lab tests is indicated **EXCEPT**
   A. Pregnancy test
   B. Hematocrit
   C. Coagulation screen

D. urinalysis
E. blood type and screen

11. A 23-year-old healthy female is being evaluated for an exploratory laparotomy for a possible unruptured ectopic pregnancy. She has no cardiac symptoms. A mid-systolic click over the mitral area is heard with no other extraneous sounds or murmurs. Thus,
A. surgery should not be performed
B. surgery should be postponed until cardiac work-up can be done
C. prophylactic antibiotics for subacute bacterial endocarditis should be given before surgery
D. a cardiac surgeon should stand by during the exploratory laparotomy
E. none of the above

12. An asymptomatic patient undergoing hysterectomy for markedly enlarged leiomyomata is most likely to have postoperative complications because of significant abnormalities of the
A. G.I. system
B. central nervous system
C. cardiovascular system
D. musculoskeletal system
E. respiratory system

13. The current recommended protocol for antibiotic prophylaxis for bacterial endocarditis is
A. 250 mg of penicillin VK, orally every 6 hours
B. cephalothin, 1 gram every 8 hours times 3 doses
C. tetracycline, 500 mg, and metronidazole, 1 gram, 1 hour before surgery
D. ceftriaxone, 250 mg IM every 6 hours times 3 doses
E. ampicillin, 2 grams, and gentamicin, 1.5 mg per kilogram, 1 hour before surgery

14. A 35-year-old woman who smokes heavily has severe stress incontinence with coughing. She is scheduled for surgical repair. For the best results in her postoperative recovery, she should be told
A. to stop smoking the day before surgery
B. to stop smoking 5 days before surgery
C. to stop smoking 10 days before surgery
D. to stop smoking 4 weeks before surgery
E. that stopping smoking will not make any difference

15. **Pulmonary** complications following surgery are most likely in a patient who
A. weighs 30% more than her ideal weight
B. is a smoker
C. has asthma
D. has had a myocardial infarction within 3 months
E. has uncontrolled diabetes mellitus

16. Two days after a vaginal hysterectomy a patient, who otherwise is doing very well, complains of continuing pain in her left knee. It hurts when flexed and there is pain on pressure in the lateral joint area. The most likely etiology is
A. septic arthritis from bacteremia
B. an anterior cruciate ligament tear
C. gouty arthritis
D. improper positioning during surgery
E. thrombophlebitis

DIRECTIONS for questions 17 - 26: For each of the questions below, ONE or MORE of the responses is correct. Select the best answer based on the following
A if 1, 2, and 3 are correct
B if only 1 and 2 are correct
C if only 2 and 3 are correct
D if only 1 is correct
E if only 3 is correct

17. The purposes of performing a preoperative evaluation on a patient include
1. evaluation of physical and mental health
2. allaying fears and anxieties
3. avoiding unanticipated findings at the time of surgery

18. A healthy 38-year-old woman is scheduled for a vaginal hysterectomy. True statements regarding prophylactic antibiotics therapy include
1. the antibiotic must be present in the tissue before the surgery
2. there is no need to kill all the bacteria in the operative site
3. prophylactic antibiotics are more cost-effective with vaginal hysterectomy than with abdominal hysterectomy

19. From a patient's point of view, a major operation is one that
1. removes a major body organ
2. involves opening the abdomen
3. is performed on her

20. Mechanical cleansing of the bowel prior to surgery is accomplished by
1. enemas (Fleets)
2. volume lavage (GoLYTELY)
3. laxatives (Dulcolax)

21. A 58-year-old patient who is scheduled for total abdominal hysterectomy and bilateral salpingo-oophorectomy is on several medications. Which of the following should be discontinued several days to several weeks prior to the procedure?
1. cortisol
2. warfarin
3. monoamine oxidase inhibitors (Nardil)

22. A 28-year-old woman has been scheduled for exploratory surgery to evaluate an anterior pelvic cystic mass palpated in clinic. Prior to the procedure a bowel prep and bladder catheterization was performed. On exam under anesthesia (EUA) no mass is palpated. Possible explanations are
    1. an ovarian cyst has ruptured
    2. a loop of bowel was mistaken for an adnexal cyst
    3. the full bladder was confused with the cyst and is now emptied
23. A 63-year-old woman with a long smoking history is scheduled for exploratory laparotomy. Tests of pulmonary function that should be obtained are
    1. arterial pO_2
    2. vital capacity
    3. FEV_1 (Forced Expiratory Volume at 1 second)
24. You wish to decrease the risk of thromboembolic disease in a healthy 60-year-old woman who is on oral replacement estrogen and is scheduled for an anterior vaginal repair. You should
    1. discontinue her replacement estrogen
    2. order prophylactic heparin
    3. ambulate her early
25. A 52-year-old diabetic woman with elevated creatinine (1.9 mg per dl) has a 8 x 9 x 10 cm pelvic mass for which you are planning exploratory surgery. This patient has no known allergies. In order to illicit the location of the ureters in relation to the mass, you should
    1. prescribe oral corticosteroids before performing an intravenous pyelogram to decrease the likelihood of an allergic response
    2. inform this patient that she has an increased risk of acute renal insufficiency following an intravenous pyelogram
    3. order an ultrasound of the kidneys, ureters, and bladder
26. A hypertensive 63-year-old woman with procidentia had a myocardial infarction 2 months ago. She has also had angina for several years. The procidentia is becoming ulcerated and is creating care problems. She wishes a surgical repair. You can correctly inform her that
    1. stable angina without myocardial infarction is not a contraindication to surgery
    2. a myocardial infarction within 3 months of surgery greatly increases the risk of recurrence perioperatively
    3. once the operation is over her immediate postoperative risk is **not** increased

ANSWERS

1. **A,** Page 722. A careful history is the most valuable portion of any evaluation, but its importance tends to be overlooked. Instead, laboratory tests or imaging techniques giving numerical or written data are often overemphasized by both the patient and the physician. An adequate history should include questions regarding the major organ systems, medications, allergies, habits, family and social history. A thoroughly performed history and physical examination form a rational basis upon which further laboratory assessment and other diagnostic aids can be obtained.
2. **E,** Page 733 and Table 23-4 (from Herbst et al). The half-life of a medication determines how long that drug will be active. Of the first and second generation cephalosporins, moxalactam has the longest half-life (120 minutes) and cephazolin has the next longest (100 minutes). Cephazolin reaches high peak serum levels (80 micrograms per ml after a 1 gram dose), but has rather high protein binding (80%, which leaves 20% free in the tissues). Moxalactam is only 50% protein bound.
3. **C,** Page 727. The rate of death from hysterectomy is 12 per 10,000. This is important when you counsel patients about the procedure in order to obtain informed consent. If the patient has other medical or surgical problems, the risk increases. For example, women with cancer have a death rate of 38 per 10,000 from hysterectomy, while those with benign disease have a rate of only 6 per 10,000. When obtaining informed consent, discussion should cover the general risks of anesthesia, hemorrhage, infection, damage to other organs, death, and failure to achieve the desired result in each case. In addition, specific risks inherent to the precise procedure contemplated should be reviewed.
4. **C,** Page 736. Five to eight percent of women will have an allergic reaction to the contrast medium used in performing an intravenous pyelogram. This is often an allergy to the iodine in the contrast. Of these, approximately one to two percent will be life-threatening, with an estimated mortality of 1 in 100,000. An intravenous pyelogram should be done for significant reasons such as large pelvic masses or pelvic malignancies, but should not be obtained routinely.
5. **C,** Page 728. The DRIPPS-American Society of Anesthesiology anesthesia risk classification is shown in Table 23-1.

   This patient with severe, but not incapacitating disease, would be a class 3. Because of

TABLE 23-1. Dripps—American Society of Anesthesiologists Classification

Class	Description
1	A normal healthy patient
2	A patient with mild-to-moderate systemic disease
3	A patient with severe systemic disease with limited activity but not incapitated
4	A patient with incapacitating, constantly life-threatening systemic disease
5	A moribund patient not expected to survive 24 hours with or without operation

Adapted from Anesthesiology 24:111. 1963. Form Jewell ER, Persson AV: Surg Clin North Am 65:4, 1985.

the emergency nature of the surgery, her anesthetic risk is doubled.

6. **E,** Page 728. MAO inhibitors should be stopped 2 or more weeks prior to surgery, as they can augment the effects of sympathetic amines to produce severe increases in blood pressure. Sympathetic amines are given to prevent hypotension during surgical procedures. There is a concomitant release of catecholamines from the stress of surgery. Other antihypertensive medications should be maintained during surgery.
7. **E,** Page 734. The dose of heparin for protection against postoperative thromboembolism is 5,000 units subcutaneously every 12 hours starting just before surgery and continuing until the patient is fully ambulatory. Heparin should never be given IM, nor should other medications be given IM when a patient is on heparin because of the high risk of hematoma formation from needle trauma to the muscle. Intermittent pressure leg wraps are as effective to prevent lower and upper leg thromboses in low risk patients.
8. **B,** Page 732. All of the factors, obesity, carcinoma of the cervix, varicose veins, age, and use of birth control pills increase this patient's risk of thromboembolism. However, the greatest risk in this patient is the malignancy. Adding to her high risk are the problems of longer surgery, immobilization after surgery, and risk for postoperative infection. Ideally, the birth control pills should be stopped for at least 4 weeks prior to the surgery. She is a candidate for minidose heparin or intermittent pressure leg wraps as prophylaxis against thrombosis.
9. **C,** Page 738. No elective surgery should be scheduled for this patient until her diabetes has been evaluated and is under better control. Her cardiovascular, renal, and neurologic systems should be evaluated by appropriate tests. Maintenance of postprandial serum glucose at less than 140 milligrams per ml should be achieved and controlled at that level over several weeks before elective surgery is scheduled. Frequent monitoring of diet, exercise, insulin, and blood sugars is necessary to maintain good control.
10. **C,** Pages 724-725. The hematocrit, urinalysis, blood typing, and screening should be obtained prior to any major surgery. Urinalysis rarely changes management, but is cheap and may reveal asymptomatic bacteriuria or unknown diabetes. Anemia should be ruled out. Knowledge that compatible blood is available in your facility before surgery is important. A coagulation screen is not indicated routinely, but should be obtained if there is a history of bleeding in either the patient's personal or family history. A pregnancy test should be obtained in any sexually active woman who does not have a regular menstrual history. In this case the possibility of an ectopic pregnancy should be considered. A barium enema and intravenous pyelogram are other tests that need not be done routinely unless the history and physical findings so dictate.
11. **E,** Page 739. Mitral prolapse with no evidence of other cardiac disease does not contraindicate surgery, nor does it require prophylactic antibiotics although some authorities suggest that they be given. If used, ampicillin, 2 grams IM or IV, and gentamicin, 1.5 milligrams per kilogram IM, should be given an hour before surgery.
12. **E,** Page 736. Mild chronic obstructive pulmonary disease, COPD, is a frequent finding, especially in obese patients or patients who smoke. Anesthesia, postoperative pain, abdominal distention, and relative immobility combine to produce symptomatic atelectasis in many patients, and this is intensified in those with preexisting pulmonary disease. Such patients need definite preoperative instructions in deep breathing, coughing, movement, and pulmonary ventilatory exercises to prevent severe pulmonary complications.
13. **E,** Page 741. The suggested regimen for bacterial endocarditis prophylaxis is ampicillin, 2 grams, and gentamicin, 1.5 milligrams per kilogram, 1 hour before surgery. If the patient is allergic to penicillin, vancomycin, 1 gram IV, may be substituted for the ampicillin.
14. **D,** Page 737. Smoking causes a six fold increase in the risk of postoperative pulmonary

complications. Smoke deposits particulate matter in the lungs and paralyzes respiratory cilia preventing normal removal of these particles. Coughing is increased. This places additional stress on the surgical repair. Therefore, it is best if the patient can stop smoking for a prolonged time, but even her willingness to stop smoking for a few days will decrease sputum production and be beneficial in the postoperative course.

15. **B,** Page 737. Common conditions can cause a marked increase in surgical risk. Obesity greater than 30% of average doubles the risk of surgery. Current smoking increases the risk of pulmonary complications six-fold even if the amount smoked is small. Asthma increases the risk of pulmonary complications fourfold. Diabetes and cardiovascular disease may cause problems because of increased cortisol, catecholamines, glucagon,and ADH released by the patient during the perioperative period, not to mention the potential stress of changing blood volumes or possible infections that may occur. Diabetics also have poor wound healing and an increased infection rate. A myocardial infarction within three months will increase the mortality rate from recurrent infarction 30% if noncardiac surgery is performed during this time.
16. **D,** Page 732. Pressure on the joint by the stirrup or by a surgeon leaning on the supported leg is most likely. Without heat or fever, a septic process is unlikely. The location and timing are wrong for thrombophlebitis. The position is also wrong for an anterior cruciate ligament tear. This would be an unusual site for gout. Remember to check for pressure points after positioning any patient at the time of surgery.
17. **A** (1, 2, 3), Pages 721-723. The evaluation of the physical and mental health of the patient is incumbent on the health care team prior to any surgical procedure. Allaying the fears and anxieties of the patient is equally important. If all these have been successfully accomplished, the surgeon is unlikely to encounter surprises either during surgery or afterward, and the patient is not likely to have expectations from the results of the surgery that are different from what actually occurs. Patient education is necessary to obtain an informed consent. The patient should know both what can and cannot be expected from a procedure.
18. **C** (2, 3), Page 730. There is no need to kill all the bacteria in the operative site, but it is necessary to reduce their numbers. Prophylactic antibiotics are more cost-effective with vaginal hysterectomy than with abdominal hysterectomy. Antibiotics should be present in the tissue within at least three hours of the tissue injury in order to provide effective prophylaxis. Usually the course is started just prior to surgery. The best antibiotic for prophylaxis has yet to be determined. However, the usual antibiotics are first or second generation cephalosporins or ampicillin or tetracycline. These are given in a single dose or a three-dose regimen. Further prolongation does not add to their prophylactic effectiveness.
19. **A** (1, 2, 3), Page 721. Patients are understandably concerned about any procedure that is performed on them. An adequate informed consent must beobtained. This implies a recognition of the risks and benefits of the procedure. Any surgical procedure entails some risk that is borne by the patient, and she has a right to understand it and regard the surgery as a major event. Even a relatively so called "minor" procedure may have severe consequences, either in its performance or its findings. For example, a D&C may lead to the diagnosis of endometrial cancer; a patient is apt to be quite anxious. Recognition of, and empathy for, the patient's concerns are parts of the art of medicine. Patients should have help in alleviating their fears and anxieties.
20. **A** (1, 2, 3), Page 735. Enemas cause direct mechanical cleansing of the bowel while laxatives work by stimulating bowel peristalsis to evacuate the contents. GoLYTELYis an oral volume lavage which causes diarrhea without significant fluid or electrolyte shifts. Antibiotics do not cause mechanical cleansing, but do cause a marked decrease in the number of bacteria found in the gut, thereby decreasing the probability of infection if the bowel is opened during the procedure.
21. **E** (3 only), Page 728. Monoamine oxidase inhibitors should be stopped. Anticoagulants and corticosteroids may be continued with adjustment in type and dosage prior to and during surgery. If anticoagulation is needed, it is better to use heparin than coumadin. Cortisol should be increased if a patient is on adrenal suppressive doses for other systemic disease. Thyroid replacement should be given until the day of surgery in its usual dose. The insulin requirement must be carefully adjusted relying upon frequent serum glucose determinations during the perioperative period.

22. **A** (1, 2, 3), Page 723. Most pelvic surgeons have discovered that suspected pathology has disappeared, or that previously unsuspected pathology was present when they did an examination under anesthesia (EUA) just prior to surgery. Therefore this examination should be routinely performed on patients who are having surgery for suspected pelvic mass(es).
23. **A** (1, 2, 3), Page 737. In an older patient with a history or physical examination suggestive of respiratory problems, an extensive evaluation of the pulmonary function is warranted. The vital capacity should be greater than 50% of the predicted normal for her age and body size, and the pO_2 should be greater than 65 mm Hg. The FEV_1 should be greater than 75% of the predicted normal volume. A chest X-ray should also be normal. If any of these findings are abnormal, further evaluation and treatment should be done before surgery is undertaken.
24. **E** (3 only), Page 734. This healthy woman is going to have a short procedure that has no high risk factors dictating the use of subcutaneous doses of heparin for prophylaxis. Replacement estrogen is not associated with increased thrombosis. However, a younger woman on birth control pills should stop them several weeks before major elective surgery. The birth control pills decrease the concentration of coagulating inhibitors (antithrombin) and elevate several clotting factors. Early ambulation is one of the best preventive measures.
25. **A** (1, 2, 3), Pages 738-739. A patient with both renal insufficiency and diabetes is at a significantly increased risk of developing acute renal insufficiency after an intravenous pyelogram. The risk of allergic reaction in any patient from an intravenous pyelogram is 5-8%. Most of these reactions are mild. Pretreatment with corticosteroids will decrease this risk. However, this risk is not a major contraindication. Knowledge concerning the ureters' position does not guarantee safety during surgery. The best way to prevent injury during surgery is to identify the ureters during the surgical procedure. An intravenous pyelogram is the best way to demonstrate a double ureter which is an uncommon event; an ultrasound will occasionally reveal a double ureter, particularly if they are distended. In this patient perhaps an ultrasound evaluation would give the needed information without the risks inherent in intravenous pyelogram.
26. **B** (1,2), Page 741. Angina of recent occurrence (within 3 months) is a high risk factor, but stable angina is not. The recent myocardial infarction is of serious concern. Patients with recent myocardial infarctions should wait at least 6 months before any elective surgical procedure is done. The risk of repeat myocardial infarction persists for several days postoperatively and about one-third occur on the third or fourth postoperative day. Therefore, the patient should be followed closely in the immediate postoperative period.

CHAPTER

24 Postoperative Complications

DIRECTIONS for questions 1 - 19: Select the one best answer or completion.

1. The initial management of moderate superficial thrombophlebitis at the site of an intravenous catheter includes all of the following except
   A. heat
   B. elevation
   C. rest
   D. ibuprofen
   E. heparin
2. The most cost-efficient modality in preventing and treating atelectasis is
   A. chest physical therapy
   B. bedside incentive spirometer
   C. intermittent positive pressure breathing
   D. aerosol therapy
   E. bronchoscopy
3. On the fifth postoperative day a patient has a fever of 102°F but does not feel sick. She does not appear as sick as her temperature would imply. She has been on intravenous Keflin for a suspected urinary tract infection for 5 days. The most likely diagnosis is
   A. atelectasis
   B. urinary tract infection
   C. wound infection
   D. drug fever
   E. pneumonia
4. Of the following, the blood component that does not carry with it the risk of hepatitis is
   A. packed cells
   B. frozen plasma
   C. cryoprecipitate
   D. platelet concentrate
   E. Factor VIII concentrate
5. The most likely sign of pulmonary emboli is
   A. tachycardia
   B. tachypnea
   C. rales
   D. cyanosis
   E. accentuation of pulmonic closure
6. A 47-year-old patient, three weeks after a vaginal hysterectomy and posterior repair, complains of ten days of involuntary passage of gas and small amounts of fecal material from the vagina, and a foul-smelling vaginal discharge. On physical examination, a 1/2 cm dark red area of what appears to be granulation tissue is seen in the lower 1/3 of the posterior vagina. At this point you would
   A. place the patient on a low-residue diet
   B. perform a sigmoidoscopy
   C. perform a barium enema
   D. schedule the patient for immediate repair
   E. schedule the patient for a diverting colostomy
7. The currently preferred method for detecting deep vein thrombophlebitis is
   A. physical examination
   B. venography
   C. fibrinogen ^{125}I scan
   D. duplex ultrasonography
   E. impedance plethysmography
8. Of the symptoms listed, the least common in cases of a documented pulmonary embolus is
   A. dyspnea
   B. chest pain
   C. apprehension
   D. hemoptysis
   E. cough
9. A 35-year-old patient has just undergone a difficult abdominal hysterectomy for large leiomyomata. During surgery it was estimated that she lost 2,000 ml of blood. Records indicate that she was given 2,000 ml of D_5 Ringers' Lactate as intravenous fluid. Currently, her BP is 90/60 and her pulse 115. Preoperatively the BP was 135/85 and during surgery it ran around 100-150/70-100. Her urine output has been 25-30 ml per hour. The patients current problem is probably due to the
   A. the sedative effect of anesthesia
   B. inadequate fluid replacement
   C. inadequate hemostasis and continued blood loss
   D. myocardial infarction

E. the physiologic release of aldosterone and antidiuretic hormone

10. The test with the greatest efficacy in detecting pulmonary emboli is
    A. pulmonary angiography
    B. ventilation-perfusion lung scan
    C. arterial blood gas determination
    D. EKG
    E. chest X-ray

11. A 35-year-old patient, 3 hours following a total abdominal hysterectomy for large leiomyomata, develops increasing tachycardia and decreasing blood pressure. The operative blood loss is estimated at 800 ml and the patient received 1500 ml of D_5 Ringer's Lactate during surgery. Initial management should include
    A. having the patient void to estimate urinary output
    B. insertion of a central venous pressure line
    C. infusion of a crystalloid solution, 3 ml for each ml of estimated blood loss
    D. immediate exploratory surgery
    E. sedation to allay anxiety

12. The most reliable early sign of hypovolemia due to postoperative intraperitoneal hemorrhage is
    A. shoulder pain
    B. cold, clammy extremities
    C. muscle rigidity
    D. decreased urine output
    E. skin pallor

13. Factors which contribute to the development of wound infection include all of the following **EXCEPT**
    A. inappropriate prophylactic antibiotics
    B. obesity
    C. use of cautery
    D. presence of a hematoma
    E. increased duration of preoperative hospitalization

14. You are called on the phone by the nurse about an obese 40-year-old patient who underwent a total abdominal hysterectomy 18 hours ago. She reports that the vital signs are a temperature of 38°C, a BP of 80/40, a pulse of 110, and respirations of 30. The nurse raises the possibility of postoperative atelectasis. The findings that support her hypothesis include all of the following **EXCEPT**
    A. temperature
    B. pulse
    C. respiratory rate
    D. blood pressure
    E. number of hours since surgery

15. The typical conditions associated with the development of femoral neuropathy following an abdominal operation are
    A. short stature, thin body habitus, transverse incision, self-retaining retractors
    B. short stature, fat body habitus, transverse incision, large Richardson retractors
    C. short stature, fat body habitus, vertical incision, self-retaining retractors
    D. tall stature, thin body habitus, vertical incision, large Richardson retractors

16. You are planning to perform a total abdominal hysterectomy, bilateral salpingoophorectomy on a 50-year-old markedly obese, hypertensive, insulin-dependent diabetic patient for symptomatic leiomyomata. Methods to reduce the risk of deep vein thrombophlebitis in this patient include the combination of
    A. subcutaneous low dose heparin and intravenous dextran
    B. subcutaneous low dose heparin and intra- and postoperative intermittent leg compression
    C. intra- and postoperative intermittent leg compression and intravenous dextran
    D. intra- and postoperative intermittent leg compression and dihydroergotamine mesylate
    E. dihydroergotamine mesylate and subcutaneous low dose heparin

17. The most accurate statement concerning the postoperative use of urinary tract catheters include
    A. a Foley catheter is associated with earlier spontaneous voiding than a suprapubic catheter
    B. suprapubic catheters are less comfortable than Foley catheters
    C. infections are more common after Foley catheter use than after intermittent straight catherization
    D. prophylactic antibiotics are recommended if urinary catheters are used
    E. symptoms associated with a catheter acquired infection are more pronounced than cystitis unrelated to a catheter

18. Three days after a total abdominal hysterectomy, bilateral salpingoophorectomy, a 35-year-old patient is found to have a hematocrit of 18%. Her preoperative hematocrit was 31%. Blood loss at surgery was estimated at 1200 ml. Vital signs are stable. She has mild, lower abdominal tenderness and a 5 cm tender fluctuant midline mass at the apex of her vaginal cuff.

Given the most likely diagnosis, you would

A. order an intravenous pyelogram
B. order an endovaginal ultrasound scan
C. order a barium enema
D. begin a transfusion of packed red blood cells
E. plan an exploratory laparotomy

19. A 30-year-old patient develops a fever to 39°C 3 weeks after a vaginal hysterectomy. Based on the timing of the onset of fever, the most likely cause of the fever is

A. pneumonia
B. cuff cellulitis
C. an ovarian abscess
D. deep vein thrombophlebitis
E. a urinary tract infection

DIRECTIONS for questions 20 - 21: For each numbered item, select the one heading most closely associated with it. Each lettered heading may be used once, more than once, or not at all.

20-21. Match the complication

(A) cuff cellulitis
(B) granulation tissue
(C) prolapsed fallopian tube
(D) lymphocyst
(E) ovarian abscess

20. consequence of pelvic node dissection
21. fatal intraperitoneal rupture

DIRECTIONS: For each numbered item 22 - 35, indicate whether it is associated with

A only (A)
B only (B)
C both (A) and (B)
D neither (A) nor (B)

22-24. Postoperative pulmonary complications

(A) atelectasis
(B) pneumonia
(C) both
(D) neither

22. predisposing factors include obesity
23. characterized by coarse rales
24. chest x-ray may show patchy infiltrate

25-27. Anticoagulant therapy

(A) heparin therapy
(B) thrombolytic (streptokinase-urokinase) therapy
(C) both
(D) neither

25. indicated for nonmassive pulmonary emboli
26. continued for 10 days
27. may be used long-term instead of warfarin

28-31. Urinary tract fistulas

(A) vesicovaginal fistula
(B) ureterovaginal fistula
(C) both
(D) neither

28. intermittent urine loss more typical than constant loss
29. IV indigo carmine causes staining of a vaginal tampon
30. transurethral methylene blue instillation causes staining of a vaginal tampon
31. surgical repair delayed at least two months

32-35. Postoperative gastrointestinal complications

(A) ileus
(B) bowel obstruction
(C) both
(D) neither

32. progressively severe crampy, abdominal pain
33. nausea and vomiting
34. absent bowel sounds
35. air-fluid levels on abdominal X-ray

DIRECTIONS for questions 36 - 41: For each of the questions below, ONE or MORE of the responses is correct. Select the best answer based on the following

A if 1, 2, and 3 are correct
B if only 1 and 2 are correct
C if only 2 and 3 are correct
D if only 1 is correct
E if only 3 is correct

36. Postoperative factors contributing to the development of atelectasis include

1. incisional pain
2. bulky abdominal dressings
3. anorexia

37. Causes of shock include

1. cardiac failure
2. sepsis
3. an anaphylactic reaction

38. The etiology of wound dehiscence is associated with

1. an incision through an area of previous incision
2. use of catgut suture
3. vertical abdominal incision

39. Sequelae of deep vein thrombophlebitis include

1. muscle atrophy
2. pain on exercise (claudication)
3. skin ulceration

40. Causes of postoperative fever include

1. malignant neoplasms
2. halothane hepatitis
3. thyroid storm

41. There is a positive correlation between the length of an operation and the

1. development of postoperative fever
2. incidence of thrombophlebitis
3. severity of postoperative ileus

ANSWERS

1. **E,** Page 760. Superficial thrombophlebitis is most commonly associated with intravenous catheters. Although the inflammation does not necessarily cease when the catheter is removed, it is recommended that this be done as soon as the diagnosis is made. Mild cases of superficial thrombophlebitis should be treated with rest, local heat, and elevation. A nonsteroidal anti-inflammatory agent such as ibuprofen may be used in cases that are more severe. The use of heparin and antibiotics is reserved for the rare case of proximal progression of inflammation.
2. **B,** Page 755. The basis for preventing atelectasis consists of simple activities that are, unfortunately, more difficult for the postoperative patient. These include taking deep breaths, walking, coughing, turning from side to side, and not lying supine. If necessary, an incentive spirometer can be used effectively to prevent or treat atelectasis. If these techniques do not clear the atelectasis, the patient should then be managed with chest physical therapy, intermittent positive pressure breathing, or aerosol therapy. Bronchoscopy may be required to remove large mucus plugs.
3. **D,** Page 752. Drug fever is often a diagnosis of exclusion. It may be suspected if eosinophilia is discovered or if the patient feels and looks better than the temperature course might suggest. Presumptive evidence of drug fever is a fever that disappears when a drug is discontinued.
4. **D,** Page 757 and Table 24-2. Platelet concentrate is the only component listed that does not expose the recipient to the risk of hepatitis. It can, however, cause Rh isoimmunization if the blood types are not compatible. Packed cells, frozen plasma, cryoprecipitate, and Factor VIII concentrate do carry the risk of hepatitis.
5. **B,** Page 768. In a national study of documented pulmonary emboli conducted by Blinder and Coleman, (Blinder RA, Coleman RE: Evaluation of pulmonary embolism. Radiol Clin North Am 23:392, 1985.) tachypnea was found in over 90% of the patients, rales were discovered in 58%, tachycardia in 44%, cyanosis in 20%, and accentuation of pulmonic closure in 53%. Shock and syncope were associated with massive pulmonary emboli.
6. **A,** Page 778. The patient described presents with the classic symptoms (involuntary loss of gas and stool, a foul-smelling vaginal discharge) of a rectovaginal fistula. It is more commonly associated with obstetric rather than gynecologic complications. Initial therapy includes low-residue diet and Lomotil. One in four will heal spontaneously. If corrective surgery must be performed, a 2-3 month delay is appropriate. Preoperative evaluation should include visualization of the entire vagina and sigmoidoscopy of the rectal mucosa to discover if there is more than one opening. A barium enema or flexible endoscopy is needed if there is suspicion of the coexistence of inflammatory bowel disease. A diverting colostomy should be used for all radiation-induced fistulas; the majority of fistulas associated with inflammatory bowel disease; and some large postoperative fistulas at the apex of the vagina, which lie above the peritoneal reflection.
7. **D,** Page 763. Although signs and symptoms of deep vein thrombophlebitis depend on the severity and extent of the process, 50% of patients are asymptomatic. Physical examination of the legs results in false positive findings' 50% of the time. In cases where signs and symptoms suggest deep vein thrombophlebitis, the diagnosis should be confirmed with an imaging technique. Venography is the most accurate current method for detecting deep vein thrombophlebitis. The diagnostic accuracy is 95% for peripheral disease and 90% for iliofemoral thrombophlebitis. Scanning with fibrinogen ^{125}I is an excellent method to screen women for occult thrombi. The test has been used extensively in research protocols. However, its clinical utility is being replaced by duplex ultrasonography. Duplex ultrasonography is a noninvasive screening test for deep venous thrombosis. Real time ultrasound imaging provides visualization of the larger veins, while simultaneous sensitive Doppler is focused on the suspicious vessel. The technology depends on changes in venous flow for a positive diagnosis. The advantages of this method are that it is not invasive, easy to use, highly accurate, objective, simple, and reproducible. The main disadvantage of duplex diagnosis is that the accuracy is limited when investigating small vessels in the calf. Impedance plethysmography is another noninvasive screening method to detect deep venous thrombosis. This method has at least

a 15% false negative rate and a 20% false positive rate. As with Doppler studies, the accuracy of this method to detect thrombi of small vessels is limited.

8. **D,** Page 768. Signs and symptoms of a pulmonary embolus are nonspecific. Chest pain, dyspnea and apprehension are the most common symptoms. In a national study conducted by Blinder and Coleman (Blinder RA, Coleman RE: Evaluation of pulmonary embolism. Radiol Clin North Am 23:392, 1985.), only 30% of patients with documented pulmonary embolus had hemoptysis. Cough was found in 53%.
9. **B,** Pages 752, 756-757. This patient has significant hypotension and tachycardia. Her reaction is more than an effect of anesthesia although hypotension in the immediate postoperative period may be secondary to the residual effects of anesthesia, over sedation, or hypothermia. The physiologic release of aldosterone and antidiuretic hormone is a response to the stress of surgery. The higher level of aldosterone produces an increase in both sodium and water retention, while increased levels of antidiuretic hormone promote free water retention. Depending on the type and amount of intraoperative and postoperative intravenous fluids, the hematocrit on the first postoperative day may be misleading and reflect fluid changes rather than postoperative hemorrhage. There is nothing in this history to suggest either myocardial infarction or continued blood loss although both are certainly possible. Tachycardia and decreased urine output are two early signs of hypovolemia. Actual measurement of intraoperative blood loss is imprecise even with extensive use of suction equipment. Studies have demonstrated that 15-45% of surgical blood loss is absorbed on the drapes, laparotomy pads, and other areas. Thus,the blood loss was probably underestimated. Even if this was a correct estimate, the three-to-one rule suggests a replacement ratio of 3 ml of crystalloid solution for every 1 ml of blood loss. This patient received 1 ml of crystalloid solution for every 1 ml of blood loss.
10. **B,** Page 768. Pulmonary angiography is the most definitive test in the detection of emboli. This test is not ordered routinely because of the potential morbidity (hypotension and cardiac arrhythmias) and risk of death associated with its use. Most deaths are directly related to pulmonary hypertension and right ventricular dysfunction. Because of potential morbidity (5%) and mortality (0.2%) associated with angiography, the ventilation-perfusion lung scan is the first imaging technique usually used to diagnose a pulmonary embolus. A negative scan essentially rules out an embolus. Findings on blood gas determination, chest X-ray, and EKG are helpful but not diagnostic.
11. **C,** Page 756. The goals in initially managing the patient who has developed presumed postoperative hemorrhage should be replacement of circulating blood volume and establishment of cellular perfusion and oxygenation. Crystalloid solution should be infused rapidly, with 3 ml being used for each 1 ml of blood loss. A Foley catheter is used in all cases to monitor urinary output. One should not rely on the patient's ability to void. The urinary output should be greater than 30 ml per hour. The pulmonary wedge pressure should be between 10 and 15 mm of mercury. Thus, a Swan-Ganz catheter should be inserted if rapid changes in fluid status and blood pressure continue. This is preferable to a central venous pressure line. Studies have demonstrated that in the supine position the volume of intravascular depletion will be severely underestimated by a central venous pressure measurement. Exploratory surgery should be promptly performed if there is evidence of postoperative bleeding, but only after adequate volume replacement has been accomplished. Although sedation may help to relieve the patient's anxiety, it is apt to make the problem worse.
12. **D,** Page 756. Tachycardia and decreased urine output are two early signs of hypovolemia due to hidden internal bleeding. Tachycardia is caused by the body's adrenergic response to hemorrhage, and the decreased urine output is caused by poor perfusion of the kidneys. With further loss of blood the patient becomes agitated, appears weak, and develops skin pallor and cold, clammy extremities. Muscle rigidity of the abdominal wall is a late sign of intraperitoneal hemorrhage and is not due to hypovolemia.
13. **A,** Page 779. There are many factors that contribute to the development of wound infection. Most significant are local factors, which include the presence of foreign bodies, necrotic tissue, hematomas, dead space, use of cautery, and decreased

tissue perfusion. Systemic factors include malnutrition, obesity, diabetes, liver disease, immunosuppression, age, and increased duration of preoperative hospitalization. Prevention is the foundation of any approach to the management of wound infections. Prophylactic antibiotics, especially in high-risk cases, definitely decrease the incidence of wound infection. Inappropriate antibiotics would neither decrease the incidence nor be a source of infection. It might be responsible for the overgrowth of endogenous bacteria.

14. **D,** Page 753-754. The classic triad of atelectasis is fever, tachypnea, and tachycardia, presenting in the first 72 postoperative hours. These findings must, however, be evaluated along with the other clinical factors. In the case described, the marked hypotension of 80/40 in an obese patient should also suggest other causes such as postoperative bleeding, and a pulmonary embolus.
15. **A,** Page 785. Factors that contribute to the development of femoral neuropathy are thinness, long retractor blades, prolonged operative times and systemic diseases such as diabetes mellitus, gout, alcoholism, and malnutrition. However, the classical patient who develops this complication is a short, thin, athletic woman who has a transverse incision in which a self-retaining retractor is used.
16. **B,** Pages 765. Women who are at high risk for deep vein thrombophlebitis should be treated with both low dose heparin and pneumatic compression devices. Embolex (dihydroergotamine mesylate plus heparin) has also been shown to be effective; however, because of its listed contraindications of sepsis, hypertension, and atherosclerotic heart disease (ASHD), it would not be advisable for this patient. Dextran is expensive, and anaphylaxis occurs in approximately 1 in 3500 patients. Dextran's method of action is not understood. It may decrease platelet adhesion, or it may decrease blood viscosity. The cost for external pneumatic compression is nearly the same as the cost for low-dose heparin, and either is about 50% of the cost for prophylactic dextran.
17. **C,** Page 771. Compared with intermittent straight catheterization and suprapubic catheterization, the use of a Foley catheter delays spontaneous voiding, is more uncomfortable, and predisposes the patient to urinary tract infection. Although systemic prophylactic antibiotics do decrease the initial incidence of infection, the effect is short-lived only. The use of prophylactic antibiotics also promotes the emergence of antibiotic-resistant bacteria. As a result, antibiotics are not recommended for catheterized patients unless they are immunocompromised. In fact, catheter-related infections are not treated with antibiotics unless the patient is febrile. The signs and symptoms associated with a catheter acquired lower tract urinary infection are **less** pronounced and less specific than cystitis that develops unrelated to catheter use.
18. **D,** Pages 752, 756. Most young, healthy women without a complicating medical illness will tolerate hematocrits of about 20% to 22% without needing a transfusion. The patient described has probably developed a postoperative cuff hematoma. The hematoma is usually the result of slow, venous oozing and is self-limited. Even if the hematoma is not infected, a low-grade fever is common because of inflammation surrounding the hematoma. The diagnosis of a retroperitoneal hematoma is usually possible by physical exam. Imaging studies are rarely necessary in this situation. Both a barium enema and an ultrasound would not contribute to either the diagnosis or management. One might consider ordering an intravenous pyelogram if the position of the hematoma suggests that a ureter might be obstructed. Hematomas less than 5 cm in diameter may be treated conservatively. Surgical management is usually not recommended unless there is evidence of persistent blood loss or infection. If needed, surgery is usually by way of the extraperitoneal route (transvaginally).
19. **C,** Pages 751, 785 and Table 24-1 (from Herbst). Only 20% of postoperative fevers are directly related to infection. It is not unusual for a hysterectomy patient to have a mild temperature elevation during the first 72 postoperative hours with no identifiable infection. Atelectasis is the cause of over 90% of fevers presenting in the first 48 hours. Pneumonia, cuff cellulitis, phlebitis, and urinary tract infections tend to cause fever after the first 48 hours. Chronologically, most ovarian abscesses appear later in the postoperative course than other retroperitoneal abscesses. Ovarian abscesses usually present 2 to 3 weeks postoperatively, but cases have been re-

ported as late as 3 to 4 months post surgery.

20-21. 20, **D**; 21, **E**; Pages 784-785. A lymphocyst is a local collection of lymphatic fluid found most frequently following pelvic node dissections. Conditions that predispose the patient to formation of a lymphocyst are previous radiation and anticoagulation. Small cysts regress spontaneously while larger ones require intermittent aspiration or insertion of an indwelling catheter. Traditional surgical management involves removing a large segment of the wall of the lymphocyst and placing a tongue of omentum in the cavity. An ovarian abscess is a potentially fatal complication of a hysterectomy. If the diagnosis is not made, intraperitoneal rupture may ensue. Ovarian abscesses arise from bacterial colonization of the ovarian cortex. This may occur either through disruption of the ovarian capsule by the presence of a corpus luteum or via an operative disruption such as cystectomy. Initial therapy is parenteral broad-spectrum antibiotics, although most patients require surgical removal of the affected adnexa.

22-24. 22, **C**; 23, **B**; 24, **C**; Pages 754-755. It is critical to be able to differentiate postoperative atelectasis from pneumonia. The two are commonly associated, and the treatments are the same except for the addition of parenteral antibiotics for the patient with pneumonia. Patients who are obese are at risk for both conditions. Atelectasis is commonly associated with tubular breathing, decreased breath sounds, and moist inspiratory rales especially over the base of the lungs. With both conditions there is fever and tachycardia. An important difference is that pneumonia also typically presents with productive, purulent sputum. The classic physical finding of pneumonia is coarse rales over the infected area. The patient usually has a higher temperature and more systemic toxicity than does a woman with atelectasis. A patchy infiltrate seen on a chest X-ray is compatible with either condition.

25-27. 25, **A**; 26, **A**; 27; **D**; Pages 768, 770. The management of most cases of pulmonary emboli is with full-dose intravenous heparin. One method of administration is to give an initial loading dose of 5000 IU, followed by an hourly infusion of 1000-1500 IU. Recently some women have been treated with thrombolytic (streptokinase-urokinase) therapy or recombinant human tissue-type plasminogen activator. However, this therapy is more expensive and more dangerous than heparin. Thrombolytic therapy is reserved for cases of massive embolus only. A thrombolytic agent is used only in the first 24 hours of therapy. Heparin is continued for 7-10 days. All patients with pulmonary emboli should have warfarin therapy for 3-6 months. Neither heparin nor thrombolytic therapy is indicated for long-term therapy.

28-31. 28, **B**; 29, **C**; 30, **A**; 31, **C**; Pages 773-774. The classic symptom of a vesicovaginal fistula is painless and almost continuous loss of urine. If this loss is intermittent and related to position, a ureterovaginal fistula should be suspected. Intravenous injection of 1-2 ml of indigo carmine will result in the blue staining of a vaginal tampon both in cases of a ureterovaginal fistula and a vesicovaginal fistula. If a vesicovaginal fistula is suspected, methylene blue is instilled into the bladder. A tampon is placed in the vagina. The tampon will be discolored blue if a vesicovaginal fistula exists, but not in the presence of a ureterovaginal fistula. The repair of both vesicovaginal and ureterovaginal fistulas should be delayed 2 - 6 months after the initial operation to allow possible spontaneous healing and if that does not occur to maximize the integrity and health of the surgical area after it has completely healed.

32-35. 32, **B**; 33, **C**; 34, **A**; 35, **C**; Page 773. Adynamic ileus probably is a result of poorly-coordinated motor activity of the small intestine. It is not easily differentiated from small bowel obstruction. The patient with an ileus is uncomfortable, but it is the patient with an obstruction that suffers from progressively severe, crampy abdominal pain. Patients with either an ileus or a small bowel obstruction have nausea and vomiting. Bowel sounds are hypoactive or absent with an ileus, whereas in obstruction peristaltic rushes and high-pitched tinkles are common. Air-fluid levels on abdominal X-ray may occur in either ileus or obstruction. In the former, they occur infrequently and if so, at the same levels. In the latter, air-fluid levels are common and demonstrate a step-ladder appearance—multiple air-fluid levels throughout the small intestine with an absence of gas in the colon and rectum.

36. **B** (1, 2), Page 753. Atelectasis develops in 10% of women who undergo pelvic surgery. It is the most common cause of post-

operative fever. Pain, the supine position, and abdominal distension deter the patient from taking deep inspirations. Deep breaths normally expand all areas of the lung, thus preventing atelectasis. Similarly, immobility and binding around the abdomen and chest cause the patient to breathe at lower lung volumes, thus predisposing to atelectasis. Obesity, smoking, age greater than 60 years, prolonged operative time, and coexisting medical problems such as cardiac disease and pulmonary infection all predispose patients to postoperative atelectasis. Anorexia per se is not known to be a direct cause of atelectasis.

37. **A** (1, 2, 3), Page 755. Shock is a condition in which circulatory insufficiency prevents adequate vascular perfusion of vital organs. The etiology of shock includes cardiac failure, sepsis, an anaphylactic reaction, and hemorrhage. Shock due to postoperative hemorrhage is usually seen within the first few hours of surgery. These cases are due primarily to inadequate hemostasis. In general, it takes a reduction of approximately 20% of the blood volume to produce shock in a woman of reproductive age.

38. **B** (1, 2), Page 780. Wound dehiscence usually implies disruption of the abdominal wound through the fascia but not through the peritoneum. Wound infection is present in half of women with a wound-disruption. As stronger synthetic absorbable sutures have replaced catgut, the incidence of dehiscence has decreased. There appears to be little effect on the incidence of dehiscence whether a vertical or horizontal incision had been made. Important mechanical factors predisposing to disruption are conditions that increase the tension on the incision line, such as abdominal distension and chronic lung disease. Other factors include obesity, the patient's age, malignant disease, prior radiation, and whether the incision was made through a previous incision. A mass closure utilizing through-and-through monofilament nylon is a commonly used abdominal closure for incisions that have broken down. An alternative closure is the Smead-Jones closure.

39. **C** (2, 3), Page 761. Deep vein thrombophlebitis is the process of venous thrombosis formation occurring in any deep vein due to blood coagulation and fibrin formation in the presence of venous stasis. In addition to pulmonary embolus, major sequelae of deep vein thrombophlebitis include chronic venous insufficiency resulting in damage to the valves of deep veins. This produces shunting of blood to superficial veins, skin ulceration, pain on exercise, and chronic edema. Deep vein thrombophlebitis has not been shown to be associated with muscle atrophy.

40. **A** (1, 2, 3), Page 752. Rare causes of postoperative fever include malignant neoplasms, pelvic thrombophlebitis, halothane hepatitis, thyroid storm, and malignant hyperthermia.

41. **B** (1, 2), Pages 751, 762, 774. Two intraoperative factors which dramatically increase the risk of postoperative fever are an operative time greater than two hours and the necessity for intraoperative transfusion. The length of the surgical procedure has an important influence on the development of thrombophlebitis. If the surgery is one to two hours approximately 15% of women develop the disease while if the surgery is longer than three hours, the risk is greater than 45%. On the other hand, the duration of the surgical procedure does not directly influence the severity of the ileus.

PART FOUR GYNECOLOGIC ONCOLOGY

Principles of Radiation Therapy and Chemotherapy in Gynecologic Cancer

DIRECTIONS for questions 1 - 10: Select the one best answer or completion.

1. The growth phase in which a cell is most sensitive to radiation damage is
   A. mitosis
   B. phase of protein synthesis
   C. phase of DNA duplication
   D. phase of RNA synthesis
   E. Resting phase
2. Three months ago, a 60-year-old woman completed a nine course treatment with Cytoxan, *cis*-platinum and Adriamycin for Stage III serous cystadenocarcinoma of the ovary. At a "second look" operation 1 year after the onset of treatment, there is no microscopic or macroscopic evidence of the disease. This response is best called a
   A. cure
   B. complete response
   C. objective response
   D. stabilization
   E. partial remission
3. Energy (such as that used to treat cancers) transmitted from a source to a target area
   A. converges as it approaches the target tissue
   B. diverges as it approaches target tissue
   C. travels parallel as it approaches target tissue, that is, neither converges nor diverges
   D. converges or diverges depending upon the energy source
   E. is transmitted as a wave form
4. Each of the following improves the effectiveness of a chemotherapeutic agent **EXCEPT** a
   A. small original tumor burden
   B. more frequent administration of the chemotherapeutic agent
   C. higher dose of chemotherapeutic agent
   D. smaller percentage of cells in G_0 (resting) phase
   E. decreased mitotic activity of tumor cells
5. The major advantage of high energy particulate radiation, such as accelerated neutrons, is that it
   A. can kill the cell directly
   B. has low linear energy transfer (LET)
   C. is most effective in well-oxygenated tissue
   D. can be administered from both external and internal sources
   E. does not decrease proportional to the distance traveled
6. When macrophages are activated and then enter into the immune response becoming cytotoxic to tumor cells, they produce a number of soluble immune mediators known as
   A. T-cells
   B. Tumor Anti-growth Factor
   C. cellular immunity
   D. cytokines
   E. beta-activators
7. As a cytokine, tumor necrosis factor (TNF) provides a theoretical advantage over standard chemotherapeutic agents due to
   A. the resistance of normal cells compared to malignant cells
   B. a lower incidence of systemic side effects
   C. its use as a replacement for potentially toxic interferons
   D. the stimulation of a higher proportion of tumor cells in the replicating phase
8. An example of an agent used to diminish the toxicity of chemotherapeutic agents is
   A. interferon
   B. interleukin
   C. T-cell activator

D. erythropoietin
E. Tumor Necrosis Factor

9. Ifosfamide has marked anti-tumor effects, but also is highly toxic to the
A. liver
B. GI tract
C. central nervous system
D. heart
E. genitourinary system

10. Each of the following potentiates the effects of radiation therapy on tumor growth **EXCEPT**
A. hyperthermia
B. hyperfractionation
C. *cis*-platinum
D. decreasing the size of the field

DIRECTIONS for questions 11 - 21: For each numbered item, select the one heading most closely associated with it. Each lettered heading may be used once, more than once, or not at all.

11-14. Methods of augmenting the immune response to tumor cells
(A) interferon
(B) BCG (bacillus Calmette-Guerin)
(C) dinitrochlorobenzene (DCNB)
(D) active specific immunotherapy
(E) passive immunity

11. nonspecific immunotherapy used to activate both cell mediated and humoral antibody
12. radiated tumor cells used to produce a vaccine
13. prevents cancer cell division by augmenting natural killer cells
14. extracts of "transfer factor" confers immunologic memory to patient's lymphocytes

15-18. Chemotherapeutic agents characteristics
(A) doxorubicin (Adriamycin)
(B) cyclophosphamide (Cytoxan)
(C) methotrexate
(D) vincristine
(E) *cis*-platinum

15. positively charged alkyl groups react with negatively charged portion of DNA
16. plant alkaloid that attacks the cell spindle during mitosis
17. enzymatic inhibitor in the synthesis of purine nucleotides
18. may cause cardiomyopathy

19-21. Match a phase of the cell cycle with each statement (see Fig. 25-1)
(A) Mitosis (M)
(B) Resting cell (G_o)
(C) Protein synthesis (G_2)
(D) DNA synthesis (S)

19. resistant to cytotoxic drugs

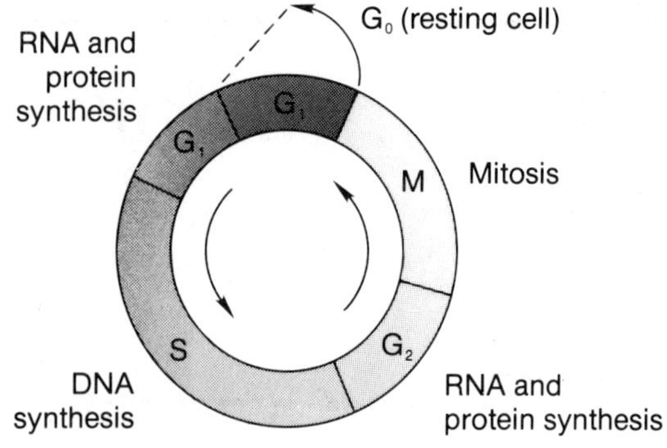

FIGURE 25-1.
Phases of the cell.
(From Droegemueller W, Herbst AL, Mishell DR, Stenchever MA: Comprehensive gynecology. St. Louis, The C.V Mosby Co., 1987.)

20. most affected by antimetabolites (methotrexate)
21. most affected by vinca alkaloids (vincristine)

DIRECTIONS: For each numbered item 22 - 27, indicate whether it is associated with
A only (A)
B only (B)
C both (A) and (B)
D neither (A) nor (B)

22-24. Use the isodose curves in Figure 25-2 to answer the following questions
(A) isodose curve for a 6 MV beatron
(B) Isodose curve for a 22 MV beatron
(C) both
(D) neither

22. more likely to treat deep pelvic nodes in a woman 5 feet 2 inches tall, weighing 240 lbs
23. high doses more likely to cause skin damage
24. used to treat 3 cm central recurrence of epidermoid carcinoma of cervix

25-27. Characteristics of radiation therapy
(A) brachytherapy
(B) teletherapy
(C) both
(D) neither

25. dose delivered to the cancer by inverse square law
26. uses radioisotopes with a defined half-life
27. uses concept of Source Axis Distance (SAD)

DIRECTIONS for questions 28 - 32: For each of the questions below, ONE or MORE of the re-

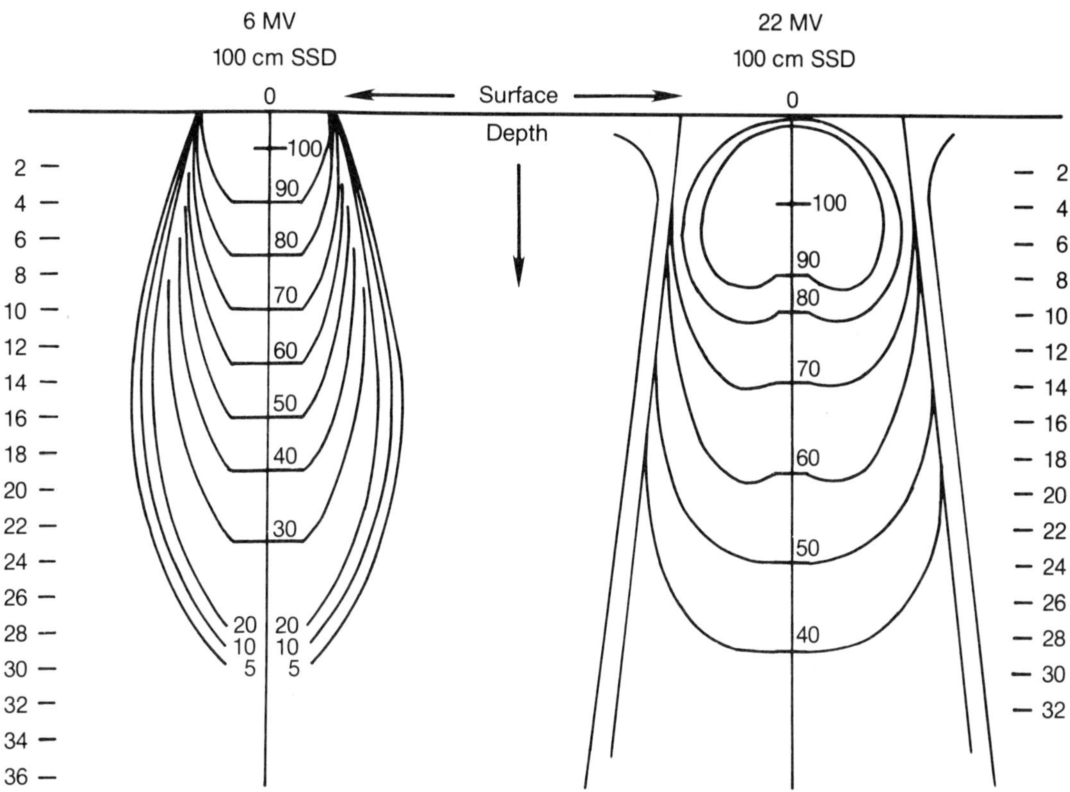

FIGURE 25-2.
Comparison of isodose curves and depth-dose distribution for 6 MV and 22 MV beatrons.
(Redrawn from DiSaia PJ, and Creasman WT: Clinical gynecologic oncology, 2nd ed. St. Louis, The C.V. Mosby Co., 1984.)

sponses is correct. Select the best answer based on the following

A if 1, 2, and 3 are correct
B if only 1 and 2 are correct
C if only 2 and 3 are correct
D if only 1 is correct
E if only 3 is correct

28. Tumor growth stimulates the host immune system and specifically has been shown to activate
    1. T-lymphocytes
    2. B-lymphocytes
    3. macrophages
29. The *growth fraction* (GF) for a given tumor
    1. determines the doubling time
    2. is faster in smaller tumors
    3. is faster after chemotherapy
30. Ionizing radiation causes cell death by
    1. directly altering the localized host immune response
    2. producing free hydroxyl radicals
    3. leading to the formation of peroxide in tissues
31. Characteristics of electromagnetic ionizing radiation used for tumor therapy include that it
    1. has no mass
    2. has no electrical charge
    3. is produced in discrete quanta
32. The resistance of large tumors to chemotherapy is due to their
    1. increased DNA synthesis
    2. heterogenous cell population
    3. lower growth fraction

ANSWERS

1. **A,** Page 804, Figure 25-2. During mitosis the cell is most sensitive to radiation. Thus, rapidly dividing cells are the most radiosensitive. Dividing radiation into a number of smaller doses (fractionation) allows for effective treatment of the tumor without increasing the complications of irradiation to the normal surrounding tissues which have a rapid turnover such as the bone marrow and the intestine.

2. **B,** Page 812. In assessing the effect of chemotherapeutic agents, a number of definitions are used to describe the response of the tumor being treated. A cure implies a permanent absence of disease for a period of 5 years or longer. A complete remission is total disappearance of the tumor for at least 1 month. An objective response is a 50% or greater reduction in the size of the tumor for at least 1 month. Stabilization is used to indicate that the disease has not changed in size. The phrase partial remission is no longer used in lieu of the term objective response.
3. **B,** Page 803. Regardless of the source of electromagnetic or photon radiation, the transmitted energy from the source diverges as the distance it travels from the source increases. This divergence causes a decrease in energy, and the relationship is described by the inverse square law. For example, the dose of radiation 2 cm from a point source is only one fourth the value of the dose at 1 cm.
4. **E,** Page 812, Figures 25-8 and 25-9. One of the reasons chemotherapy appears to affect cancer tissue more than normal tissue is that malignant tumor cells have a higher growth fraction in comparison to normal cells. The ability of a chemotherapeutic agent to destroy a greater number of cancer cells more effectively is enhanced if the agent can be given more frequently or in larger doses per unit time. However, dose and frequency are limited by tolerance of normal tissue. A higher percentage of cells in the G_0 or resting phase will limit chemotherapeutic effectiveness. Increased, not decreased, mitotic activity of tumor cells will render them more susceptible to successful chemotherapy.
5. **A,** Page 803. With particulate radiation using heavy particles such as neutrons, the ionization is known as high linear energy transfer. That is, the rate of energy loss as it traverses a unit length of tissue is greater than with photon irradiation. This form of radiation produces high energy recoil protons which kill the cell directly upon impact and are independent of oxygenation. Currently, systems are being developed that use neutron generators as a form of external beam therapy. This type of energy cannot be generated by internal sources. Even though this is a high energy source, the principle of the inverse square law still applies with this type of radiation.
6. **D,** Page 816. T-lymphocytes are cells that confer cell mediated immunity, while Beta lymphocytes are cells associated with antibody production and humoral immunity. Macrophages also act directly on tumor cells and when activated they can enter into the immune response and become cytotoxic to tumor cells. This activation process produces a number of soluble immune mediators known as cytokines or lymphokines. With the development of recombinant DNA technology, these substances can be synthesized and a number of them are being evaluated for their potential in tumor therapy.
7. **A,** Page 817. Tumor necrosis factor (TNF) is a cytokine which induces necrosis of tumor cells in vitro and appears to act synergistically with interferons. TNF appears to be selective for tumor cells and this provides a theoretical advantage over classical chemotherapeutic agents insofar as approximately 100-10,000 times the concentration of TNF is needed to affect normal cells in comparison to malignant cells in vitro. However, its administration has also been accompanied by severe toxicity including shock-like symptoms, fever and hypotension.
8. **D,** Page 816. Stimulators of the hematopoietic system are being used to diminish the toxicity of chemotherapeutic agents. This includes the use of erythropoietin (EPO) to overcome the chronic anemia that often occurs with chemotherapy. T-cells are cells that confer cell mediated immunity and interferon and interleukin are forms of cytokines which release humoral factors which enhance tumor cell damage.
9. **E,** page 813. Ifosfamide is highly toxic to the bladder and uroepithelium with reports of severe hemorrhagic cystitis. This drug is a relative of cyclophosphamide which has long been known to be associated with hemorrhagic cystitis. A urinary metabolite, acrolein, causes the damage. This can be prevented by the prophylactic administration of Mexna which binds to acrolein and prevents urotoxicity.
10. **D,** Pages 807-808, Figure 25-6. Larger fields of radiation contain more scattered radiation, which leads to a greater dose at a given depth. Recently, there has been experimental work evaluating hyperfractionation which involves smaller multiple doses given more frequently two or three times per day rather than the traditional once a day exposure. Of late a number of

pharmacologic agents such as hydroxyurea and metronidazole have been investigated for their abilities to potentiate the sensitivity to radiation. These are not yet used routinely although certain chemotherapeutic agents such as *cis*-platinum are being tested with radiation treatment to improve response rates. Hyperthermia is also being explored to potentiate the therapeutic effectiveness of radiation.

11-14. 11, **B**; 12, **D**; 13, **A**; 14, **E**. Pages 816-818. A number of approaches have been taken to augment the immune response to human tumors. Most of these remain investigational, but the clinician should be aware that it is this field of tumor biology which shows the most promise for successful cancer treatment. Interferon has been found to prevent cancer cell division by augmenting the action of natural killer cells. By preventing the replication of cancer cells, the treatment should gradually lead to tumor regression, especially if used as an adjunctive treatment. Active specific immunotherapy involves the use of tumor cells and their antigens to reproduce specific tumor immunity. These cells are usually modified by chemotherapy or radiation and grown in media to produce a vaccine. Passive immunity may be conferred through transferring specific immunityusing extracts of lymphocytes sensitized to tumor antigens. These "transfer factors" may lead to a type of adaptive immunotherapy by transfer or "immunologic memory" to the patient's own lymphocytes. Nonspecific immunotherapy involves the use of adjuvant agents, usually of microbiologic origin. These are used to simulate cell-mediated and humoral immunity as well as to activate macrophages. The most commonly cited example of this is the use of BCG (bacillus Calmette-Guerin). This agent produces a marked proliferation of lymphocytes, but its use as effective therapy in gynecologic malignancies has not yet been identified.

15-18. 15, **B**; 16, **D**; 17, **C**; 18, **A**. Pages 814-815. This series of questions addresses characteristics of commonly used cytotoxic agents in gynecologic malignancy. They represent different classes of drugs with generally different mechanisms of action. Although a single drug characteristic out of context may not seem important, a general knowledge of the classes of cytotoxic agents is important in determining rational therapy for gynecologic malignancy. The alkylating agents, of which chlorambucil and cyclophosphamide are examples, interfere directly with DNA replication and function. Cross-linking of DNA also occurs. These agents may be administered either intravenously or orally, and they are particularly toxic to bone marrow. Vinblastine and vincristine are plant alkaloids. They attack the cell during mitosis and cause toxic destruction of the mitotic spindle. However, this can result in synchronization of the cell cycle for those cells surviving therapy, and therefore these agents are often given as part of a combination treatment to cause a greater sensitivity to other agents. There is little bone marrow suppression with this group of drugs, but they can be severely neurotoxic. Methotrexate has been used longer than any of the above chemotherapeutic agents and is an enzyme inhibitor. Metabolic transfer of one carbon unit is prevented, thereby inhibiting the synthesis of thymidylic acid as well as different purine nucleotides. Side effects of this treatment may be overcome by administration of folinic acid (citrovorum factor) which replenishes the tetrahydrofolate. The antitumor antibiotics most commonly used in gynecologic malignancy are doxorubicin (Adriamycin) and Actinomycin D. Myelosuppression occurs regularly with both of these agents; they are often used as part of multiple agent protocols. Adriamycin in particular can cause cardiomyopathy, so cardiac function should be monitored by ultrasound evaluation or radionuclide scans. Other chemotherapeutic agents include the heavy metal derivatives, such as *cis*-platinum, and hormones such as progesterone derivatives.

19-21. 19, **B**; 20, **D**; 21, **A**. Pages 810-831 including Figure 25-1. This series of questions refers to the use of chemotherapy relative to its mechanism of action in the cell replication cycle. Knowledge of cell kinetics is important in understanding the rational use of various chemotherapeutic agents. Knowledge of cell type, size of tumor, and previous treatment are all important in determining chemotherapeutic agents. A problem with larger tumors is that they contain a higher proportion of cells in the resting or G_0 phase of the cell cycle. These cells are resistant to cytotoxic drugs and may become a source of future growth when they leave the G_0 phase to enter the cell replication cycle. Thus smaller tumors, those with a higher growth fraction, and those with a shorter doubling time are the most sensitive to cytotoxic agents.

22-24. 22, **B**; 23, **A**; 24, **C.** Pages 805-807, Figure 25-5. An isodose curve is a line that connects points in the tissue that receive equivalent doses or irradiation. Figure 25-2 contrasts the isodose curves for 6 MV and 22 MV machines. With the 6 MV machine the maximum dose is near the surface, with more rapid fall off in the deeper tissues, while with the 22 MV machine the maximum dose is well beneath the surface. Thus, at any given depth, a higher dose of radiation can be achieved with the 22 MV, sparing the effects of radiation on the skin. These high-energy machines are particularly useful for treating deep tumors and for treating obese patients. Either of these sources could be used for treating a central recurrence. This choice is dependent on factors such as the size of the patient and the size of the field being treated. Larger fields contain more scattered radiation, which leads to greater dose at a given depth. Thus, the radiation dose delivered to a point within the tumor is affected by the energy source, the depth of the tumor beneath the surface,and the size of the field undergoing irradiation.

25-27. 25, **C**; 26, **A**; 27, **B.** Pages 804-805. In general, two techniques are used in radiation treatment: brachytherapy (internal) and teletherapy (external). Both of these radiation techniques rely on the principle of the inverse square law to determine treatment doses. Since brachytherapy refers to the radiation source being placed within or adjacent to the target tissue, these systems use radioisotopes with defined half-lives. Examples include interstitial needles, afterloading systems placed in the vagina and cervix, and the intraperitoneal instillation of radioactive liquids. Since teletherapy refers to the placement of the radioactive source at a distance from the patient, consideration of the source-to-tumor distance is important in determining overall dosage and avoiding unnecessary damage to normal tissues. With the use of different angles and ports of treatment, the concept of source axis distance (SAD) has been introduced; it denotes the distance from the radiation source to the central axis of the machine rotation. Treatment ports are arranged around this axis to optimize tumor dose and minimize damage to normal tissues.

28. **A** (1, 2, 3). Page 816. It has been shown that many experimental animal tumors are able to elicit an immune response. However, specific antigens unique to a given gynecologic tumor have not been identified as yet. It appears that tumor growth stimulates the major cells of the immune system, including the T-lymphocyte, B-lymphocyte, and macrophages. T-lymphocytes confer cell-mediated immunity, B-lymphocytes are responsible for antibody production and humoral immunity, and macrophages provide direct action against tumor cells.

29. **A** (1, 2, 3). Pages 810-812. The proportion of cells actually involved in the proliferation of a tumor is known as the *growth fraction* (GF). It is this proportion that determines the doubling time of a given tumor. In general, smaller tumors and metastatic lesions grow more rapidly than larger tumors. An increase in the growth rate also appears to be operative following the administration of cytotoxic agents. These agents reduce the mass of the tumor, but cellreplication then appears to proceed at a faster rate.

30. **C** (2, 3). Page 804. Ionizing radiation causes cell death by dislodging orbital electrons from the atoms of the medium or tissue through which they pass. This produces secondary electrons and free hydroxyl radicals, which damage the cell and the normal DNA replication process. In addition, free hydroxyl radicals may react with molecular oxygen to form peroxide in the tissues. This adds to the lethal effect of radiation. Although there may be a change in the host immune response based on extensive radiation therapy, there is no known change in local immune response of the target tissues. Further, whereas oxygen is important for the tissue effects of photon irradiation, the oxygen tension of target tissue is not increased. In fact, since cancerous tissue frequently has decreased oxygenation, the effects of photon irradiation in these relatively hypoxic areas are often diminished.

31. **A**, (1, 2, 3). Page 803. One form of ionizing radiation is electromagnetic, which refers to x-rays or gamma rays. These sources of energy have no mass and no electrical charge. They are produced in discrete quanta or photons, and their energy is proportional to their frequency;

that is, higher energies are transmitted at a higher frequency of electromagnetic radiation. Since the frequency of a photon is inversely proportional to the wavelength, electromagnetic radiation with shorter wavelengths has a higher frequency and thus higher energy. Examples of these types of energy sources used to treat tumors include both external beam therapy and radiation caused by decay of radioactive isotopes. Examples of the use of isotopes are internal systems, such as cesium applicators.

32. **C** (2, 3). Page 810. Although some tumors may have their origins in a single (stem) cell, clinically evident malignancies are composed of a heterogenous population of cells with different cell cycle lengths and varying growth fractions. Larger tumors are more likely to contain cells resistant to a single cytotoxic agent. An additional problem with larger tumors is their lower growth fraction, meaning a larger proportion of cells in their resting or G_0 phase of the cell cycle. These cells are more resistant to cytotoxic drugs. As a larger proportion of these cells are in the resting phase, during which there is decreased DNA and RNA synthesis, they do not respond to chemotherapy.

CHAPTER 26

Intraepithelial Neoplasia of the Cervix

DIRECTIONS for questions 1 - 15: Select the one best answer or completion.

1. A 35-year-old patient has had two pap smears that were consistent with severe dysplasia and a colposcopically-directed biopsy showing CIN (Cervical Intraepithelial Neoplasia) I. The ECC (endocervical curettage) is negative. The management of choice is
   A. repeat the pap smear every 3 months
   B. conization
   C. repeat the colposcopy and directed biopsy
   D. cryocautery
   E. laser ablation
2. The difference between leukoplakia and acetowhite epithelium is
   A. acetowhite epithelium is white and leukoplakia is not
   B. leukoplakia appears white without acetic acid
   C. leukoplakia is a clinical description and acetowhite epithelium is a histological description
   D. leukoplakia is precancerous and acetowhite epithelium is not
   E. acetowhite epithelium is a clinical diagnosis and leukoplakia is a histologic diagnosis
3. The risk of developing cervical cancer for a woman marrying a man whose first wife had cervical cancer compared to a woman who is marrying a man whose first wife did **not** have carcinoma of the cervix is
   A. 0.3
   B. 0.5
   C. 1.0
   D. 2.0
   E. 3.0
4. What is the purpose of a routinely processed endocervical curettage? To
   A. identify which part of the cervical canal has cancer
   B. rule out an endocervical human papilloma virus infection
   C. ascertain with high reliability whether a neoplasm exists in the endocervical canal
   D. document chlamydial cervicitis
   E. detect accurately tubal or ovarian carcinoma
5. A 32-year-old woman has a colposcopically-directed excisional biopsy revealing a single focus of microinvasive carcinoma with clear margins. An ECC is negative. She should have
   A. no further treatment
   B. a cervical conization
   C. a vaginal hysterectomy
   D. a radical hysterectomy
   E. cryocautery
6. In performing cryotherapy on a patient with a negative ECC and an adequate colposcopy after multiple directed cervical biopsies have diagnosed CIN II, the best technique is a
   A. single 1-minute freeze
   B. single 3-minute freeze
   C. single 5-minute freeze
   D. double 1-minute freeze
   E. double 3-minute freeze
7. A 24-year-old gravida 1 woman has had cervical conization for CIN III. On pathologic review, the proximal margins of the cone were involved with CIN III. The patient wants to retain her child-bearing capability. The best immediate course of action is
   A. electrocautery
   B. cryocautery
   C. laser treatment
   D. repeat the cervical conization
   E. follow with pap smears and colposcopy
8. A 24-year-old woman at 10 weeks of gestation is found to have an abnormal pap smear consistent with CIN III. Immediate management should include
   A. conization
   B. colposcopy and biopsy
   C. suction D&C
   D. repeat pap smear
   E. hysterectomy
9. Punctation is
   A. the area between the squamous epithelium of the cervical portio and the columnar epithelium of the endocervix

B. a colposcopic pattern that contains white epithelium with stippling due to blood vessels seen on end
C. a name for cells with perinuclear cavitation
D. a colposcopic pattern that reveals acetowhite areas outlined by blood vessels
E. the pattern of native squamous epithelium

10. All of the following HPV (Human papillomavirus) types have been associated with cervical carcinoma **EXCEPT**
A. 2
B. 6
C. 11
D. 16
E. 18

11. A PCR (polymerase chain reaction) is a(n)
A. enzyme that reproduces itself
B. method of amplifying DNA
C. atomic reaction
D. standard step in performing Southern Blot analysis
E. test limited to finding HPV 16 & 18

12. The greatest risk of developing cervical cancer is predicted by
A. coitarche at age 17
B. an atypical PAP smear
C. CIN II at the margin of a cervical cone
D. HPV 16 found on cervical smear
E. persistent abnormal cytology after cryocautery for dysplasia

13. Using the Bethesda system for reporting a PAP smear result, a patient who is found to have a smear consistent with an HPV infection would be classified as
A. high grade SIL
B. low grade SIL
C. reactive inflammatory change
D. atypical type undetermined
E. infection

14. A 50 year old woman has CIN III on cervical biopsy, an inadequate colposcopy, and an ECC positive for dysplastic fragments. The cervix sounds to 2 cm. How long should the cone be?
A. 5 mm
B. 7 mm
C. 10 mm
D. 15 mm
E. 20 mm

15. The most common complication of conization is
A. infertility
B. cervical stenosis
C. bleeding
D. an incompetent cervix
E. an infection

DIRECTIONS for questions 16 - 22: For each numbered item, select the one heading most closely associated with it. Each lettered heading may be used once, more than once, or not at all.

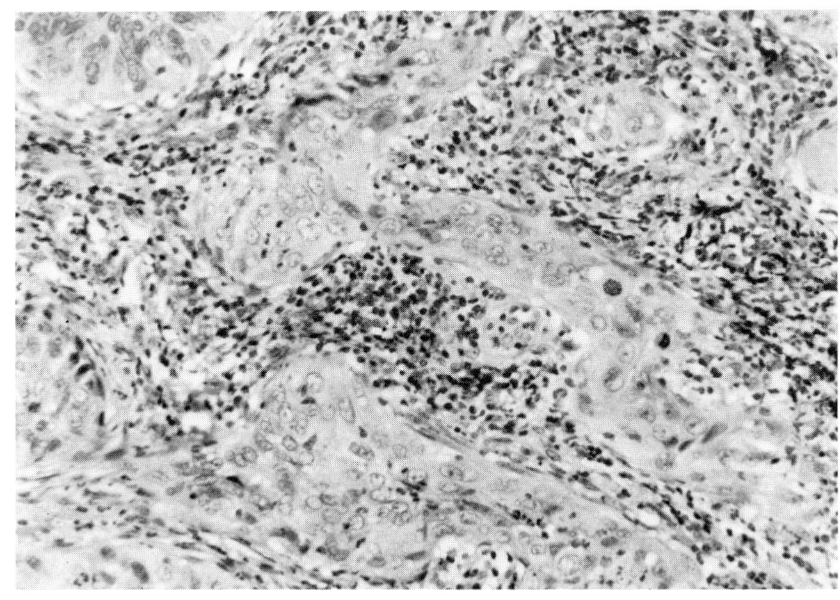

FIGURE 26-1.

(From Droegemueller W, Herbst AL, Mishell DR, Stenchever MA: Comprehensive gynecology, St. Louis, The C.V. Mosby Co, 1987.)

16-18. Choose the most appropriate interval between pap smears for the following patients
(A) annually
(B) annually until two negative tests, then stop
(C) every 3 to 5 years
(D) every 6 to 8 years
(E) testing may be stopped
16. a sexually active 14-year-old female
17. a 42-year-old female who had a hysterectomy 1 year ago for CIN III
18. a 33-year-old female who had a hysterectomy 1 year ago for leiomyomata

19-22. Match the histologic picture with the correct diagnosis
(A) Figure 26-1
(B) Figure 26-2
(C) Figure 26-3
(D) Figure 26-4
(E) Figure 26-5
19. cervical intraepithelial neoplasia (CIN I)
20. cervical intraepithelial neoplasia (CIN III)
21. moderate dysplasia of the cervix (CIN II)

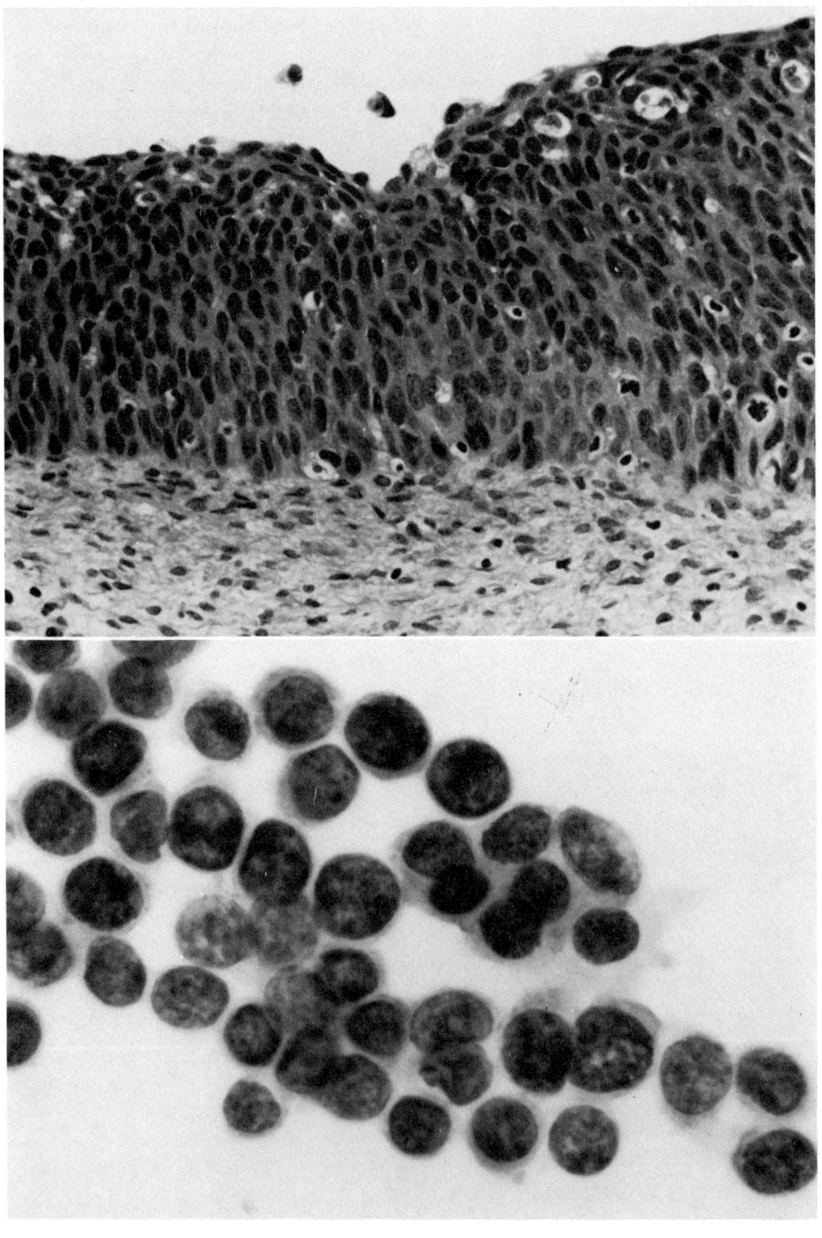

FIGURE 26-2.

(From Droegemueller W, Herbst AL, Mishell DR, Stenchever MA: Comprehensive gynecology, St. Louis, The C.V. Mosby Co, 1987.)

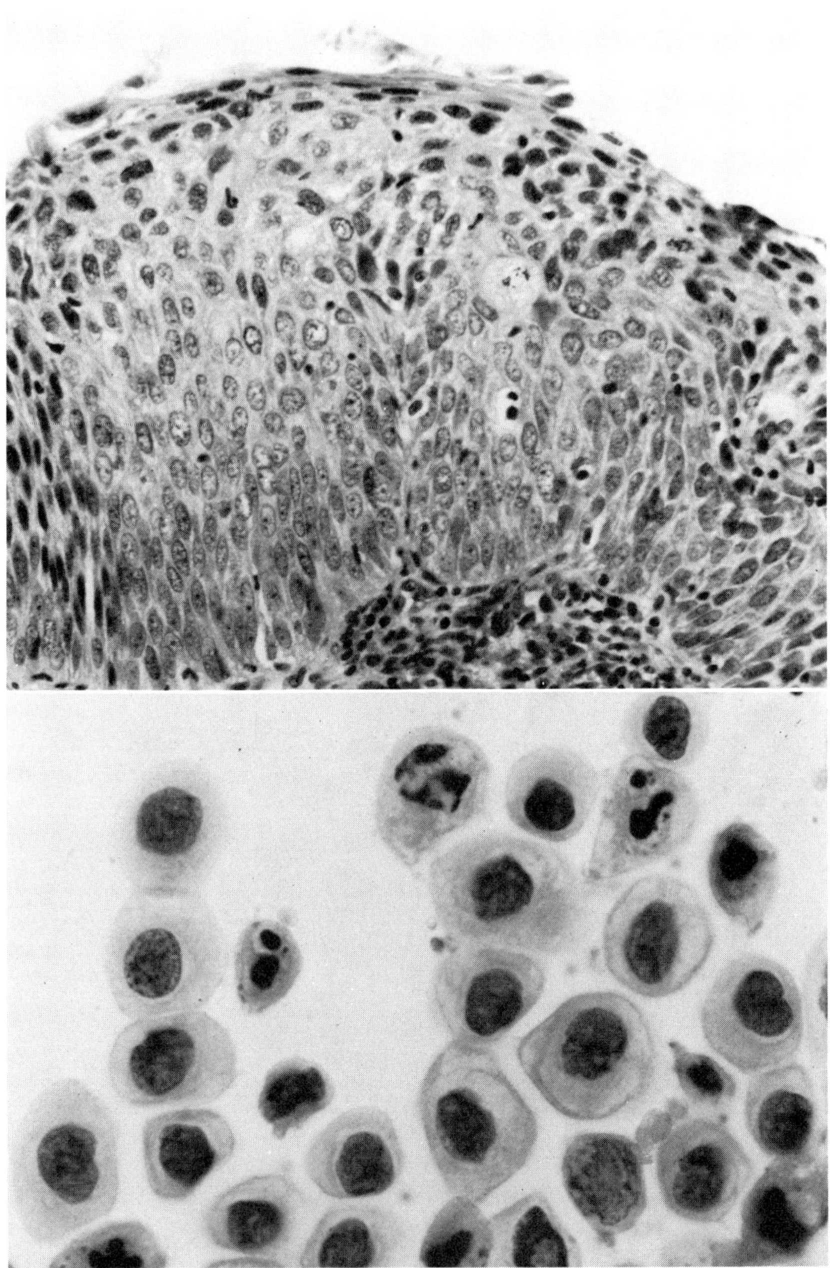

FIGURE 26-3.
(From Droegemueller W, Herbst AL, Mishell DR, Stenchever MA: Comprehensive gynecology, St. Louis, The C.V. Mosby Co, 1987.)

22. invasive squamous cell carcinoma of the cervix

DIRECTIONS: For each numbered item 23 - 25, indicate whether it is associated with

A only (A)
B only (B)
C both (A) and (B)
D neither (A) nor (B)

23-25. Characteristic of
(A) cervical intraepithelial neoplasia (CIN)
(B) human papillomavirus (HPV) infection
(C) both
(D) either

23. stains acetowhite on colposcopy
24. a cause of atypia on pap smears
25. koilocytosis

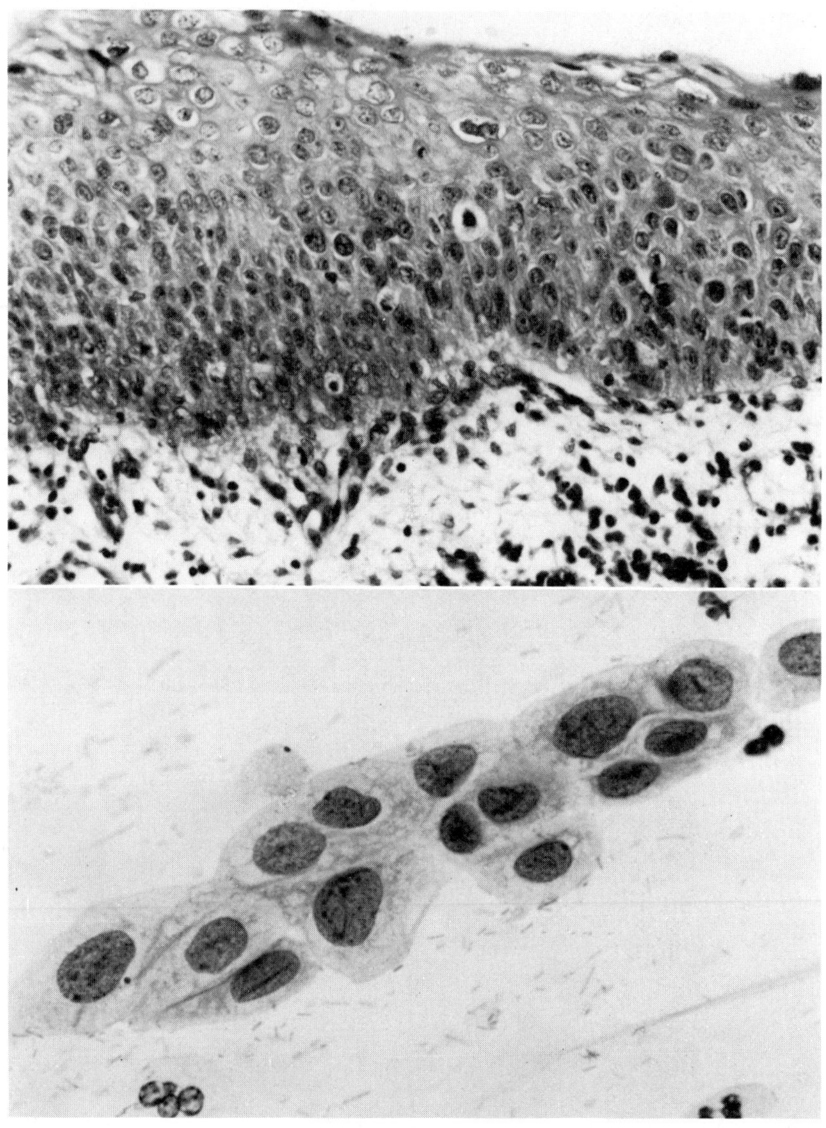

FIGURE 26-4.

(From Droegemueller W, Herbst AL, Mishell DR, Stenchever MA: Comprehensive gynecology, St. Louis, The C.V. Mosby Co, 1987.)

DIRECTIONS for questions 26 - 30: For each of the questions below, ONE or MORE of the responses is correct. Select the best answer based on the following

A if 1, 2, and 3 are correct
B if only 1 and 2 are correct
C if only 2 and 3 are correct
D if only 1 is correct
E if only 3 is correct

26. Factors known to increase the risk of squamous cell carcinoma of the cervix are
    1. multiple sexual partners
    2. smoking
    3. intrauterine diethylstilbesterol (DES) exposure
27. Suspicious findings for significant dysplasia on colposcopy include
    1. wide, irregular intercapillary distances
    2. irregular surface pattern
    3. large, abnormal transformation zone
28. The requirements for adequate colposcopy include
    1. endocervical curettage
    2. demonstration of white epithelium
    3. visualization of the entire transformation zone
29. A patient with extensive CIN III has the di-

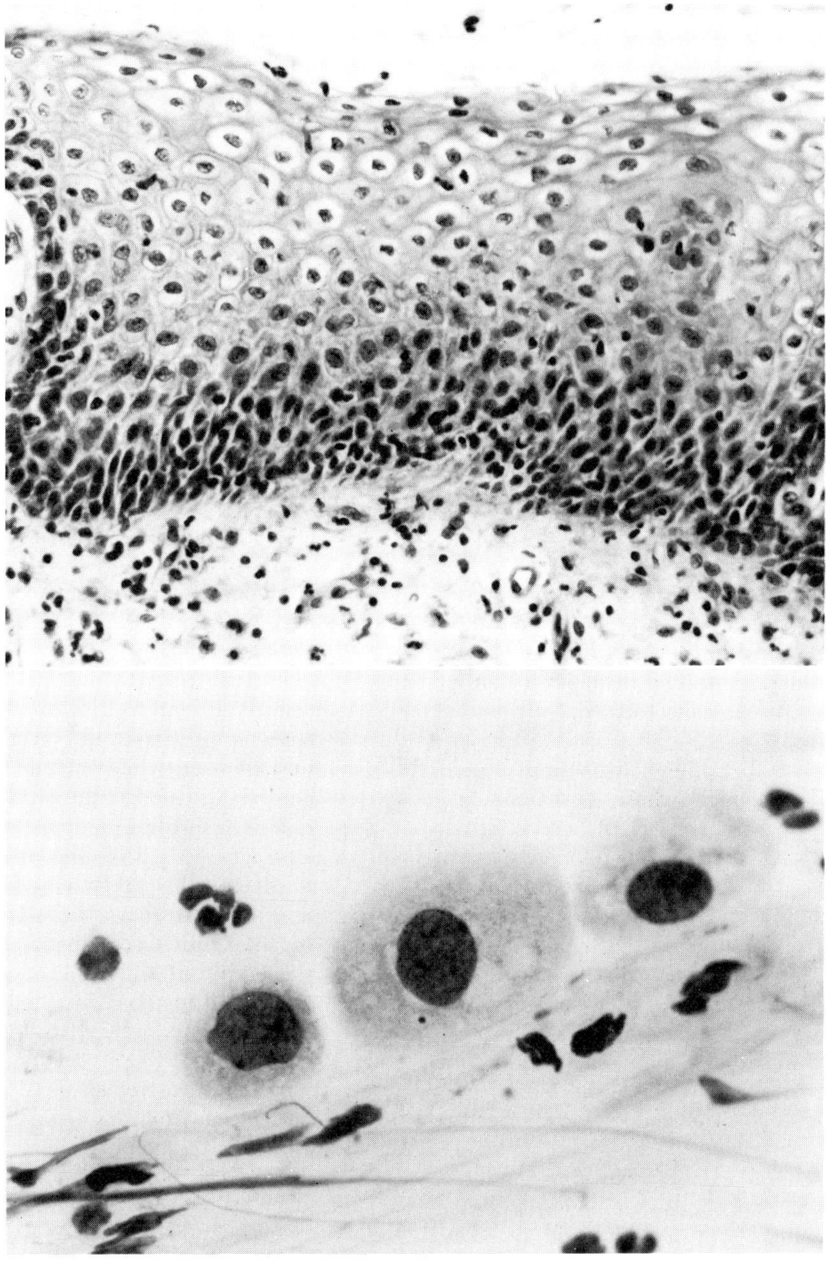

FIGURE 26-5.
(From Droegemueller W, Herbst AL, Mishell DR, Stenchever MA: Comprehensive gynecology, St. Louis, The C.V. Mosby Co, 1987.)

agnosis made by multiple colposcopically-directed biopsies. The endocervical curettage was negative. All abnormal areas were completely visualized. This patient can be treated appropriately by

1. laser ablation
2. conization
3. electrocautery

30. A 30-year-old woman with a pap smear consistent with CIN II and an endocervical curettage showing dysplasia is being counseled regarding cervical conization for treatment. The possible adverse consequences associated with this procedure include

1. cervical stenosis
2. bleeding
3. infertility

ANSWERS

1. **B,** Pages 843, 847. Specific indications for cervical conization are: 1) unsatisfactory colposcopy; 2) a positive ECC (endocervical curettage); 3) cells on the pap smear that are not adequately explained by histology on biopsy; 4) microinvasive cancer; 5) clinical uncertainty regarding the presence of invasive disease. It has also been suggested that conization should be done in patients over the age of 50 if a biopsy diagnosis of carcinoma in situ is made because of the incidence of unsuspected invasion is high beyond this age. The purpose of conization in such a case is to rule out invasive cancer.
2. **B,** Pages 821, 841. Leukoplakia and acetowhite epithelium are both clinical descriptive terms. Leukoplakia is white before the application of acetic acid, while acetowhite epithelium looks normal initially and becomes white after application of acetic acid. Neither term defines a precancerous lesion. The histology of either one may be precancerous, but not necessarily so.
3. **E,** Page 830. Epidemiologic studies indicate that women whose husbands' first wives had carcinoma of the cervix are at three times the risk of developing cervical cancer when compared to women whose husbands' first wives did not have cervical cancer. This supports the hypothesis that a factor causing cervical cancer may be sexually transmitted. Some other factors that increase the risk of cervical cancer are related to sexual activity, such as multiple sex partners and venereal disease.
4. **C,** Page 840. The endocervical curettage (ECC) is designed to find whether or not endocervical neoplasia exists. It can detect dysplasia, squamous carcinoma, and adenocarcinoma. An ECC should be done whenever a biopsy is taken from the cervix. The ECC cannot identify which part of the cervical canal has cancer, rule out endocervical human papilloma virus infection, or document chlamydial cervicitis. Although cells from ovarian or other upper abdominal carcinoma can be found on either pap smears or ECC specimens, neither of these modalities provides an accurate way of making the diagnosis of upper genital tract or other abdominal carcinoma.
5. **B,** Page 850. A biopsy diagnosis of microinvasive cancer of the cervix requires conization to rule out invasive disease. A radical hysterectomy may be too much treatment if no invasion exists, and a total hysterectomy is too little treatment if it does. Cryocautery should not be done for this lesion. Further study and appropriate treatment are mandatory depending upon the eventual diagnosis. If the cone is negative and she desires more children, the conization can be considered treatment at this time.
6. **E,** Pages 845-846. A double 3-minute freeze will cure approximately 90% of CIN lesions in which the initial evaluation is adequate, which it was in this patient. The double freeze will destroy most of the transformation zone in cervical crypts. However, close follow-up with a pap smear every 6 months for 1 or 2 years, followed by annual pap smears, is needed to assure that the dysplastic process has been eliminated. These women should always have pap smears done at least annually.
7. **E,** Page 850. Studies have shown that even with positive margins on a cervical conization, up to 70% of these patients have no recurrence at 5 years. With careful follow-up, which includes endocervical pap smears, most of these patients may retain their fertility.
8. **B,** Pages 851, 853. There is no need to terminate the pregnancy for CIN. The first step is to have the patient evaluated by an experienced colposcopist. That physician will do a biopsy if indicated. Often the transformation zone and endocervical canal are seen better because of the cervical eversion which occurs during pregnancy. If invasive cancer is not found, the patient may delivery vaginally. Conization would be done only if there is suspicion of invasion by either cytology or colposcopy which is not confirmed on biopsy. This is a rare situation.
9. **B,** Page 822. Mosaicism, punctation, and transformation zone are all terms used to describe colposcopic findings. Respectively, they refer to a colposcopic pattern in which acetowhite areas are outlined by blood vessels; a pattern that contains stippling due to blood vessels seen on end in acetowhite areas; and the expanse of epithelium at the junction between the squamous epithelium of the cervix and the columnar epithelium of the endocervix. Native squamous epithelium is the original squamous epithelium found on the portio of the cervix and in the vagina.
10. **A,** Page 834. Although certain HPV types

have been more frequently associated with cervical cancer than others, use of more sensitive tests has shown a high prevalence of these so called high risk types in women who have negative cervical cytology. Currently the use of HPV typing has not proven helpful clinically. Type 2 has not been associated with cervical carcinoma.

11. **B,** Page 833. A PCR (polymerase chain reaction) is a highly sensitive method of enzymatically reproducing segments of DNA so that very small amounts can be amplified and the segment can be easily identified and studied. It is a useful technique for many situations because it is possible to detect a single DNA fragment in a million cells. Care must be exercised in its use to prevent amplification of a contaminant, thereby yielding false positive results.
12. **E,** Page 831. Persistent abnormal cervical cytology after treatment for dysplasia is a bad prognostic sign. For this reason, all patients should be followed with PAP smears after treatment for cervical dysplasia. A finding of positive margins after a cone biopsy has a low rate of more severe disease developing, but must be followed closely. Young age of first coitus and mildly abnormal cytology are risk factors, but not as significant as persistent positive cytology after treatment. The finding of HPV 16 in the cervix of an otherwise normal woman requires follow-up smears.
13. **B,** Pages 836-837. The Bethesda system first requires a statement regarding the adequacy of the cytologic preparation for diagnosis. It classifies HPV as a low grade squamous intraepithelial lesion. (SIL). Changes consistent with CIN I are also classified as low grade SIL. Other infections are noted separately. Such smears without neoplastic change can be repeated in 6 months.
14. **E,** Page 848 (Boonstra, H., et al., *Minimum extension and appropriate topographic position of tissue destruction for treatment of cervical intraepithelial neoplasia.* Obstet Gynecol, 1990. **75**(2): p. 227-31). Boonstra's data on 65 specimens showed that CIN III lesions had a maximum depth of crypt involvement of 4.5 mm and a maximum length of involvement of 17.6 mm. The depth and extent of gland involvement increases in older women. There is a greater risk of cancer in this older age group which is why this cone should remove most of the endocervix. In this population reproduction is no longer an issue. A larger cone is associated with a small increase in risk in return for a better diagnostic sample. The cone size should be tailored to the patient and clinical situation. In laser ablation a common practice is to obliterate the tissue surrounding the endocervical canal to a depth of 5 to 7 mm, which is not deep enough to include the extent of lesions as defined by other studies, especially in the older population.
15. **C,** Page 849. Although infertility and an incompetent cervix may occur, the risk is small. In woman near or past menopause these are not risks. Bleeding, both immediate and late (7-14 days) is the major complication. Stenosis may be decreased by sounding the cervix at 1-3 weeks post cone. Other rare complications are infection, damage to nearby organs, and uterine perforation.

16-18. 16, **A;** 17, **A;** 18, **C;** Page 838; Table 26-2 (from Herbst). Different reports list different intervals at which pap smears are recommended. However, all agree that young, sexually active women should have annual smears until at least two smears are negative and then have a smear every year. Most also state that high risk women should continue to have annual smears. High risk women are those who began sexual intercourse at an early age, have had multiple sexual partners, or have had abnormal pap smears, HPV or HSV infections in the past. A woman who has had a hysterectomy for dysplastic disease remains at high risk for dysplasia or carcinoma at the vaginal apex. Women who had hysterectomy for benign disease should still have pap smears, but the interval between them can safely be extended to 3 to 5 years. The pelvic exam done in conjunction with obtaining a pap smear in any woman is also a good clinical screening tool for such entities as vaginitis, cervicitis, ovarian tumors, and other pelvic pathology. It also brings the patient to the physician for other health maintenance measures such as mammography.

19-22. 19, **E;** 20, **C;** 21, **D;** 22, **A;** Pages 823, 825. The concept of dysplastic changes of the cervical epithelium progressing to invasive carcinoma is well established. Various terms have been used to describe the histology of the dysplastic changes in the cervix. Cervical intraepithelial neoplasia (CIN) is designated as I, II, or III. CIN I and II are described as having the same histologic findings as mild and moderate dysplasia, respectively. CIN III refers to the same histologic patterns found in either severe dysplasia or carcinoma in situ. As the treatment for severe dysplasia or carcinoma in situ is the same, the term CIN III has been used to describe both of these entities. As degrees of CIN or dysplasia lie on a continuum, the distinctions may be interpreted differently by different observers, especially at the less severe end of the spectrum. Fig 26-2 shows changes consistent with HPV infection which could be called CIN I by some pathologists.

23-25. 23, **C**; 24, **C**; 25, **B**; Pages 829, 837. Both CIN and some HPV stain acetowhite with the application of acetic acid. Both may result in atypical cells appearing on the pap smear. For these reasons, colposcopically-directed biopsies must be taken to rule out dysplasia when abnormal findings are reported on pap smear or seen with the colposcope. It is difficult, if not impossible, to make the diagnosis of dysplasia by pap smear or colposcopy only. Koilocytes are specific for HPV. They may be found in areas of dysplasia (CIN) as well, but they imply a concomitant HPV infection. If dysplastic cells occur through the entire thickness of the cervical epithelium, the diagnosis is carcinoma in situ, which is included in the diagnosis of CIN III. CIN III may also be associated with HPV infection. In cases of obvious dysplasia, the presence or absence of HPV infection is disregarded for purposes of therapy.

26. **B** (1, 2), Pages 829-830. Multiple sex partners and immunosuppression have been implicated epidemiologically with an increased incidence of cervical carcinoma. In some studies, birth control pill use has not been found to increase the risk of cervical carcinoma independent from the risk associated with increased sex partners, whereas in other studies, it appears to be a risk factor. Smoking appears to increase the relative risk of cervical carcinoma by 1.5. Intrauterine diethylstilbesterol (DES) exposure has not proven to increase the risk of carcinoma of the cervix, although concern exists about this possibility.

27. **A** (1, 2, 3), Page 841. On colposcopic examination, the main criteria used to detect dysplastic lesions are the vascular pattern, the distance between capillaries, the sharpness of the borders, the intensity of the color, and the size of the abnormal transformation zone.

28. **E** (3 only), Pages 841-842. Colposcopy is used to detect an abnormality and to determine the best site for biopsy. To do this adequately, the entire transformation zone must be seen. White epithelium and/or leukoplakia may define abnormalities, but do not indicate whether the colposcopic exam was adequate or inadequate. An endocervical curettage is usually done to complete the evaluation of the patient, but is not required for adequate colposcopy.

29. **A** (1, 2, 3), Pages 845-847. The purpose behind the treatment of CIN is to eradicate the dysplastic epithelium completely. Electrocautery, laser, cold knife conization, or cryocautery can all destroy the dysplasia. Conization has the advantage of complete removal and provision of a histologic specimen. The techniques employed must be done properly and long-term follow-up is required. The chance of developing new sites of CIN is greater in this patient than in the general population because she has demonstrated a propensity to develop CIN.

30. **A** (1, 2, 3), Page 849. The risks of any surgical procedure include problems with anesthesia, infection, hemorrhage, damage to surrounding organs, and failure to achieve the desired result. With cervical conizations, specific complications are infertility and cervical stenosis. An incompetent cervix may also occur but is quite rare. These are not common complications but should be outlined when counseling a patient.

CHAPTER

27 Malignant Disease of the Cervix

DIRECTIONS for questions 1 - 6: Select the one best answer or completion.

1. A patient with a diagnosis of a stage Ib adenocarcinoma of the cervix would have the greatest chance for survival with an initial treatment of
   A. combined radiation and surgery
   B. surgery
   C. radiation
   D. chemotherapy
   E. surgery and immunotherapy
2. A 49-year-old woman has had squamous cell carcinoma of the cervix diagnosed by biopsy. On examination under anesthesia she is found to have a tumor in the upper third of the vagina and in the parametria. An intravenous pyelogram reveals obstruction of the left ureter. The stage of her tumor is
   A. Ib
   B. IIa
   C. IIIa
   D. IIIb
   E. IV
3. Of the following, the most virulent form of carcinoma of the cervix is
   A. large cell, non keratinizing
   B. adenosquamous
   C. basaloid
   D. verrucous
   E. glassy cell
4. A 52-year-old patient who had a supracervical hysterectomy in the past now has stage IIb carcinoma of the cervix. The treatment of choice is
   A. external radiation
   B. intracavitary radiation
   C. radical surgery
   D. chemotherapy
   E. trachelectomy
5. A 60-year-old woman presents with a firm nodule above her left clavicle. Her history reveals slight weight loss and mild vaginal spotting for 6 months. She has not had a physical examination or pap smear for many years. On pelvic exam she has a large bulky cervix with firm induration extending to the pelvic side walls. A biopsy of the cervix reveals invasive squamous cell carcinoma. Chest x-ray and intravenous pyelogram are normal. The next step in her care should be
   A. external radiation to 50 Gy
   B. total abdominal hysterectomy and bilateral salpingo-oophorectomy
   C. radical hysterectomy and pelvic lymph node dissection
   D. 500 mg hours of cervical brachytherapy
   E. scalene node biopsy
6. A patient had had cervical carcinoma diagnosed by conization. The maximum depth of the tumor from the base of the epithelium was between 6-7 mm and there was no lateral extension greater than 5 mm. There was no parametrial, nodal or metastatic involvement. According to the 1985 FIGO the lesion would be classified as
   A. O
   B. Ia_1
   C. Ia_2
   D. Ib
   E. III

DIRECTIONS for questions 7 - 13: For each numbered item, select the one heading most closely associated with it. Each lettered heading may be used once, more than once, or not at all.

7-10. Match the patient with the most likely 5-year percent survival
   (A) 8%
   (B) 31%
   (C) 57%
   (D) 70%
   (E) 78%

7. 28-year-old woman with stage I squamous cell carcinoma of the cervix
8. 42-year-old woman with invasive carcinoma of the cervix discovered in an operative specimen after a vaginal hysterectomy for prolapse
9. 42-year-old woman with stage III carcinoma of the cervix
10. 28-year-old woman with stage II carci-

noma of the cervix discovered during the second trimester of pregnancy

11-13. Match the description with the most likely source
- (A) Vulvar
- (B) Cervical
- (C) Endometrial
- (D) Ovarian
- (E) Vaginal

11. female genital tract cancer causing the greatest number of deaths
12. most common female genital tract-type cancer
13. the genital tract cancer whose frequency is steadily decreasing as a result of population screening

DIRECTIONS: For each numbered item 14 - 30, indicate whether it is associated with

A only (A)
B only (B)
C both (A) and (B)
D neither (A) nor (B)

14-17. Match the therapeutic modality
- (A) brachytherapy
- (B) teletherapy
- (C) both
- (D) neither

14. form of radiation therapy
15. employs colpostats
16. Fletcher-Suit applicator
17. surgical procedure which severs nerves to prevent pain

18-20. Match the tumor
- (A) endophytic cervical carcinoma
- (B) exophytic cervical carcinoma
- (C) both
- (D) neither

18. barrel-shaped cervix
19. associated with early abnormal bleeding and staining
20. primary path of distant spread is through lymphatics to regional lymph nodes

21-23. Match the type of hysterectomy with the description
- (A) radical hysterectomy
- (B) total abdominal hysterectomy
- (C) both
- (D) neither

21. includes surgical removal of the paraaortic nodes
22. includes surgical removal of the pelvic nodes
23. includes surgical removal of the ovaries

24-26. Cervical carcinoma treatment
- (A) point A
- (B) point B
- (C) both
- (D) neither

24. defined anatomical location used in calculating dosage of pelvic irradiation
25. located on the lateral pelvic sidewall
26. receives 85 Gray total radiation with standard therapy for invasive carcinoma

27-30. Match the complications
- (A) complication of radical hysterectomy for cervical cancer
- (B) complication of radiation treatment for cervical cancer
- (C) both
- (D) neither

27. urinary fistula
28. bladder dysfunction
29. shrinkage of vaginal apex
30. hemorrhagic cystitis

DIRECTIONS for questions 31 - 34: For each of the questions below, ONE or MORE of the responses is correct. Select the best answer based on the following

A if 1, 2, and 3 are correct
B if only 1 and 2 are correct
C if only 2 and 3 are correct
D if only 1 is correct
E if only 3 is correct

31. The major advantage(s) of **surgery** in the treatment of carcinoma of the cervix Stage Ib or IIa is/are
    1. preservation of the ovaries
    2. less vaginal fibrosis
    3. better cure rate
32. When compared to squamous cell carcinoma, adenocarcinoma of the cervix
    1. is less apt to be cured by radiation therapy
    2. is more frequently found in older women
    3. runs a course that may be predicted by CA 125
33. Pelvic node metastases from cervical cancer has been shown to independently correlate with
    1. age
    2. vascular space involvement
    3. depth of invasion
34. True statements about recurrent carcinoma of the cervix include
    1. recurrent carcinoma is defined as reappearing within 6 months after therapy
    2. half of all recurrences are in the pelvis
    3. current chemotherapeutic regimens which include CIS-platinum are the most effective.

ANSWERS

1. **A,** Pages 877, 882. Recent reports suggest that patients with early stages of **adeno-**

carcinoma of the cervix have a better survival rate if treated with partial irradiation by local implants of radium in the cervix and vagina followed by radical surgery. The approach of radiation followed by surgery is also used in stage Ib barrel-shaped squamous cell carcinoma of the cervix. Radiation alone is used for Stage IIb or greater cases of carcinoma of the cervix.

2. **D,** Pages 862, 882. Stage is defined by the greatest extent of tumor spread which in this case is the ureteral obstruction as demonstrated by the intravenous pyelogram. Currently, in contrast to ovarian carcinoma, the staging of cervical cancer is done by physical exam and a few specialized tests such as an intravenous pyelogram and a chest x-ray. Once the stage is determined, it does not change even if the operative findings reveal that it is more or less advanced than determined initially. The staging criteria for cervical cancer should be committed to memory.
3. **E,** Page 867. Glassy cell carcinoma is a virulent subtype of adenosquamous cervical cancer. It is highly malignant and has a predilection for early metastases. Small cell cancer is also quite malignant, while verrucous and large cell variants are less so. Other rare cell types include adenoma malignum, adenoid cystic, and basaloid.
4. **A,** Page 885. Supracervical hysterectomies are not often done now but were common several years ago. Although radical surgery may be considered for stage I or IIa disease, stage IIb presents a more advanced tumor that is not amenable to surgical therapy. Brachytherapy is difficult because the uterine fundus is removed, which makes it difficult to place intracavitary radiation sources. Therefore, external radiation is the best choice. Chemotherapy as an initial treatment for carcinoma of the cervix is not satisfactory and trachelectomy is inadequate treatment.
5. **E,** Page 877. A patient with a large supraclavicular node, weight loss and proven invasive carcinoma of the cervix is apt to have metastases via the pelvic and paraaortic nodes to the supraclavicular node. The presence or absence of metastases should be evaluated before any form of therapy is begun, because the presence of a positive supraclavicular node would change both the prognosis and therapy.
6. **D,** Page 869. The staging is Ib because it exceeds 5 mm in depth. As there is no parametrial, side wall, ureteral, or metastatic involvement, it would not be a Stage II tumor. Vascular space involvement should be separately mentioned.

7-10. 7, **E;** 8, **D;** 9, **B;** 10, **C;** Pages 873-875. Although individual reports may give somewhat different figures, the worldwide statistics from FIGO in 1985 showed a 5-year survival for stage I carcinoma of the cervix to be approximately 78%, stage II approximately 57%, stage III approximately 31%, and stage IV 7.8% (see Table 27-1).

Patients with carcinoma of the cervix in pregnancy have the same survival rate, stage for stage, as patients who are not pregnant. Overall survival of early carcinoma discovered inadvertently after hysterectomy performed for another reason is approximately 70%, whether either additional surgery or adjunctive radiation therapy is employed.

11-13. 11, **D;** 12, **C;** 13, **B;** Page 862. Endometrial carcinoma is the most frequent of the genital tract cancers, but causes relatively fewer deaths than either ovarian or cervical cancer because it is often found and treated early. Ovarian cancer is less common, but because of its silent early course, it is often not discovered until it has already metastasized. The incidence of cervical carcinoma has been decreasing, in part, because ofearly detection of dysplastic lesions by routine pap smears.

14-17. 14, **C;** 15, **A;** 16, **A;** 17, **D;** Pages 861, 880. Brachytherapy and teletherapy are both forms of radiation therapy. With brachytherapy, the radiation source is placed close to the tumor employing interstitial needles, intracervical tandems, or vaginal ovoid applicators. A Fletcher-Suit applica-

TABLE 27-1. Carcinoma of the Cervix Uteri: Distribution by Stage and Five-Year Survival Rates*

	Patients Treated*		5-Year Survival	
Stage	No.	%	No.	%
I	10,791	33.3	8,430	78.1
II	11,599	35.8	6,610	57.0
III	8,623	26.6	2,671	31.0
IV	1,377	4.3	107	7.8
No stage	9	0.0	4	—
Total	32,428	100.0	17,843	55.0

Modified from Pettersson F, et al: Nineteenth annual report on the results of treatment in gynecological cancer. Stockholm, International Federation of Gynecologists and Obstetricians, 1985.

*Patients treated in 1976 to 1978.

tor is a specific vaginal ovoid applicator to deliver brachytherapy. With teletherapy, the radiation source is at a distance from the patient and is usually called external therapy. Surgery severing the lateral spinothalamic tract to prevent pain is called a cordotomy.

18-20. 18, **A**; 19, **B**; 20, **C**; Page 871-872. Cervical carcinoma can develop as an ulcer, a cauliflower like growth on the outside of the cervix, or a silent, penetrating tumor growing into the cervical stoma. The ulcer or cauliflower (exophytic) type tends to present with irregular bleeding, while the internally growing tumor (endophytic) is asymptomatic for a long time during which metastases often occur. The endophytic tumor often causes a large, bulky barrel-shaped cervix. The most common mode of spread of all cervical cancer is through the cervical lymphatics into regional nodes. Blood-borne metastases occur much less frequently.

21-23. 21, **D**; 22, **D**; 23, **D**; Pages 861, 877-878. A radical hysterectomy removes the uterine cervix, upper vagina, and paracervical-parametrial tissue. A total hysterectomy removes the entire uterus (cervix and fundus). Neither removes the tubes, ovaries, or the pelvic lymph nodes. If any of these structures are removed, the surgery is identified by stating what is done (for example, bilateral salpingo-oophorectomy, pelvic lymphadenectomy, paraaortic node dissection). Many patients do not realize the difference between these two procedures. Before surgery, the patients should know exactly what is to be done. This requires time for careful counseling to assure that the patient understands.

24-26. 24, **C**; 25, **B**; 26, **A**; Page 878. See Figure 27-1.

Points A and B are defined positions in the pelvis used for calculating radiation dosage. Point A is 2 cm cephalad to the vaginal fornix and 2 cm lateral to the cervical canal. Point B is 3 cm lateral to point A. Because point A is closer to the source of brachytherapy, it receives a higher dose of ionizing radiation (approximately 85 Gray) than point B (approximately 50 to 60 Gray) during standard radiation therapy for invasive cervical carcinoma.

27-30. 27, **C**; 28, **C**; 29, **B**; 30, **B**; Pages 880, 883-884. Surgical complications usually occur soon after the operation and include genital urinary fistula, bladder dysfunction, and a loss of sensation that is usually temporary. Radiation complications can occur during treatment or at any later date, al-

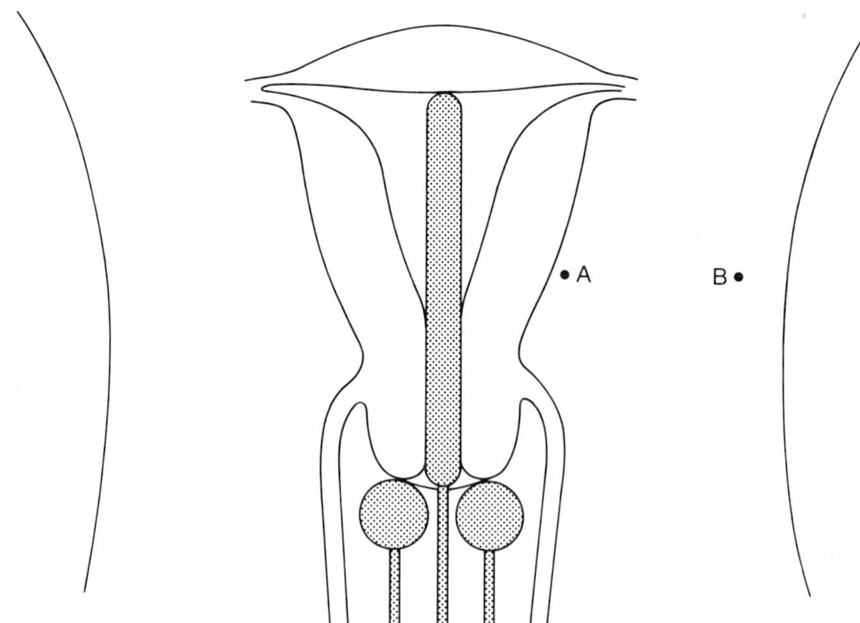

FIGURE 27-1.
Points A and B with central stem (tandem) and 2 ovoids in place.
(From Droegemueller W, Herbst AL, Mishell DR, Stenchever, MA: Comprehensive gynecology, St. Louis, The C.V. Mosby Co, 1987.)

though most are within 1 or 2 years. Ulcerations of the vagina and cervix may occur. Postradiation cystitis (hemorrhagic cystitis) may cause frequency, dysuria and bleeding. Fibrosis of the vagina and/or the ureters may be major problems for sexual and urinary function, respectively. Urinary fistulas also occur after radiation, but with modern treatment are quite uncommon. They occur most frequently in those cases where there is bulky tumor involvement near the bladder. Bowel fistulas, diarrhea, and rectal bleeding also occur and are more common than urinary complications. The risk of radiation complications increase with increased radiation dose, and as the frequency of cure increases, the rate of complication from the radiation also increases.

31. **B** (1, 2), Page 877. In young women, the preservation of ovarian and sexual function is very important and the ability to sample nodes for spread is also a distinct advantage in determining the need for further treatment. These are advantages of surgery. However, the cure rate is similar for surgery and irradiation in Stage Ib and IIa cervical carcinoma.
32. **A** (1, 2, 3), Page 875. Women with adenocarcinoma of the cervix tend to be nulliparous, older, and more often diabetic than women with squamous cell cervical carcinoma. Cervical clear cell adenocarcinoma is rare, but the incidence is increased in women with prior DES exposure in utero. Adenocarcinoma generally has a poorer prognosis than any comparable stage of squamous cell carcinoma. Just like adenocarcinoma of the ovary, the course of adenocarcinoma of the cervix may be predicted by CA 125 levels.
33. **A** (1, 2, 3), Page 875. There is independent correlation of pelvic node metastasis with the age of the patient (younger women have a poorer prognosis), the presence of tumor in lymphatic or vascular spaces in the cervix and the depth of invasion. The latter two factors are obvious intuitively.
34. **C** (2, 3), Pages 887-888. The definition of recurrence of cervical cancer is that it reappears 6 months or more after the time of therapy. If the tumor reappears within 6 months, it is considered a persistent. Approximately 50% of recurrences will be in the pelvis. Chemotherapy for recurrent cervical cancer is not very effective, but the best response rate occurs with multiple-agent regimens that include CIS-platinum. These regimens have been used with an increased survival in patients with positive nodes after radical hysterectomy.

CHAPTER

28 Neoplastic Diseases of the Uterus

DIRECTIONS for questions 1 - 17: Select the one best answer or completion.

1. A 68-year-old woman complains of vaginal spotting. On examination she has an atrophic vagina, a clean cervix with a closed os, and a normal-sized uterus. No masses are felt. A pap smear is obtained from the exocervix. If this patient has endometrial carcinoma, in what percent of cases will the obtained pap smear detect it?
   A. 10%
   B. 25%
   C. 50%
   D. 75%
   E. 90%
2. A 53-year-old woman has a D&C for postmenopausal bleeding. The pathology report states she has a malignant glandular epithelium with areas of squamous metaplasia in the endometrium. What is the most likely diagnosis?
   A. adenocarcinoma
   B. adenoacanthoma
   C. adenosquamous carcinoma
   D. atypical adenematous hyperplasia
   E. endolymphatic stromal myosis
3. A 63-year-old has a D&C for abnormal vaginal bleeding. On review of the pathology from the D&C, you see the pattern shown in Figure 28-1 Many sections appear similar and no mitotic figures are seen. What is the diagnosis?
   A. clear cell adenocarcinoma
   B. cellular leiomyoma
   C. cystic endometrial hyperplasia
   D. malignant mixed mullerian tumor
   E. atypical adenomatous hyperplasia
4. A 36-year-old woman has had a D&C for irregular bleeding. It reveals adenomatous hyperplasia without atypia (complex hyperplasia). What can you tell the patient?
   A. most (more than 50%) will progress to carcinoma within 8 to 12 years
   B. treatment should be hysterectomy
   C. induction of ovulation is contraindicated
   D. cyclic progestin therapy should promote monthly withdrawal
   E. repeat endometrial sampling is not necessary
5. A 61 year old woman with irregular uterine bleeding had severe, atypical, endometrial hyperplasia on D&C. Her risk of having carcinoma in her uterus, when the specimen is examined after hysterectomy, is approximately
   A. 1%
   B. 10%
   C. 25%
   D. 50%
   E. 75%
6. A 47-year-old woman has a poorly differentiated endometrial carcinoma and a uterine cavity that measures 10 cm in depth. The endocervix has stromal invasion of endometrial carcinoma, but no other structure is involved. What is the stage of her endometrial cancer?
   A. IA
   B. IB
   C. IC
   D. IIA
   E. IIB
7. Of the following rare primary tumors of the endometrium, which has the worst prognosis?
   A. clear cell adenocarcinoma
   B. papillary serous carcinoma
   C. secretory carcinoma
   D. mucinous carcinoma
   E. squamous cell carcinoma
8. A 52 year old woman with moderately differentiated endometrial cancer was surgically staged. Her uterus had sounded to 12 cm and had no cervical involvement. The cancer was limited to the endometrium. Peritoneal cytology, pelvic and periaortic nodes were negative. Using the most recent (1988) FIGO uterine corpus cancer staging, the stage of the above case would be:
   A. IA
   B. IB
   C. IC

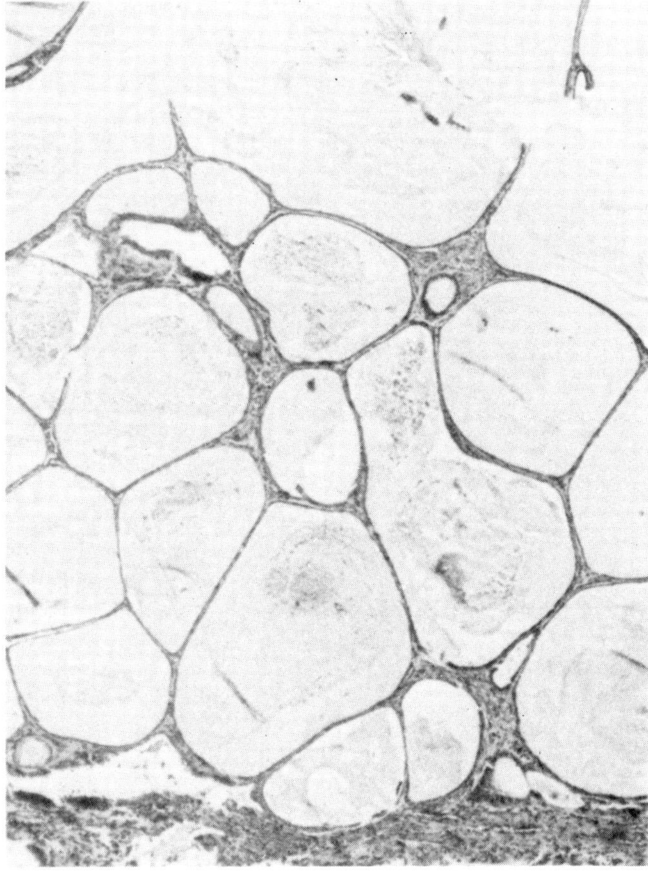

FIGURE 28-1.

(From Christopherson WM and Gray LA: In Coppleson M, ed: Gynecologic oncology, Edinburgh, Churchill-Livingstone, 1981.)

D. IIA
E. IIB

9. Which is the most common malignancy of the female genital tract?
   A. endometrial carcinoma
   B. cervical carcinoma
   C. tubal carcinoma
   D. vulvar carcinoma
   E. ovarian carcinoma
10. Which Stage III tumor is most likely to respond to progesterone therapy?
   A. carcinoma of the cervix
   B. ovarian carcinoma
   C. endometrial carcinoma
   D. vulvar carcinoma
   E. vaginal carcinoma
11. In endometrial carcinoma, estrogen receptors would be found in greatest number in which lesion?
   A. Stage I, G1
   B. Stage II, G3
   C. Stage III, G2
   D. Stage III, G3
   E. Stage IV, G3
12. Of the following cytotoxic chemotherapeutic agents, which would be *least likely* to be used in a patient who had persistence or recurrence of Stage III endometrial adenocarcinoma?
   A. cyclophosphamide (Cytoxan)
   B. doxorubicin HCL (Adriamycin)
   C. cis-platinum (Platinol)
   D. 5-FU (Adrucil)
   E. mitomycin (Mutamycin)
13. A 57-year-old woman has homologous uterine sarcoma. What is the current recommended primary treatment?
   A. radiation
   B. chemotherapy
   C. surgery
   D. surgery and chemotherapy
   E. surgery and irradiation
14. Ninety percent of adenocarcinomas of the

endometrium that recur do so within approximately
A. 1 year
B. 3 years
C. 5 years
D. 10 years
E. 20 years

15. Which is the most common sarcoma of the uterus?
A. endometrial stromal sarcoma
B. rhabdomyosarcoma
C. liposarcoma
D. endolymphatic stroma myosis
E. leiomyosarcoma

16. A 56-year-old patient is found to have both an endometrial adenocarcinoma and a rhabdomyosarcoma of the uterus. The tumor would be best described as a
A. heterologous sarcoma
B. endometrial stromal sarcoma
C. homologous sarcoma
D. carcinosarcoma
E. malignant mixed mullerian tumor

17. The International Society of Gynecologic Pathologists have developed new terms to classify endometrial hyperplasias. In this system the term complex hyperplasia refers to
A. atypical adenomatous hyperplasia
B. cystic hyperplasia
C. adenomatous hyperplasia
D. carcinoma in situ
E. hyperplasia combined with squamous metaplasia

DIRECTIONS for questions 18 - 25: For each numbered item, select the one heading most closely associated with it. Each lettered heading may be used once, more than once, or not at all.

18-20. Match the following women with the most appropriate treatment:
(A) No further treatment
(B) Provera 10 mg daily on a cyclic basis
(C) Clomid 50 mg on days 1-5
(D) Megace 40-320 mg per day
(E) Hysterectomy with bilateral salpingoophorectomy

18. A 28-year-old with complex endometrial hyperplasia found on D&C
19. A 58-year-old with atypical (adenomatous) endometrial hyperplasia
20. A 30-year-old anovulatory woman who wants a pregnancy now but who has mild atypical (adenomatous) endometrial hyperplasia

21-25. Match the following photomicrographs with the appropriate diagnosis.
(A) Figure 28-2
(B) Figure 28-3
(C) Figure 28-4
(D) Figure 28-5
(E) Figure 28-6

21. adenomatous hyperplasia
22. papillary serous carcinoma

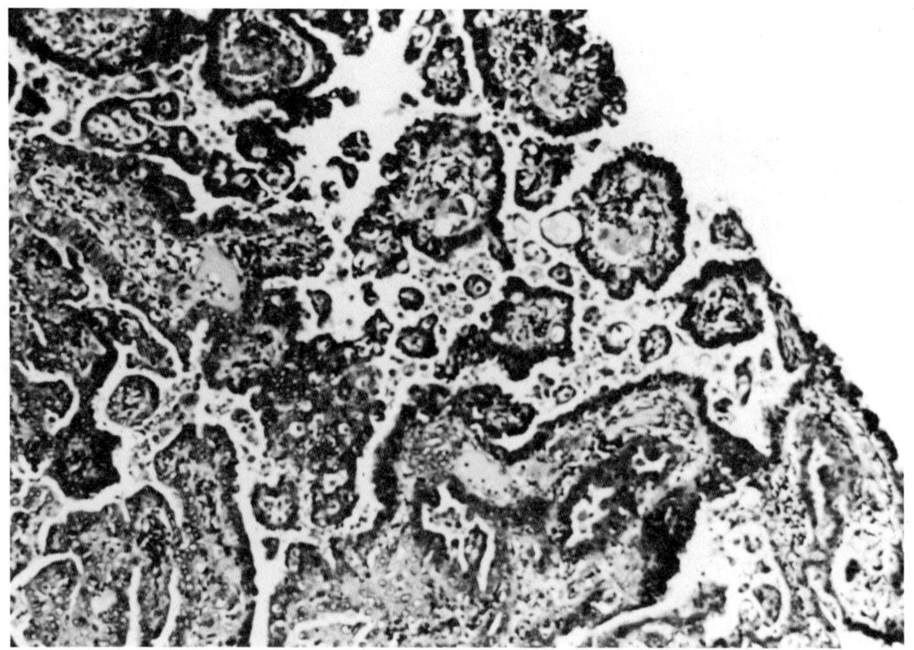

FIGURE 28-2.

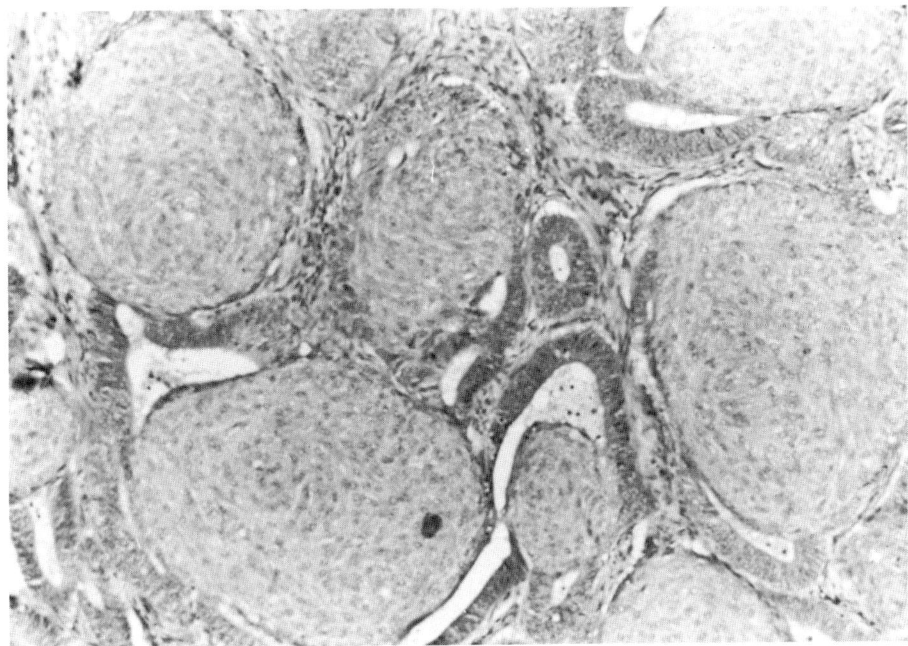

FIGURE 28-3.

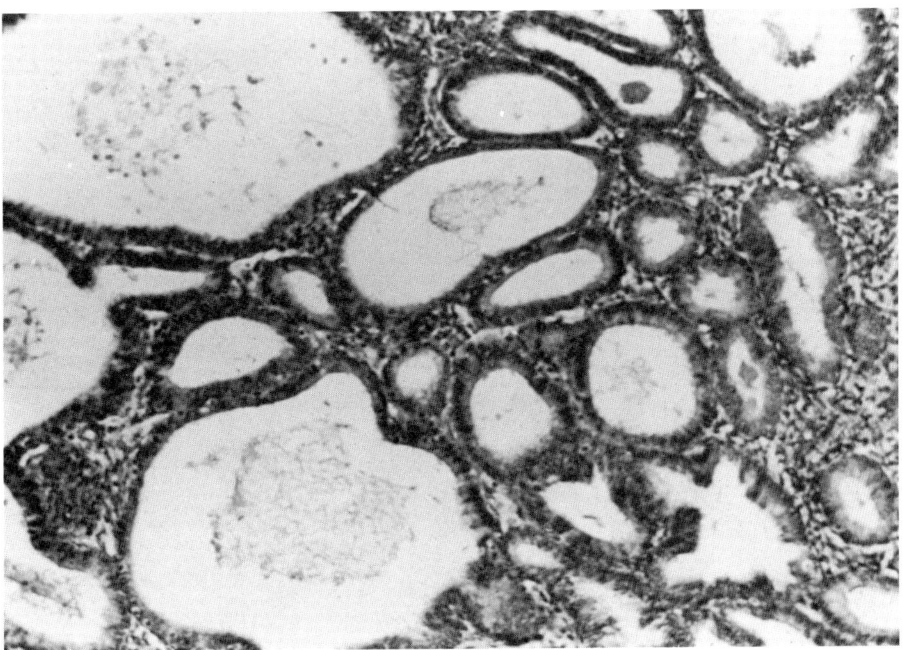

FIGURE 28-4.

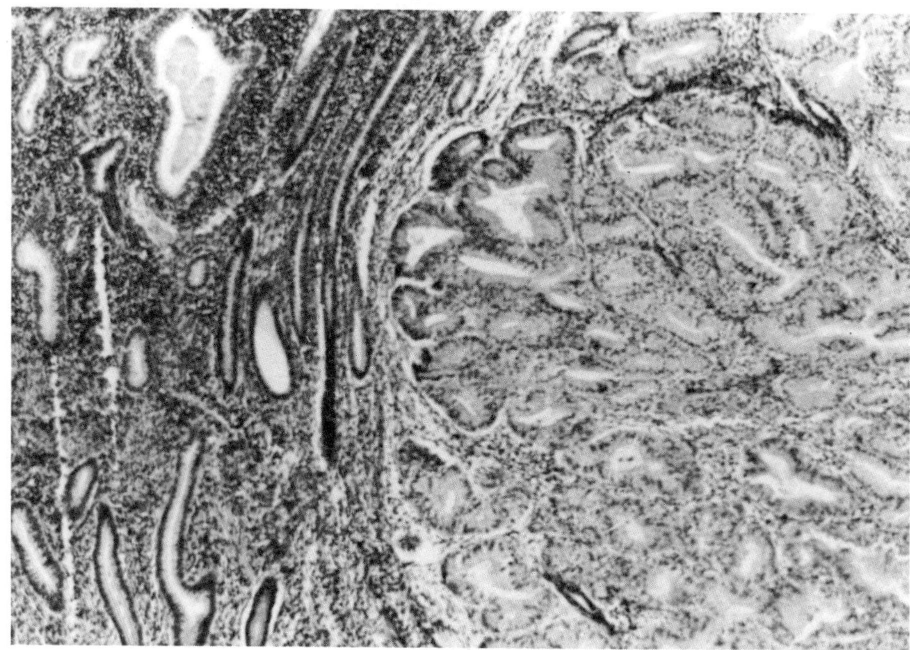

FIGURE 28-5.

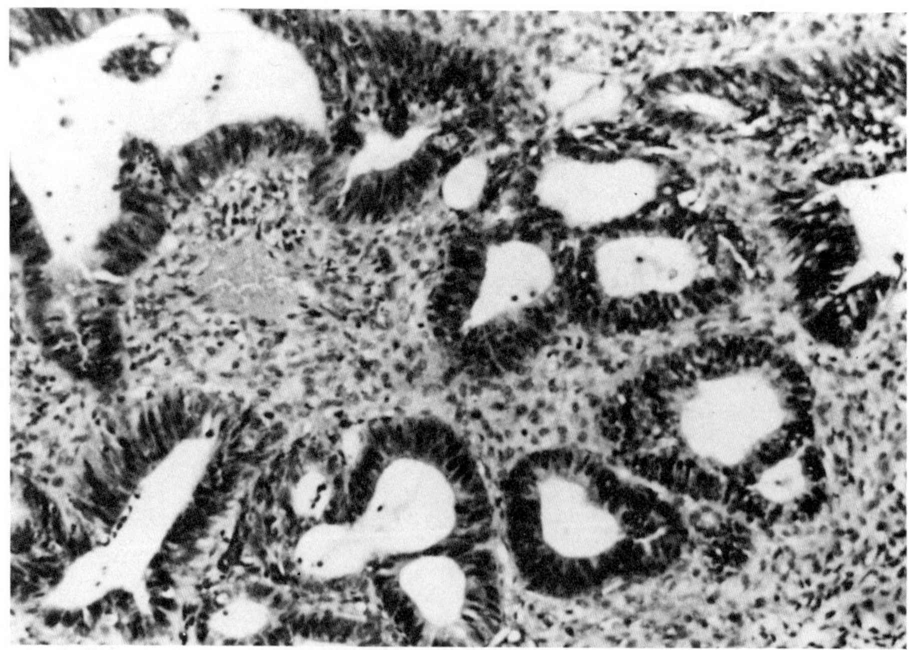

FIGURE 28-6.
(Courtesy of Robert C. Maier, MD, Medical College of Georgia)

23. atypical (adenomatous) hyperplasia
24. adenoacanthoma
25. adenocarcinoma of the endometrium

DIRECTIONS for questions 26 - 30: For each of the questions below, ONE or MORE of the responses is correct. Select the best answer based on the following

A if 1, 2, and 3 are correct
B if only 1 and 2 are correct
C if only 2 and 3 are correct
D if only 1 is correct
E if only 3 is correct

26. A 46-year-old woman complains of irregular periods and some spotting between periods not associated with coitus. General examination is within normal limits. The vagina and uterus have no evidence of abnormalities or lesions. You suggest an office D&C to evaluate the endometrium. Which of the following are true statements?
    1. oral prostaglandin synthetase inhibitors may decrease uterine cramping
    2. suction curettage yields good samples
    3. endometrial polyps and small subserous fibromas are easily detected by office D&C
27. During her routine annual examination, a 58-year-old woman asks about the risk of developing uterine cancer. True statements include:
    1. the prevalence of cancer of the endometrium is greatest between the age of 55 and 65
    2. late menopause is a risk factor
    3. hypertension is a risk factor
28. Tamoxifen therapy has been shown to increase the risk of
    1. endometrial cancer
    2. breast cancer
    3. ovarian cancer
29. Which modalities are used in the initial treatment for Stage II adenocarcinoma of the endometrium?
    1. surgery
    2. brachytherapy
    3. external Irradiation
30. In which of the following cases of endometrial adenocarcinoma should paraaortic and pelvic node sampling be done?
    1. Stage I, grade 1
    2. Stage I, grade 2
    3. Stage II

ANSWERS

1. **C**, Page 905. A pap smear has a false negative rate of about 20% for cervical cancer and at least a 50% false negative rate for endometrial cancer. Obviously it is not a good test for endometrial cancer. To rule out endometrial cancer, one must thoroughly sample the endometrium by curettage, preferably with separate samples from the endometrium and the endocervix. Approximately 14% of patients with postmenopausal bleeding will have that symptom due to endometrial carcinoma.
2. **B**, Page 905. Malignant glandular epithelium in the uterus is adenocarcinoma. A mixture of benign squamous epithelium with malignant glandular epithelium is called an adenoacanthoma. An adenoacanthoma has approximately the same prognosis as adenocarcinoma of the same grade and stage and should be treated similarly. If both adenomatous and squamous components were malignant, the tumor would be an adenosquamous carcinoma. Atypical adenomatous hyperplasia is a premalignant lesion in which there is crowding of glands and cytologic atypia. Endolymphatic stromal myosis is a low-grade stromal sarcoma.
3. **C**, Page 905; Figure 28-2 (from Herbst). The glands are dilated, but the cellular architecture is benign and there is no invasion. There is a classic benign Swiss-cheese configuration; therefore, the diagnosis is cystic endometrial hyperplasia or simple hyperplasia. Clear cell adenocarcinoma has many malignant cells with clear cytoplasm. A cellular leiomyoma would have whorls of connective tissue cells. A mixed mullerian tumor would have mitotic figures in connective tissue cells. Adenomatous hyperplasia has a crowded glandular architecture with no invasion.
4. **D**, Pages 898-899. Progression of adenomatous hyperplasia is slow and occurs in only a small number of cases. Usually the D&C will be therapeutic, but either progestin, if no pregnancy is wanted, or Clomid for ovulation induction, if pregnancy is desired, are proven treatments. Hysterectomy is not warranted for adenomatous hyperplasia alone. Repeat endometrial curettage is advised to assess completeness of cure.
5. **C**, Page 905. Older women with atypical hyperplasia are at risk both for having carcinoma already present (approximately 28%), or developing carcinoma (25%). For this reason the postmenopausal patient with proven atypical hyperplasia is best treated by hysterectomy.

6. **E,** Page 910. The involvement of the cervical stroma by invasive endometrial carcinoma makes the endometrial carcinoma a stage IIB. Depth of the uterus does not influence surgical staging, but is used if only radiation therapy is selected. The reason for doing a fractional D & C during the diagnostic process is to rule out cervical extension of endometrial invasive tumor and to rule out primary cervical carcinoma. Stage IIA would involve only the endocervical glands.
7. **E,** Pages 905-906. (Also see White A J et al: Primary squamous cell carcinoma of the endometrium, *Obstet Gynecol* 41:912. 1973.) Squamous cell carcinoma is a rare form of cancer of the endometrium with a poor prognosis. It is usually associated with pyometra. White's study has documented no 5-year survival. The other tumors of the endometrium such as clear cell adenocarcinoma, papillary serous carcinoma, secretory carcinoma, and mucinous carcinoma are also rare. Secretory and mucinous carcinoma have a relatively good prognosis, while clear cell and papillary serous carcinomas have a poor prognosis.
8. **A,** Page 910. The most recent uterine corpus cancer staging relies on operative evaluation. The older staging is used if irradiation treatment is chosen because depth of invasion and cytologic washings cannot be evaluated. Depth of the uterine cavity is not a factor in surgical staging, but the extent of proven invasion of the uterus is a factor. In this case, though the uterus was large, the cancer only involved the endometrium and therefore was stage IA. Becauseit was moderately differentiated (G2) node sampling should be done.
9. **A,** Page 896. Although the most common malignancy of the female genital tract is endometrial adenocarcinoma, fewer deaths occur from it than from either ovarian or cervical cancer. This is largely because it is detected and treated in an early stage. Early detection is possible because irregular uterine bleeding occurs early and is the most common presenting symptom.
10. **C,** Pages 921-922. Progesterone is used in the management of both recurrences and metastasis of endometrial carcinoma. The tumor is more likely to respond if it is well differentiated. Response rates of 10% to 30% have been reported and seem to be higher in patients whose tumors have the largest number of progesterone receptors. Other forms of cytotoxic chemotherapy also have been used. Cytotoxic drugs seem to have a better response rate if the tumor is undifferentiated.
11. **A,** Page 914. Estrogen receptors are found in the nuclei of well differentiated cancer cells. It was previously thought that estrogen receptors were found in the cytoplasm (cytosol). This misconception was an artifact of the receptor analysis procedure. As endometrial cancer cells become more undifferentiated they lose their estrogen receptors.
12. **E,** Pages 921-922. The primary chemotherapeutic agent used in endometrial adenocarcinoma is a progestin. Tamoxifen has also been used as it seems to increase the number of progesterone receptors in the tumor tissue. Neither of these are cytotoxic however. In the cytotoxic group, cyclophosphamide, doxorubicin, cis-platinum, and 5-FU are frequently used in combination for endometrial carcinoma. Mitomycin has been used primarily in gastric cancer.
13. **C,** Page 925. The treatment for homologous uterine sarcoma is surgical. Metastases or recurrences are usually treated with multiple-agent chemotherapy. Radiation has not been shown to increase survival significantly, although it appears to decrease the risk of pelvic recurrence. Distant metastases are frequent and most often occur in the lungs or abdomen. Chemotherapy has been used, but has not improved survival.
14. **C,** Page 921. Ninety percent of the adenocarcinomas of the endometrium that recur do so within 5 years, but as 10% recur later, prolonged follow-up is important. The most frequent site of recurrence is in the pelvis(approximately 50%), followed by lung (17%).
15. **E,** Page 923. Leiomyosarcomas comprise nearly 50% of all uterine sarcomas. They are diagnosed if the tumor contains over five mitoses per 10 high-power fields. The more mitoses present, the worse the prognosis. Endolymphatic stroma myosis is a more benign form of endometrial stromal sarcoma, both of which are rare. The heterologous rhabdomyosarcoma, liposarcoma, chondrosarcoma, and osteosarcoma are less common than the homologous types. In total, sarcomas comprise less than 5% of all uterine malignancies.

16. **E,** Pages 928-929. If a uterine sarcoma forms mesenchymal tissue normally found in the uterus, it is called a homologous sarcoma. If it forms mesenchymal tissue not normally found in the uterus, such as bone, fat, striated muscle, and cartilage, it is called heterologous. If the heterologous sarcoma is in combination with adenocarcinoma, it is called a malignant mullerian mixed tumor (MMMT). Prior pelvic radiation therapy is a predisposing factor, having been performed in approximately 12% of patients with MMMT. If an adenocarcinoma and a homologous sarcoma coexist, this tumor may be called a carcinosarcoma. Endolymphatic stromal myosis is a rare low-grade sarcoma made up of cells resembling the endometrial stroma. These are most often found in premenopausal females. Endometrial stromal sarcoma is a more malignant version of the same cell type.

17. **C,** Pages 898-899. Pathologists frequently change terminology. Clinicians must keep abreast of these changes so the changes add rather than detract from patient care. Complex hyperplasia refers to adenomatous hyperplasia without atypia.

18-20. 18, **B;** 19, **E;** 20, **C;** Pages 904-905. A young woman with benign endometrial hyperplasia could be managed by long term followup or may be given cyclic progestins (for example, Provera 10 mg for 10 to 14 days each month) which will induce monthly withdrawal bleeding. A postmenopausal woman with atypical endometrial hyperplasia (called CIS, Carcinoma insitu, by some pathologists) should have definitive treatment with removal of the uterus unless medically contraindicated. A young anovulatory woman who desires pregnancy but who has atypical endometrial hyperplasia may be treated with clomiphene citrate to induce ovulation if it is not occurring spontaneously. If successful, this therapy will interrupt the continuous unopposed estrogen that had previously stimulated her endometrium.

21-25. 21, **C;** Page 899. Adenomatous hyperplasia is identified by crowded irregular glands without significant cytologic atypia.

22. **A;** Page 909. Papillary serous carcinoma is a highly malignant form of endometrial carcinoma that has a papillary form resembling papillary serous adenocarcinoma of the ovary.

23. **E;** Page 899. Atypical adenomatous hyperplasia is a premalignant variant of endometrial hyperplasia. There is cytologic atypica but no invasion.

24. **B;** Page 908. An adenoacanthoma is an endometrial carcinoma that has islands of benign squamous cells.

25. **D;** Page 899. There is an invasive carcinoma of the endometrium on the right side of the figure. It is moderately differentiated adenocarcinoma and has crowded glands and cellular atypia with stromal invasion.

26. **B** (1 & 2), Page 903; Table 28-3 (from Herbst). Office aspiration, or suction curettage, can adequately sample the endometrium in most cases. If the patient continues to have bleeding or other symptoms, a repeat D&C may be indicated. The office procedure usually can be done under paracervical block and some patients benefit from an oral prostaglandin synthetase inhibitor taken 30 minutes before the procedure. A disadvantage of office curettage using a small suction curet is the possibility of missing other uterine pathology, such as polyps or small submucous leiomyomata.

27. **B** (1 & 2), Page 896; Table 28-1. (from Herbst) The prevalence of cancer of the endometrium is greatest between the ages of 55 and 65. Risk factors include unopposed estrogen from any source, such as estrogen-producing ovarian tumors, polycystic ovary disease, late menopause and obesity, or oral intake of estrogens. Unopposed estrogen, whether from exogenous or endogenous sources, provides prolonged estrogen effect on the endometrium. Progestins or progesterone decreases estrogen receptor formation, stimulates the conversion of estradiol to estrone, and promotes sloughing of the endometrium when it is withdrawn. Hypertension, by itself and unrelated to obesity, is not a risk factor for endometrial carcinoma.

28. **D** (1 only), Page 896. Women who take tamoxifen for breast carcinoma are at increased risk to develop endometrial cancer.

29. **A** (All), Pages 918-919. The mainstay of therapy for stage II adenocarcinoma of the endometrium is surgery if the patient is able to tolerate it. Uterine and vaginal brachytherapy has been used before surgery in some cases and external irradiation to 40 Gray (Gy) has been given after surgery in others. Progesterone or progestins are generally used for stage III disease and for recurrences.

30. **C** (2, 3), Page 918. The spread to nodes in Stage I, grade 1 adenocarcinoma is less than 2%, while with Stage I, grade 2 the risk is approximately 11% and rises to 25 to 30% in Stage I, grade 3 adenocarcinoma. Stage II carries increased risk of pelvic node spread because there is cervical involvement. In Stage I, grade 1 carcinoma of the endometrium, the risk of nodal involvement is so low that routine sampling is not warranted.

CHAPTER

29 Neoplastic Diseases of the Ovary

DIRECTIONS for questions 1 - 16: Select the one best answer or completion.

1. A 55 year-old woman has an asymptomatic ovarian carcinoma in one ovary. Although her peritoneal cavity is free of tumor, she has retroperitoneal nodes positive for the malignancy. The stage of her ovarian tumor is
   A. I-A
   B. II-A
   C. II-B
   D. III
   E. IV
2. The approximate age at which the peak death rate from ovarian cancer occurs is
   A. 40
   B. 50
   C. 60
   D. 70
   E. 80
3. Pseudomyxoma peritonei typically is the result of a rupture of
   A. a mucinous borderline tumor
   B. a serous tumor
   C. a dysgerminoma
   D. a mature teratoma
   E. an immature teratoma
4. The cell origin of the most common type of ovarian neoplasm is
   A. germ cells
   B. epithelial cells
   C. stromal cells
   D. lipoid cells
   E. sex cord cells
5. A rare virilizing tumor of the ovary is
   A. polyembryoma
   B. mucinous cystadenocarcinoma
   C. fibroma
   D. dysgerminoma
   E. Sertoli Leydig cell tumor

Questions 6-7

6. A 65 year-old women has a 3 cm. right adnexal cyst noted on routine pelvic exam. The appropriate management is to
   A. offer reassurance
   B. repeat the exam in 2 to 3 months
   C. suppress the ovary with cyclic estrogen and progesterone
   D. order a transvaginal ultrasound
   E. perform a laparotomy
7. In the patient referred to in question 6, the additional blood test which might aid in determining management is a
   A. carcinoembryonic antigen (CEA)
   B. CA-125
   C. quantitative human chorionic gonadotropins (β-hCG)
   D. serum estrogen
   E. α-fetoprotein (AFP)
8. A 67 year-old woman has a breast mass and firm, bilaterally-enlarged ovaries. A breast biopsy reveals a mucin-secreting carcinoma. The most likely ovarian diagnosis is
   A. normal ovaries
   B. dysgerminoma
   C. clear cell carcinoma
   D. Brenner tumor
   E. Krukenberg tumor
9. A 30 year-old woman comes to you for a routine gynecologic evaluation and renewal of her birth control pills. On an otherwise normal pelvic examination, you discover a 6 cm left ovarian cyst. This patient should
   A. have her next exam in a year
   B. be re-evaluated in 2 to 3 months
   C. take 2 birth control pills a day and return in 2 to 3 months
   D. have a CT scan of the abdomen and pelvis
   E. be scheduled for laparoscopy
10. The most common type of epithelial tumor is
   A. mucinous
   B. endometrioid
   C. serous
   D. clear cell
   E. Brenner
11. After complete resection of a stage II ovarian carcinoma, chemotherapy using Alkeran is considered. A major long-term side effect is
   A. destruction of lymphocytes
   B. cardiac toxicity
   C. increased risk of leukemia

D. stomatitis
E. pulmonary fibrosis

12. A 60 year-old woman who is on no medications develops postmenopausal bleeding. On pelvic examination, she has a pink, rugated vagina and a 5 x 6 x 4 cm firm right ovarian mass. Office curettage reveals adenomatous endometrial hyperplasia without atypia. The ovarian tumor which would best account for these findings is a
    A. serous cystadenoma
    B. mucinous cystadenocarcinoma
    C. teratoma
    D. dysgerminoma
    E. granulosa cell tumor
13. A "second look" procedure in the management of an ovarian neoplasm refers to a
    A. laparoscopy done after primary debulking
    B. laparoscopy done after one year of chemotherapy when no clinical evidence of disease exists
    C. laparotomy done after one year of chemotherapy when no clinical evidence of disease exists
    D. laparoscopy for staging after an initial course of chemotherapy
    E. laparotomy done after the tumor has reoccurred
14. The second most common type of ovarian neoplasm is
    A. epithelial
    B. germ cell
    C. stromal
    D. lipoid
    E. gonadoblastoma
15. In a 22 year-old, the recommended initial treatment of a pure dysgerminoma, 6 cm in diameter, confined to one ovary is
    A. chemotherapy
    B. radiation therapy to the pelvis
    C. a radical hysterectomy and bilateral salpingo-oophorectomy
    D. a total abdominal hysterectomy, bilateral salpingo-oophorectomy and omentectomy
    E. a unilateral salpingo-oophorectomy
16. A 24 year-old gravida 0 is undergoing a laparotomy for a 6 cm adnexal mass. The mass is shelled out of the ovary and submitted for frozen section. The latter is not definitive in ruling out a malignancy. The most appropriate next step is to
    A. close the ovary and close the abdomen without removing any additional ovarian tissue
    B. proceed to a unilateral oophorectomy
    C. proceed to a unilateral salpingo-oophorectomy
    D. proceed to a total abdominal hysterectomy, bilateral salpingo-oophorectomy
    E. proceed to a total abdominal hys-

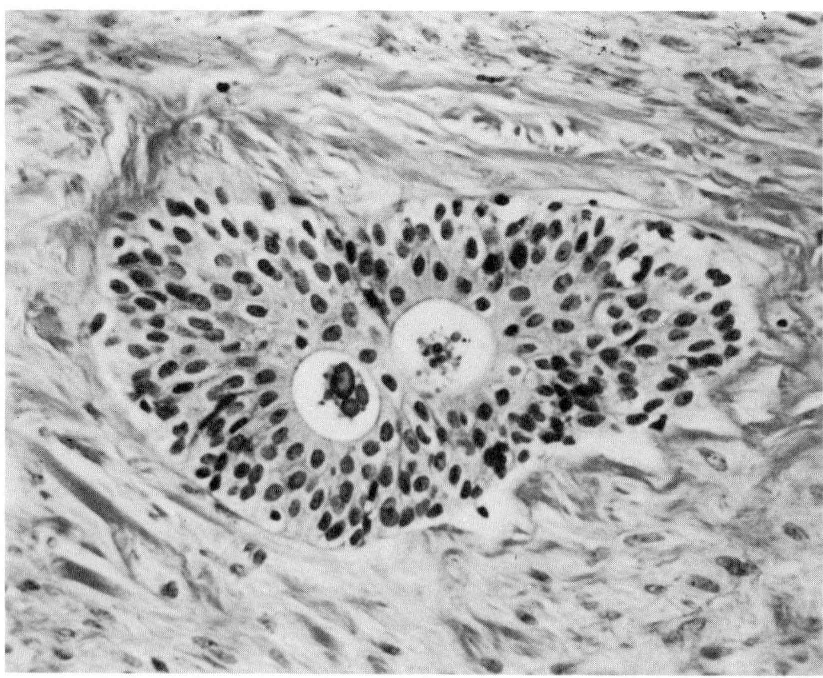

FIGURE 29-1.

terectomy, unilateral salpingo-oophorectomy

DIRECTIONS for questions 17-23: For each numbered item, select the one heading most closely associated with it. Each lettered heading may be used once, more than once, or not at all.

17-19. Match the following photomicrographs with the appropriate ovarian epithelial neoplasm
(A) serous cystadenoma
(B) mucinous cystadenoma
(C) endometrioid carcinoma
(D) clear cell adenocarcinoma
(E) Brenner cell tumor

17. Figure 29-1
18. Figure 29-2
19. Figure 29-3

20-23. Match the following photomicrographs with the appropriate ovarian neoplasm
(A) benign cystic teratoma
(B) dysgerminoma
(C) granulosa cell tumor
(D) Krukenberg tumor
(E) endodermal sinus tumor

20. Figure 29-4
21. Figure 29-5
22. Figure 29-6
23. Figure 29-7

DIRECTIONS For each numbered item 24 - 26, indicate whether it is associated with
A only (A)
B only (B)
C both (A) and (B)
D neither (A) nor (B)

24-26. Characteristic of the listed ovarian tumors
(A) germ cell tumors
(B) epithelial tumors
(C) both
(D) neither

24. produce α-fetoprotein
25. eighty percent produce CA-125
26. often contain tissue from more than one embryonic cell layer

DIRECTIONS for questions 27 - 32: For each of the questions below, ONE or MORE of the responses is correct. Select the best answer based on the following
A if 1, 2, and 3 are correct
B if only 1 and 2 are correct
C if only 2 and 3 are correct
D if only 1 is correct
E if only 3 is correct

27. Complications associated with ovarian carcinoma include
1. hydrothorax
2. malnutrition
3. bowel obstruction
28. Factors that influence the occurrence of ovarian carcinoma include
1. frequency of ovulation
2. eating a fatty diet
3. living in an industrialized country
29. Surgery for ovarian carcinoma in a 55 year-old patient includes total abdominal hysterectomy with bilateral salpingo-oophorectomy and
1. a transverse incision
2. peritoneal washings for cytology
3. periaortic node biopsy
30. The prognosis in cases of ovarian malignancy is related to the
1. stage of the tumor
2. cell type
3. patient's age

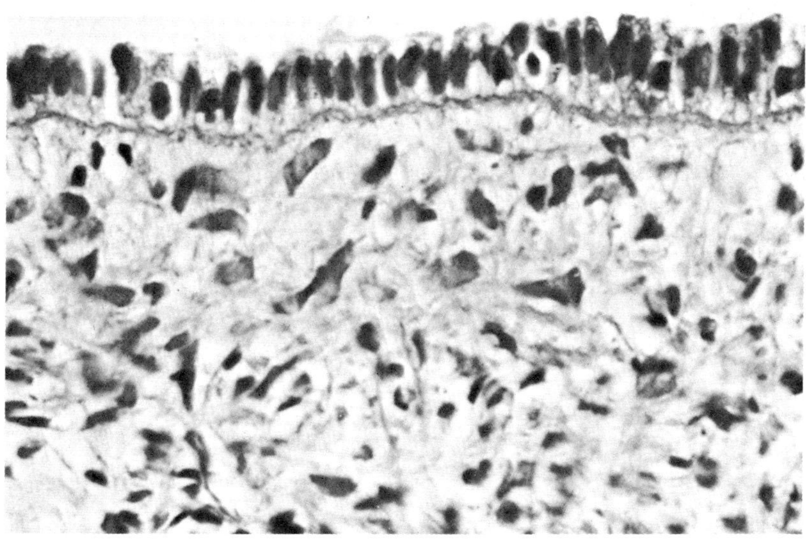

FIGURE 29-2.

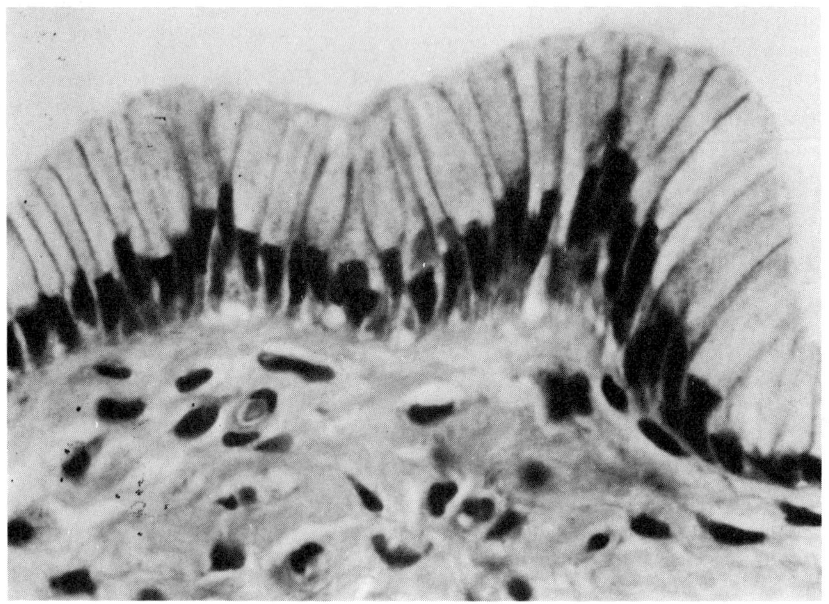

FIGURE 29-3.

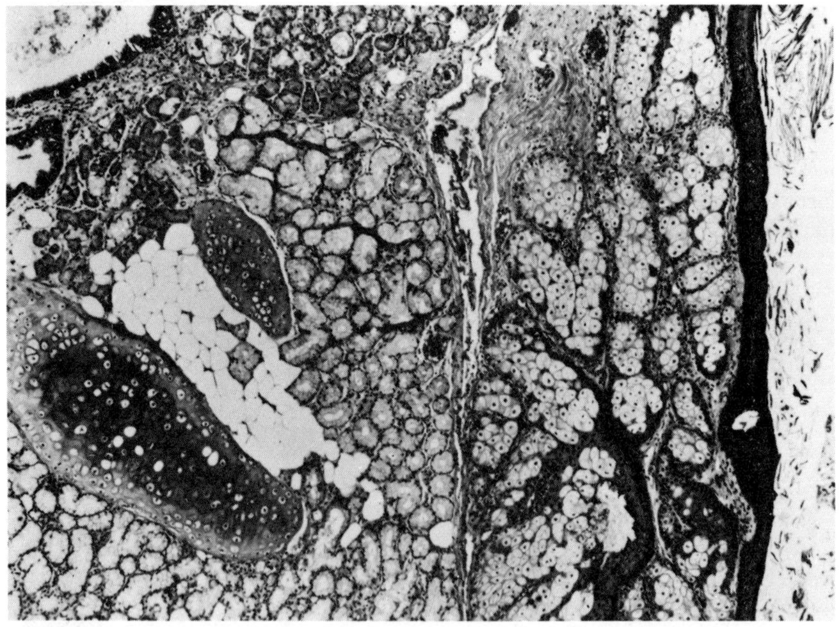

FIGURE 29-4.

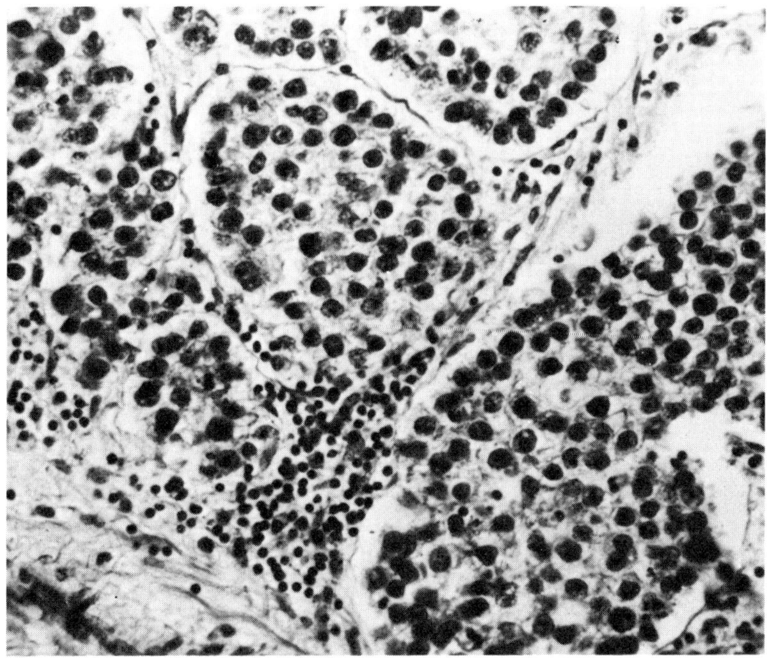

FIGURE 29-5.

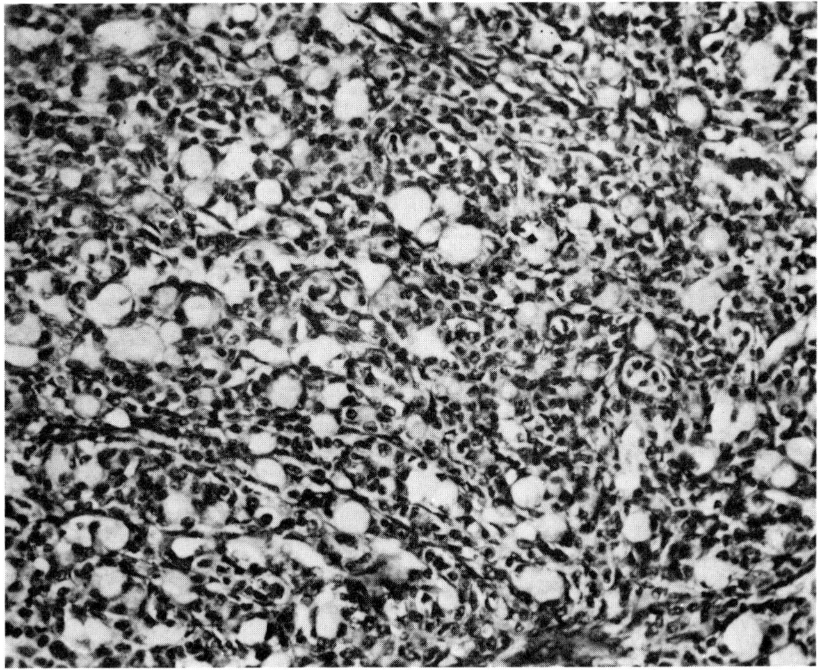

FIGURE 29-6.

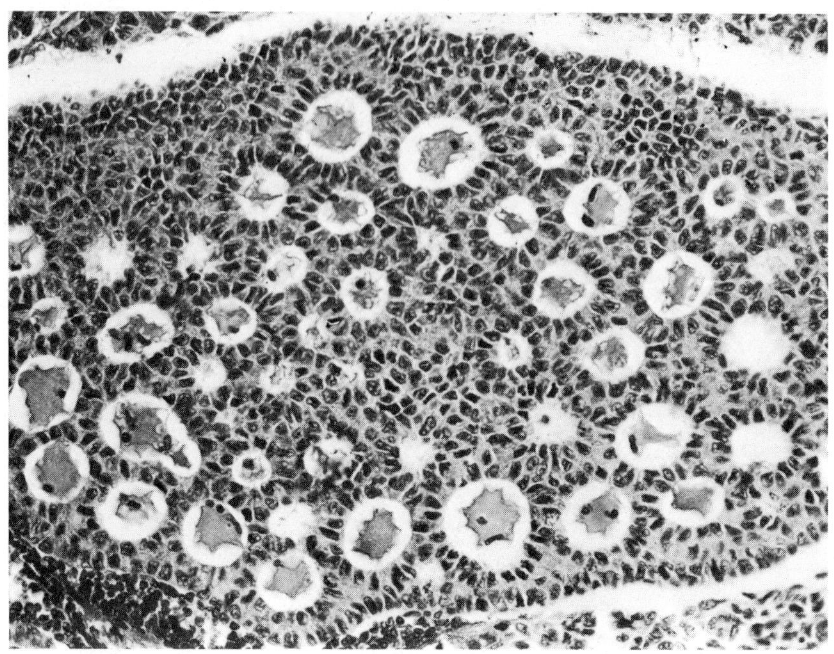

FIGURE 29-7.

31. The work-up of a 58 year-old patient with a persistent left adnexal mass should include
    1. a CT scan
    2. a barium enema
    3. cystoscopy
32. Unilateral oophorectomy alone for borderline ovarian tumors is adequate therapy if
    1. the contralateral ovary is normal
    2. peritoneal cytology is negative
    3. the tumor is stage I-A

ANSWERS

1. **D,** Page 950, Table 29-4 (from Herbst). Staging of ovarian cancer is based on the findings of the clinical examination and the surgical exploration including the histology of the specimen and cytology of fluids. In this case, the extension of the tumor to the retroperitoneal nodes places the patient in stage III. About 10 to 20% of women with carcinoma apparently confined to one ovary have been found to have retroperitoneal lymph node involvement at the time of surgery. The five year survival for stage III ovarian carcinoma is approximately 15%.
2. **E,** Page 939, Figure 29-1. Ovarian cancer causes more deaths in women than any other genital malignancy. This is due to a lack of symptoms early in the disease. Until the tumor is widespread, patients are asymptomatic. Therefore, ovarian malignancies are detected and treated late in the course of their progression. The highest death rate is in patients in their late 70's and early 80's.
3. **A,** Page 956. The rupture of a borderline mucinous tumor allows the spread of mucin-producing cells in the abdomen. They yield a large amount of mucinous material and their growth often leads to bowel obstruction. The intra-abdominal accumulation of mucin is called pseudomyxoma peritonei and can cause disability and death though it is not frankly malignant. The mucin is very difficult to remove surgically although this attempt may be aided by a copious lavage with 5% dextrose in water. Residual cells may respond to cytoxan, adriamycin and cis-platinum combination chemotherapy.
4. **B,** Page 940. Ovarian neoplasms are formed from tissues that constitute the normal ovary. These include the epithelial lining (which is the most common source of tumors), germ cells, sex cord cells and stroma. Very rarely, tumors will arise from lymphatics, blood vessels, or nerves within the ovary. Occasionally, carcinoma originating in other organs will metastasize to the ovary.
5. **E,** Pages 978-979. Sertoli Leydig tumors are the male homologue of granulosa theca

cell tumors. They may produce androgens which cause virilization in young women. Most behave as low grade malignancies with five year survivals of 70 to 90%. Higher survival rates occur when the tumor is better differentiated. Polyembryomas and dysgerminomas are both rare malignancies of germ cell origin. A mucinous tumor is derived from the epithelium of the ovary and a fibroma arises from nonfunctioning stroma.

6. **D,** Pages 947-948. The ovary decreases in size in the postmenopausal years and should be no larger than 1.5 centimeters in the greatest diameter. At this age, no physiologic enlargement should occur. Direct visualization by surgery should be accomplished if the mass is over 5 cm in diameter. Recent studies suggest that a simple cystic mass under 5 cm in size in postmenopausal patients can be followed. The use of ultrasound will aid in determining whether there are solid areas or papillations, both indications for surgical intervention.
7. **B,** Page 948. It has been reported that the addition of CA-125 may aid in the management of postmenopausal women with adnexal masses. Levels above the normal of 35 U/ml appear to indicate a higher likelihood of malignancy. They are also associated with benign conditions such as endometriosis, but utilizing this serum assay in conjunction with ultrasound, appears to help determine when surgical intervention is appropriate in the **postmenopausal** patient.
8. **E,** Page 980. Krukenburg tumors of the ovary contain mucin-producing signet ring cells and are usually metastatic from the GI tract (most commonly) or the breast. In this case, with a known mucin-secreting tumor of the breast, bilateral ovarian metastases are most likely. Dysgerminomas may occur in the elderly but are most common in young women, and are also rarely bilateral. Fibromas and Brenner tumors are also rarely bilateral, and clear cell carcinomas are relatively rare malignant ovarian epithelial tumors. In this case it would be extremely unwise to dismiss the ovaries, which are described as enlarged, as being normal.
9. **E,** Page 948. In a reproductive aged woman on no birth control pills or other ovarian suppressive treatment, the development of physiologic ovarian cysts is common and requires only observation for a short period of time. Most physiologic ovarian cysts resolve within one cycle. However, as birth control pills containing 50 micrograms of ethinyl estradiol have been felt to suppress physiologic ovarian cysts, any cyst that occurs while on oral contraceptives is much more likely to be a neoplasm. Therefore, these patients should be evaluated surgically. A CT scan or ultrasound cannot reliably distinguish between physiologic or neoplastic lesions, although identification of anything other than a simple cyst would increase the need for surgical exploration. With the advent of pelviscopic surgical techniques, many experts prefer laparoscopy over laparotomy.
10. **C,** Page 941. Epithelial tumors are the most common neoplasms of the ovary, and serous tumors are the most common of the epithelial tumors. Like most ovarian neoplasms, they can be either benign or malignant. Malignant serous tumor have the worst prognosis of all the epithelial tumors. They are bilateral in 33% to 66% of the cases.
11. **C,** Page 959. Alkeran causes bone marrow depression within two weeks. It also has the long-term side effect of increasing the risk of leukemia. This risk may range from 2% to as high as 10% within eight years of therapy. It is, therefore, important to give Alkeran only if the benefits of its use are significant. Stomatitis is more commonly seen as an acute side effect with the antimetabolites. Pulmonary fibrosis is found with bleomycin and cardiac toxicity with adriamycin. Renal damage is of significant concern with *cis*-platinum.
12. **E,** Page 977. Sex cord stromal tumors account for about 6% of all ovarian neoplasms. Some of these produce hormones. This woman has signs of an estrogen effect without being on any replacement hormones or medications. Such symptoms together with a firm adnexal mass make the possibility of a granulosa or theca cell tumor quite likely. These tumors behave as low grade carcinomas and are primarily treated surgically. A total abdominal hysterectomy and bilateral salpingo-oophorectomy should be performed in a patient of this age with such a tumor.
13. **C,** Page 962. A second-look procedure is a **laparotomy** done after a year of chemotherapy when no clinical evidence of tumor exists. It is therefore done in a patient who is in clinical remission. This pro-

cedure includes extensive biopsy and cytologic sampling of the peritoneal cavity including the retroperitoneal nodes. It is done to determine the need to continue or ability to discontinue chemotherapy. If the second look procedure is negative, the five year survival in patients with epithelial ovarian cancer is approximately 80%. The use of this approach remains controversial, as does the role of laparoscopy prior to the second look laparotomy.

14. **B,** Page 967. Physiologic cysts are the most common cause of ovarian enlargement. Of the neoplasms, epithelial tumors are the most common (approximately 65%) while germ cell derived tumors are the second most common (approximately 20 to 25%). The most frequent germ cell tumor is the benign cystic teratoma which, as its name implies, is benign and can be treated by simple removal. Only 2 to 3% of germ cell tumors are malignant. These include some very rare tumors such as the polyembryoma, the embryonal carcinoma, endodermal sinus tumors and the relatively more common dysgerminoma.
15. **E,** Pages 973-974. Insofar as patients with dysgerminoma are young, preservation of the childbearing function is desirable, if possible. The tumor can spread within the peritoneal cavity and to retroperitoneal nodes, a more likely occurrence with larger dysgerminomas. If the tumor is confined to one ovary, a unilateral salpingo-oophorectomy should be performed and the abdomen thoroughly explored to determine the presence of intraperitoneal and retroperitoneal spread. Pelvic, and paraaortic nodes should be sampled and any enlarged nodes excised. The contralateral ovary should have a wedge biopsy even if it appears normal. If frozen section indicates pure dysgerminoma and there is no evidence of spread outside the primary tumor, only a unilateral salpingo-oophorectomy is indicated The 5-year survival is in excess of 90%. Approximately 20% will recur but they can be treated by chemotherapy, radiotherapy or additional surgery. These tumors are extremely radiosensitive.
16. **A,** Page 947. In the 24 year-old patient described, if the frozen section obtained at the time of laparotomy for a suspected ovarian tumor cannot confirm the diagnosis of malignancy, the procedure should be terminated after removal of the ovarian tumor alone. A second procedure can subsequently be performed if malignancy is confirmed after detailed evaluation of the permanent sections. This is preferable to performing an unnecessary hysterectomy or other procedure in a patient who otherwise might desire to preserve her childbearing potential.

17-19. 17, **E;** 18, **A;** 19, **B;** Pages 942-943, 947; Figure 29-1, From Atlas of tumor pathology, Fascicle 16, 2nd series. Washington, DC, Armed Forces Institute of Pathology, 1979; Figure 29-2 and Figure 29-3, From Serov SF, Scully RE, Sobin LH: Histologic typing of ovarian tumors. Geneva, World Health Organization, 1973. Serous cystadenomas, mucinous cystadenomas, endometrioid carcinomas, clear cell carcinomas, and Brenner cell tumors are the five cell types that comprise the epithelial tumors of the ovary. They may form tumors that are either benign or malignant. Serous tumors are the most common neoplasm and also are the most common of the malignancies. Their lining epithelium resembles tubal epithelium. Mucinous tumors resemble endocervical mucinous cells and endometrioid tumors resemble the endometrium. The Brenner cell tumor has island of cells that resemble the Walthard cell nests of the ovary or the transitional epithelium of the bladder. A lot of ovarian stroma is found between these islands of epithelial cells. It is a rare tumor and is almost always benign. Clear cell tumors are found in the endometrium, as well as the ovary, and are malignant. They have a clear cell and a hobnail pattern.

20-23. 20, **A;** 21, **B;** 22, **D;** 23, **C;** Pages 973, 977, 980; Figure 29-4, From Serov SF, Scully RE, Sobin LH: Histologic typing of ovarian tumors. Geneva, World Health Organization, 1973: Figure 29-5, From Scully RE: Germ cell tumors of the ovary and fallopian tube. In Meigs JV, Sturgis SH, eds: Progress in Gynecology, vol. 4. New York, Grune & Stratton, 1963; Figure 29-6, From Droegemueller W, Herbst AL, Mishell DR, Stenchever MA: Comprehensive Gynecology, St. Louis. The CV Mosby Co, 1987; Figure 29-7, From Scully RE, Morris J: Functioning ovarian tumors In Meigs JV, Sturgis SH, eds: Progress in Gynecology, vol. 3. New York, Grune & Stratton, 1957; Benign, mature, cystic teratomas (dermoids) contain cells derived from all germ layers. They can occur at any time, but are most common during the reproductive age. There is histologic differentiation into different adult tissues. Cystic teratomas may even contain functional glands such as thyroid (struma ovarii). The histology shown is that of benign adult tissue. The rare malignant variants usually are associated with differentiation of the squamous components. The ovarian dysgerminoma consists of multiple germ cells with a stroma infiltrated by lymphocytes. It is analogous to the seminoma in the male. Dysgerminomas are most common in women under the age of 30 and are bilateral in about 10% of the cases. The Krukenberg tumor contains mucin-filled signet-ring malignant cells. They are metastatic to the ovary usually from the GI tract or breast. Therefore, if one is found in the ovary, a careful search for the primary lesion should be undertaken. Granulosa cell tumors are made up of granulosa cells from the specialized stroma of the ovary. They contain some fibroblasts and theca cells in varying proportions. The histopathological section shown also contains Call-Exner bodies. These are eosinophilic bodies surrounded by granulosa cells. Call-Exner bodies are also found in normal follicles. Granulosa cell tumors are quite rare, but they are mentioned infrequently because they can secrete hormones (primarily estrogen) and cause premature puberty and postmenopausal bleeding. Granulosa cell tumors behave as low grade malignancies and have a greater than 90% 10-year survival.

24-26. 24, **A**; 25, **B**; 26, **A**; Pages 949, 967. Approximately 80% of patients with epithelial ovarian cancer have increased amounts of the ovarian antibody designated CA-125 levels, which can be used to monitor the development of recurrent disease. However, as this test has a high false negative rate, it cannot be the only method used for monitoring. Germ cell tumors are derived from the toti potential germ cell, and therefore, are capable of producing many of the proteins found during the development of the embryo such as α-fetoprotein, which is produced by endodermal sinus tumors. Germ cell tumors may differentiate to mimic the three developmental layers of the embryo, namely the ectoderm, endoderm and mesoderm.

27. **A** (1, 2, 3), Page 949. A malignant or benign hydrothorax or ascites can occur with ovarian carcinoma. The fluid tends to reaccumulate especially if the tumor is malignant. Bowel obstruction and malnutrition are common late sequelae of ovarian cancer. Bowel obstruction may be treated by resection and malnutrition may be treated by hyperalimentation.

28. **A** (1, 2, 3), Pages 939-940. Women who ovulate less frequently, either because they took birth control pills or were often pregnant, appear to be less prone to develop ovarian carcinoma. Factors that increase the risk of ovarian carcinoma are living in an industrialized country, and eating a diet high in animal fat. A familial occurrence of ovarian cancer has also been reported.

29. **C** (2, 3), Page 958. When performing surgery for suspected ovarian carcinoma, a **vertical** incision should be used. Peritoneal washings or ascitic fluid should be sent for cytology. A total abdominal hysterectomy and bilateral salpingo-oophorectomy plus omentectomy should be done, as well as biopsy of peritoneal surfaces and sampling of periaortic nodes. An attempt should be made to reduce the tumor to the smallest residual mass. The patient's response to postoperative therapy is improved if residual masses are less than 2 cm in diameter.

30. **B** (1, 2), Pages 949-950. The higher the stage and grade of the ovarian tumor, the poorer the prognosis. Cell type is also important with undifferentiated and serous tumors having the worst prognosis. The amount of residual tumor after maximum removal is a factor in prognosis. The greater the amount of residual tumor, the less well the patient responds to chemotherapy. The age of the patient at the time of surgery is not a prognostic indicator.

31. **B** (1, 2), Page 949. A patient with a suspected ovarian malignancy (which must be considered in any post menopausal woman with an adnexal mass) should have, in addition to a thorough history and physical, a chest x-ray, hematocrit, white blood cell count and blood chemistry. She should also have a CT scan of the abdomen to look for retroperitoneal node involvement. A barium enema is important to rule out bowel carcinoma and to establish a baseline of bowel integrity in the event of future radiation treatment. Sigmoidoscopy is indicated if there is gastrointestinal bleeding. Cystoscopy need only be done if bladder involvement is suspected.

32. **A** (1, 2, 3), Page 955. Conservative ther-

apy for borderline tumors with preservation of childbearing function may be carried out by performing unilateral oophorectomy under the following conditions: (1) the tumor is confirmed to be stage I-A; (2) a histologic sampling of the tumor confirms that it is grade 0 (borderline); (3) the contralateral ovary appears normal; (4) the biopsy specimens of omentum and peritoneum are negative; (5) peritoneal cytologic tests are negative.

CHAPTER 30

Premalignant and Malignant Diseases of the Vulva

DIRECTIONS for questions 1 - 20: Select the one best answer or completion.

1. One of the primary histologic differences between vulvar intraepithelial neoplasia and vulvar squamous hyperplasia is
   A. a difference in the degree of nuclear enlargement
   B. the thickness of the surface hyperkeratosis
   C. the depth of rete ridges
   D. the presence of perinuclear halo
   E. an intraepithelial inflammatory cell infiltrate
2. The chromosome distribution of vulvar intraepithelial neoplasia grade III (carcinoma in situ) is most likely to be
   A. haploid
   B. diploid
   C. triploid
   D. aneuploid
   E. mosaic
3. A 52 year-old woman presents to your office with a six month history of vulvar pruritus. Examination reveals diffuse whitish plaque-like areas extending from the perineal body along the lower one half on the left labium majus. There is obvious excoriation around these lesions. Vulvar biopsy reveals histologic findings shown in figure 30-1. Treatment of this patient should be
   A. wide local excision
   B. laser vaporization
   C. topical testosterone propionate
   D. topical fluorinated corticosteroids
   E. topical 5-fluorouracil
4. Taken as a whole, progression of all grades of vulvar intraepithelial neoplasia (VIN) to invasive carcinoma is estimated to be
   A. 6%
   B. 12%
   C. 19%
   D. 24%
   E. 30%
5. The most common human papilloma virus (HPV) subtypes found in benign vulvar warts are
   A. 6 and 11
   B. 16 and 18
   C. 31 and 33
   D. 35 and 37
   E. 40 and 41
6. In a 42 year-old patient with VIN-III (carcinoma in situ) involving the lower one half of the left labium majus (approximately one quarter of the vulvar circumference), the best treatment is
   A. total vulvectomy
   B. total subcutaneous vulvectomy
   C. wide local excision of the involved area
   D. cryocautery with liquid nitrogen
   E. topical 5-fluorouracil cream
7. The main lymphatic drainage for a unilateral malignant lesion of the vulva occurring in the anterior one third of the vulva is
   A. through the ipsilateral inguinal-femoral nodes
   B. through the contralateral inguinal-femoral nodes
   C. directly into the ipsilateral deep pelvic nodes
   D. directly into the contralateral deep pelvic nodes
8. The curve in Figure 30-2 that most likely illustrates the survival of a stage II vulvar epidermoid carcinoma is
   A. line A
   B. line B
   C. line C
   D. line D
9. Microinvasive carcinoma of the vulva may be defined as
   A. contained within the basement membrane
   B. extending within 1 mm beyond the basement membrane
   C. extending within 3 mm beyond the basement membrane
   D. extending within 5 mm beyond the basement membrane
   E. stage 1A
10. The optimal therapy for a 78 year-old patient who has diabetes mellitus, severe atherosclerotic heart disease and a stage III squamous carcinoma of the left labium majus is

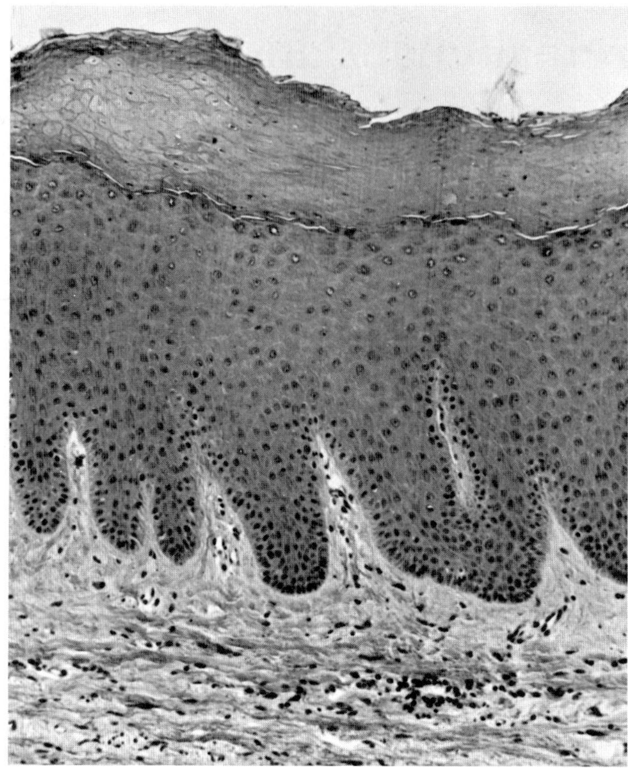

FIGURE 30-1.

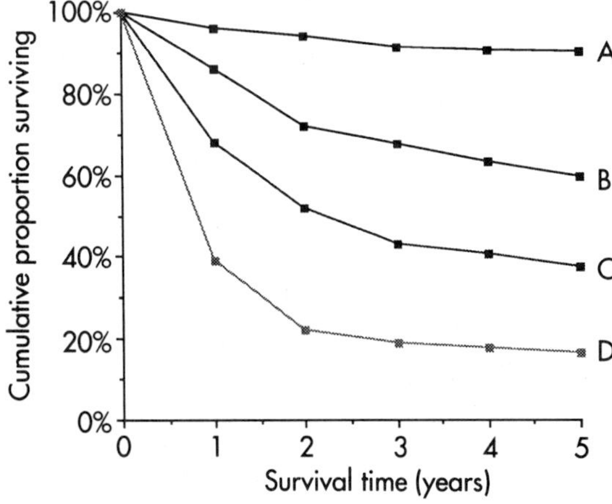

FIGURE 30-2.

A. radical left hemivulvectomy with regional lymph node irradiation
B. radical total vulvectomy with regional lymph node irradiation
C. radiation therapy of the primary lesion alone
D. combination radiotherapy and chemotherapy using intravenous 5-fluorouracil
E. systemic chemotherapy alone using intravenous 5-fluorouracil

11. A 68 year-old patient has had a wide local excision (2 cm margins) for what is interpreted to be a Clark's level II superficial spreading melanoma of the vulva. The expected five year survival is
    A. 10%
    B. 25%
    C. 50%
    D. 75%
    E. 100%
12. A "sore" is noted on the the left side of the clitoris. The biopsy diagnosis is squamous carcinoma with penetration to 5 mm and capillary space and lymphatic involvement. It is determined that this is a stage I lesion using the 1988 FIGO recommendations. The optimal treatment would be
    A. radical vulvectomy with bilateral inguinal-femoral node dissection
    B. radical vulvectomy with left inguinal-femoral node dissection
    C. radical vulvectomy alone
    D. laser excision of the visible lesion
    E. radiation therapy of the visible lesion
13. During a lymphadenectomy of the inguinal-femoral nodes performed as part

of the therapy for a 1988 FIGO stage II carcinoma of the vulva, the surgeon recognizes that several of the nodes contain tumor. Therapy now should include

A. an ipsilateral deep pelvic lymphadenectomy
B. a bilateral deep pelvic lymphadenectomy
C. radiotherapy to ipsilateral deep pelvic nodes
D. radiotherapy to bilateral deep pelvic nodes
E. triple-agent chemotherapy

14. A 28 year-old woman has biopsy proven carcinoma in situ of a 2 x 3 cm acuminate lesion on the posterior fourchette. The best treatment for this patient is
A. a total vulvectomy
B. a skinning vulvectomy
C. topical 5-fluorouracil
D. multiple trichloroacetic acid applications
E. a wide local excision

15. A 62 year-old woman has a lesion on the left labium majus that is biopsied. It is a stage 1A carcinoma of the vulva based on International Society for the Study of Vulvar Disease (ISSVD) criteria. Treatment should consist of
A. wide local excision
B. topical 5-fluorouracil
C. simple vulvectomy
D. radical vulvectomy
E. primary radiation therapy

16. A 72 year-old woman presents with a 9-month history of progressive vulvar pruritus. Examination of the vulva reveals diffuse erythema with excoriations and a 1 1/2 cm, slightly raised lesion of the posterior left labium majus. The next step in her management should be
A. Excision of the raised lesion
B. Podophyllin to the raised lesion
C. Prescribe topical corticosteroid cream
D. Office laser vaporization of the raised lesion
E. Office cryocautery of the raised lesion

17. A 71 year-old woman comes to your office with a "swelling" in her vagina for the past 4 months. Pelvic examination is unremarkable except for a 4 x 4 cm, slightly tender, moderately firm mass in the inferior medial portion of the right labium majus. The overlying skin appears normal for a woman in this age group. Your next step would be
A. vulvar colposcopy (vulvoscopy)
B. to treat with topical fluorinated steroids as a diagnostic trial
C. to incise and drain
D. to biopsy the mass
E. to ablate the mass with laser

18. Biopsy of a 9 cm condylomatous mass on the left labium majus of a 48 year-old woman reveals a verrucous carcinoma. This tumor is best managed by
A. laser ablation
B. wide local excision
C. radical vulvectomy
D. radical vulvectomy with ipsilateral inguinal-femoral lymphadenectomy
E. radical vulvectomy with bilateral inguinal-femoral lymphadenectomy

Questions 19-20

19. A 71 year-old woman with a 2-year history of progressive vulvar itching presents for treatment. The vulva has a homogeneous "onion skin" appearance. A vulvar biopsy obtained as part of your evaluation is shown in Figure 30-3. The correct diagnosis is
A. squamous hyperplasia
B. vulvar intraepithelial neoplasia (VIN) II
C. Paget's disease
D. carcinoma in situ
E. lichen sclerosus

20. The next step in your management of this patient should be

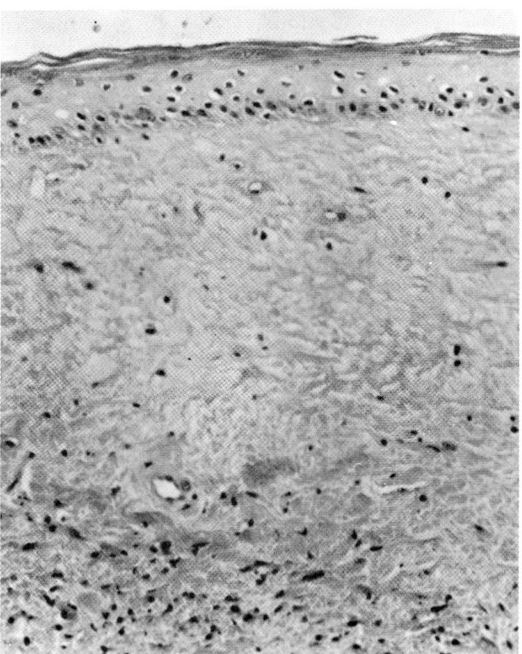

FIGURE 30-3.

(From Friedrich EG, Wilkinson EJ: The vulva. In Blaustein A, ed: Pathology of the female genital tract, 2nd ed. New York, Springer-Verlag, 1982.)

A. oral conjugated estrogen
B. topical estrogen cream
C. vulvar colposcopy
D. simple vulvectomy
E. topical testosterone cream

DIRECTIONS for questions 21 - 22: For each numbered item, select the one heading most closely associated with it. Each lettered heading may be used once, more than once, or not at all.

21-22. Match figures 30-4 and 30-5 with the most likely diagnosis
(A) Paget's disease
(B) lichen sclerosis
(C) verrucous carcinoma
(D) squamous hyperplasia
(E) melanoma

21. figure 30-4
22. figure 30-5

DIRECTIONS for questions 23 - 29: For each of the questions below, ONE or MORE of the responses is correct. Select the best answer based on the following

A if 1, 2, and 3 are correct
B if only 1 and 2 are correct
C if only 2 and 3 are correct
D if only 1 is correct
E if only 3 is correct

23. A 68 year-old woman has just had surgery for stage 1B carcinoma of the vulva. She has positive inguinal-femoral nodes. Factors important in determining chance of long term survival include the
    1. number of metastatic nodes
    2. size of metastatic nodes
    3. proximity of metastatic nodes to the primary tumor
24. A 72 year-old woman presents with an 18 month history of progressive pruritus. The vulvar skin has a diffuse, reddened eczematoid appearance. The vulvar biopsy you obtained is reproduced in Figure 30-6. This patient should have
    1. her stool tested for blood
    2. mammography
    3. a total vulvectomy
25. Excisional biopsy of a 4 mm pigmented, ulcerated lesion is performed on the left labium minus, near the clitoral hood of a 52 year-old woman. Histologic diagnosis confirms malignant melanoma. Correct observations regarding this lesion include
    1. a melanoma is the most frequent non squamous malignancy of the vulva.
    2. melanomas arises from compound nevi.
    3. local excision is adequate treatment.
26. A 68 year-old patient is evaluated for a

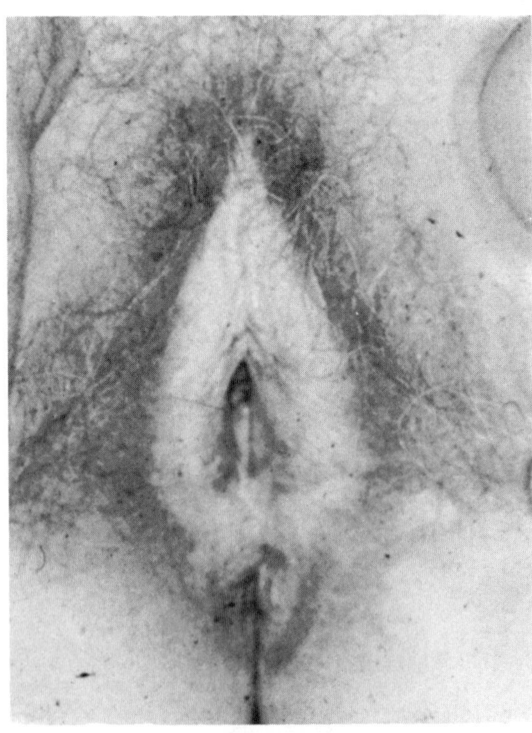

FIGURE 30-4.

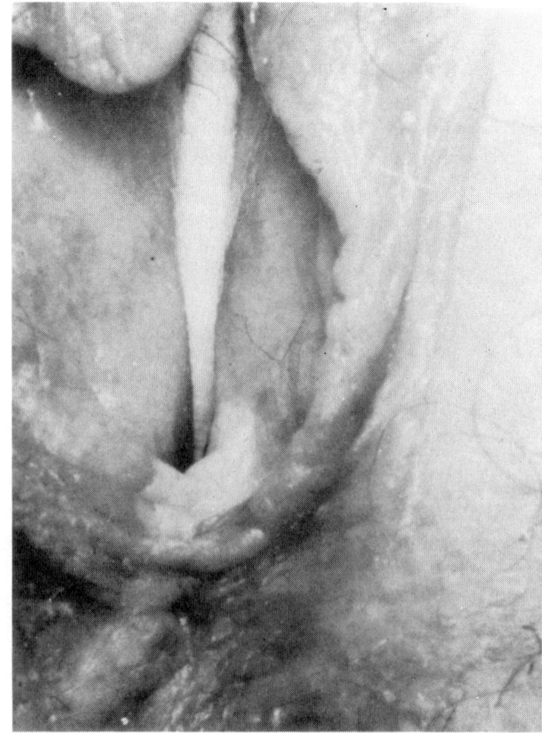

FIGURE 30-5.

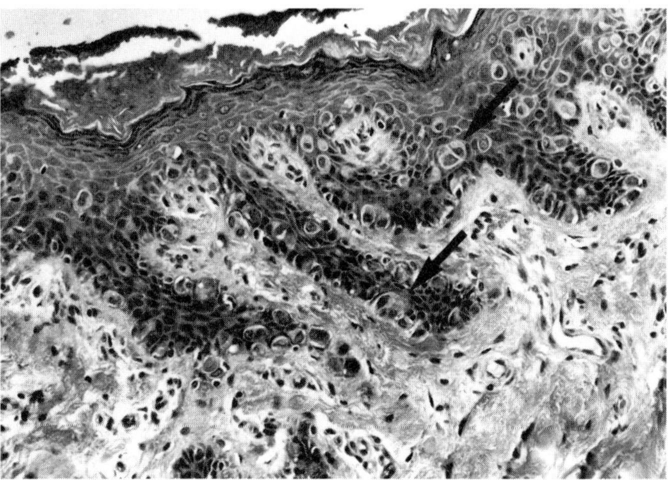

FIGURE 30-6.
Vulvar epidermis with Paget's disease. Malignamt cells *(arrows)* are seen infiltrating the epidermis and spreading along the dermal-epidermal junction. (H&E × 160.) (Courtesy Dr. Anthony Montag, The University of Chicago.)

one year history of vulvar pruritus. On physical examination she has diffuse patchy hyperkeratoticwhite lesions scattered around the posterior two thirds of the vulva. Based on physical exam assessment alone, the correct term or terms that may be applied to these lesions include
1. leukoplakia
2. leukoplakic vulvitus
3. vulvar atypia

27. In assessing suspected vulvar atypia, solutions which can be used to highlight abnormal areas include
    1. Lugol's solution
    2. toluidine blue
    3. acetic acid
28. True statements regarding the likelihood that vulvar intraepithelial neoplasia (VIN) will progress to invasive carcinoma embody
    1. the progression of VIN to invasive carcinoma is rare
    2. the risk of progression of VIN to invasive cancer is higher in older patients
    3. the risk of invasion is higher in those with raised lesions
29. Factors related to the prognosis of invasive squamous cell carcinoma include the
    1. location of the lesion
    2. size of the lesion
    3. tumor thickness

ANSWERS

1. **A,** Page 991. Nomenclature has changed in describing vulvar disease processes. Currently nonmalignant vulvar disease is classified as vulvar intraepithelial neoplasia (VIN); lichen sclerosis, which has not changed; squamous hyperplasia not otherwise specified, was previously referred to as hyperplastic dystrophy; and miscellaneous diagnoses including dermatoses and Paget's disease. The main difference between simple squamous hyperplasia and vulvar intraepithelial neoplasia is the degree of nuclear enlargement. VIN of the vulva almost always contains nuclei which have a fourfold or greater difference in size, while differences in the sizeof nuclei in condyloma or non-neoplastic epithelia are threefold or less. Depth or confluence of the rete ridges, degree of hyperkeratosis, inflammatory cells infiltrate, and perinuclear halo do not relate to the degree of atypia. Abnormal mitoses are usually observed in vulvar intraepithelial neoplasia.
2. **D,** Page 993. Nuclear characteristics of carcinoma in situ of the vulva shares similarities with the cervix. In many lesions there are multinucleated cells, abnormal mitoses, and increased density in cells as well as an increase in the nuclear to cytoplasmic ratio. Studies of the chromosome distribution of these lesions have indicated

that they are aneuploid as measured by DNA analysis.

3. **D,** Page 993; Figure 30-1 from Friedrich EG and Wilkinson EJ: The vulva. In Blaustein A, editor: Pathology of the female genital tract, New York, 1982, Springer-Verlag. Areas of squamous hyperplasia frequently appear as whitish lesions which appear thickened in focal or multifocal areas rather than the diffuse "onion skin" appearance of lichen sclerosis. Biopsy is necessary to establish the diagnosis. The histologic appearance seen in figure 30-1 is characteristic. This shows benign hyperplastic dystrophy, hyperkeratosis, acanthosis, and mild inflammation. In addition to local measures to diminish irritation, topical fluorinated corticosteroids are helpful to control the itching. Frequently used preparations are 0.025% or 0.1% triamcinaolone acetonide (Aristocort, Kenalog), fluorocinolone acetonide (Synalar), or betamethazone valerate (Valisone). These are usually applied twice daily to control the itching, which is relieved in one or two weeks. Since prolonged use of these relatively strong topical corticosteroids may be associated with vulvar atrophy, long term control of symptoms may be effected by intermittent use of 1% hydrocortisone.
4. **A,** Page 1000. Progression of VIN to invasive carcinoma is rare and has been estimated to occur in about 6% of all cases. A comparable proportion of VIN spontaneously regresses. Although VIN is being diagnosed more commonly in younger women, the risk of progression to invasivecancer is higher for those who are older as well as those who are immunosuppressed.
5. **A,** Page 1001. The potential role of human papilloma virus (HPV) has begun to be extensively studied in cases of VIN. HPV vulvar infection is widespread and is associated histologically with koilocytosis as well as intraepithelial neoplasia in some patients. Currently, HPV types 6 and 11 are generally recognized as being found more frequently in benign vulvar warts whereas HPV type 16, 18, 31, 33, and 35 are more frequently associated with intraepithelial neoplasia and even invasive carcinoma.
6. **C,** Pages 1001-1002. Management of vulvar intraepithelial neoplasia is particularly complicated and requires long-term follow-up. Many lesions are multifocal with widely separated areas being involved. Most lesions of intraepithelial neoplasia tend to be posterior predominantly in the perianal or lower labial areas. Types of therapy have changed in the last few years. In the past simple vulvectomy was widely used. This was then replaced by a "skinning vulvectomy". Both of these operations are disfiguring and probably unnecessary unless the entire vulva is covered with these lesions. Wide local excision of the affected area can be used with approximately 70% of patients not experiencing a recurrence. This is comparable to either a total or "skinning vulvectomy." If topical ablation is to be used, laser vaporization is preferable to liquid nitrogen cryotherapy. Although topical 5-fluorouracil cream has been used, it is associated with particularly bothersome complications over a prolonged period of time. It is generally not prescribed.
7. **A,** Page 1005, Figure 30-15. Tumors located in the anterior third or middle of either labium tend to drain initially into the ipsilateral inguinal-femoral nodes whereas perineal or clitoral tumors may spread into either right or left side. Although there has been concern in the past that tumors in the clitoral-urethral area would spread directly to the deep pelvic nodes, current evidence indicates that this rarely, if ever, occurs.
8. **B,** Page 1006. Figure 30-2 has been adapted from Herbst et al. Figure 30-16 which wasadapted from the 20th Report of End Results of Therapy of Gynecologic Malignancies, Stockholm, 1988, International Federation of Gynecology and Obstetrics. Nothing unusual exists regarding the information about five year survival rates of vulvar cancer patients. The graph shows a typical five year survival plot, based on stage of disease, with better survival occurring in earlier stages. Line A represents stage I, line B stage II, line C stage III, and line D stage IV. Although there are quantitative differences in other gynecologic malignancies, invariably other gynecologic malignancies can be represented in this general graphic format.
9. **E,** Page 1007. The term microinvasive carcinoma of the vulva has no uniformly accepted definition. Part of the confusion is due to different points from which the depth of invasion is measured, that is, from the surface of the tumor or from the basement membrane. The International

Society for the Study of Vulvar Disease (ISSVD) has recommended that the term microinvasion be dropped and the designation stage 1A be used for tumors less than 2 cm in diameter with depth of invasion less than 1 mm from the dermal stromal junction (basement membrane).

10. **D,** Page 1012. Combined use of chemotherapy and radiation has been introduced as a new and apparently effective means of treating recurrent and occasionally large primary vulvar carcinomas, particularly in patients who are not good operative candidates. Thus, the patient illustrated in this case as having atherosclerotic heart disease and diabetes might be such a candidate. This type of combined chemotherapy and radiation therapy is being used more widely in the treatment of squamous cell carcinomas of the lower genital tract and is described further in chapter 27 of Herbst et al.
11. **E,** Page 1014.

    The prognosis for vulvar melanoma has improved in part because most of them are of the superficialspreading (good prognosis) variety rather than the nodular (poor prognosis) variety. Although firm recommendations from available data are not possible, a reasonable approach is to excise a melanoma with a 2 cm margin without node dissection for tumors that are less than 2 mm thick. Long-term results for lesions that correspond to Clark level I or II suggest five year survivals in the vicinity of 100%.
12. **A,** Page 1010. Effective therapy for stage I or II and some early stage III vulvar carcinomas can be accomplished with a radical vulvectomy and bilateral inguinal-femoral node dissection. Previous doctrine suggested that because of the patterns of lymphatic drainage, it is important with all invasive vulvar carcinomas to perform bilateral groin dissection. In view of recent evidence that suggests that deep pelvic nodes are virtually never involved unless the inguinal nodes are also involved, most oncologists now remove only the inguinal-femoral nodes at the time of primary surgery. Likewise, unless the lesion is **central,** such as clitoral, most would perform only an ipsilateral dissection. Laser excision or primary radiation is unacceptable

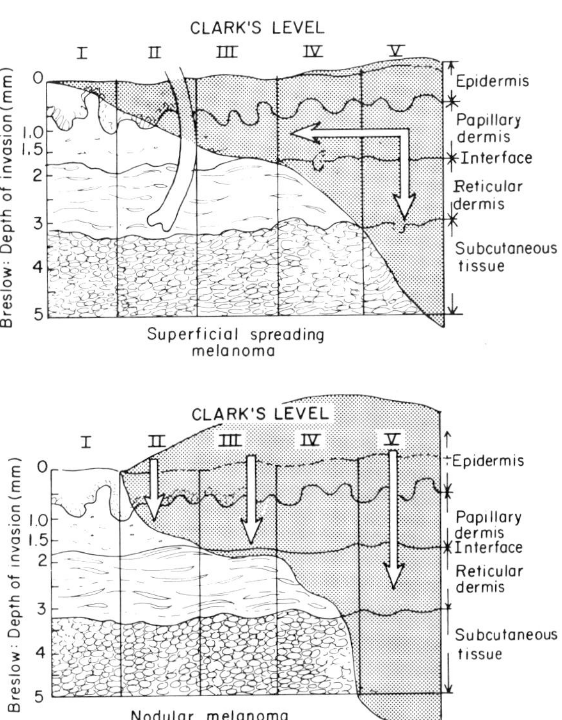

FIGURE 30-7.

Level of invasion for superficial spreading melanoma and nodular melanoma.

From Podratz KC, Gaffey TA, Symmonds RE, et al: Gynecol Oncol 16:153, 1983.)

treatment. A deep pelvic node dissection can be done if, in the frozen or permanent section of histologic specimen, the inguinal-femoral nodes are found to be involved with tumor.

13. **D,** Page 1011. A recent national cooperative randomized study suggested that radiation therapy to the deep pelvic nodes is superior to surgical therapy when it is known that the inguinal-femoral nodes contain tumor. This report indicated improved survival associated with less morbidity for those patients who received radiation of 4500 to 5000 rads. Although chemotherapy may be used for disseminated disease as a palliative measure, no chemotherapeutic regimen has been successful in treating this disease.
14. **E,** Page 1009. Wide local excision is the best treatment for a patient with an isolated lesion of the posterior fourchette that proves to be carcinoma in situ. In the past, simple vulvectomy was widely practiced to treat carcinoma in situ of the vulva, but this disfiguring operation is now infrequently used and has been shown to be unnecessary. This is particularly true in youngerwomen. Skinning vulvectomy has been advocated, followed by split-thickness vulvar skin grafting. In this case, with a small lesion, such a procedure would constitute more treatment than is necessary. 5-Fluorouracil cream has also been used to treat carcinoma in situ of the vulva. It is successful in approximately 75% of cases. However, this treatment causes severe vulvar edema and pain over a prolonged period of time and usually is not prescribed for isolated lesions. Concentrated trichloroacetic acid applications are used to treat condyloma acuminata when they are **not** associated with severe vulvar intraepithelial neoplasia. This treatment is unacceptable for true cases of carcinoma in situ.
15. **A,** Page 1011. For stage 1A lesions as defined by the International Society for the Study of Vulvar Disease (ISSVD), therapy may be less extensive than is usually employed for invasive vulvar carcinoma. Based on currently available evidence, treatment for this lesion is controversial. Protocols are being developed to evaluate the best therapy. It would appear that most patients with stage 1A carcinoma of the vulva would no longer be treated with a modified radical or radical vulvectomy. The lymph node dissection is omitted or deferred depending on the final pathologic evaluation of the primary tumor. A wide local excision appears to be adequate therapy.
16. **A,** Page 1010. A typical invasive vulvar carcinoma usually appears as a slightly raised or polyploid mass. The patient frequently complains of a "sore" that has not healed. Prolonged vulvar pruritus is frequently associated with this disease. Delay in diagnosis is common because older patients fail to seek prompt medical attention and often, when they do, a biopsy is not initially performed. In patients with this presentation, it is mandatory that an office biopsy be performed immediately and certainly before initiating treatment. If possible this should be a wide local excision, as this well may be adequate treatment. Topical treatment with corticosteroids or podophyllin is contraindicated before a tissue diagnosis is made. Both laser vaporization and office cryocautery of lesions such as this are also contraindicated until a specific diagnosis is made.
17. **D,** Page 1012. Bartholin's gland carcinoma is an adenocarcinoma and comprises 1% to 2% of vulvar cancers. An enlargement of the Bartholin's gland in a postmenopausal woman should raise the suspicion for this malignancy. Since this complaint is rarely associated with acute inflammation in a postmenopausal women, one should biopsy all such masses in this age group. Empiric treatment with laser or topical agents is not warranted unless indicated by the biopsy results. Exam with a magnifying device such as a colposcopy would not be useful in this patient since the lesion is below the epithelium. Simple incision and drainage is not appropriate unless representative samples of tissue are submitted for pathologic examination first. These tumors are treated similarly to primary squamous cell carcinoma of the vulva; radical vulvectomy with bilateral inguinal-femoral lymphadenectomy is the treatment of choice.
18. **B,** Pages 1012-1013. Verrucous carcinoma is a rare tumor that may attain considerable size, but is generally indolent in its behavior. Wide local excision is usually effective therapy. Radical vulvectomy, and radical vulvectomy with either ipsilateral or bilateral inguinal lymphadenectomy are not necessary. Laser ablation is insufficient to remove the deeper tissues. Radiation therapy is ineffective, can worsen the

prognosis, and is therefore, contraindicated.

19. **E,** Pages 991-992. The changes shown in this photomicrograph are typical for lichen sclerosus. Usually the epithelium becomes markedly thinner with the loss or blunting of the rete ridges. The superficial portion of the dermis is hyalinized while the deep portion contains a lymphocytic infiltrate. This is not a premalignant condition, but it tends to be multifocal and usually reoccurs.
20. **E,** Page 998. The next step in managing a patient with lichen sclerosus would be topical testosterone cream. The efficacy of testosterone is excellent. It should be remembered that estrogen does not significantly affect changes in vulvar skin, although it promotes maturation and thickening of the vaginal epithelium. Vulvar colposcopy (vulvoscopy) is difficult and non-essential since the vulva has a homogeneous appearance. If it is readily available and will not drive up the cost ofcare, its use cannot be criticized. Simple vulvectomy is unnecessary as the condition is benign.

21-22. 21, **B;** 22, **D;** Page 997; Figures 30-8 and 30-9 from Herbst et al. Originally from Kaufman RH, Gardner HL, and Merrill JA: Diseases of the vulva and vagina. In Romney SL, et al, editors: Gynecology and obstetrics, New York, 1980, McGraw-Hill Book Co. A clinical diagnosis must not replace a histologic diagnosis. Lesions of the vulva should be biopsied. Figure 30-4 depicts tissue of the labia minora and perineum which has a white, brittle "cigarette paper" appearance. Figure 30-5 depicts squamous hyperplasia which in the past has been labelled hyperplastic dystrophy. Note the sharply demarcated, raised, white area at lower tip of white pointer. These lesions usually appear thickened and the process tends to be more focal or multifocal than diffuse. A biopsy is necessary to establish the diagnosis.

23. **B** (1, 2), Page 1011. Survival of patients with vulvar carcinoma is directly related to the presence of metastatic disease in regional lymph nodes. After radical vulvectomy and bilateral node dissection, there is about a 95% 5-year survival for patients with negative regional lymph nodes. As the number of metastatic nodes increase, the 5-year survival diminishes progressively. There is also a direct correlation between survival and metastatic nodal size. Those lesions associated with higher nodal tumor volume are generally associated with earlier recurrence and decreased survival rates.
24. **A** (1, 2, 3), Page 996. This is a patient with Paget's disease, which is a disease of the vulva generally seen in postmenopausal women with a long history of vulvar pruritus. It is frequently associated with other invasive carcinomas. These may present as squamous carcinoma of the vulva or cervix, adenocarcinoma of the sweat glands of the vulva, or as Bartholin's gland carcinoma. Cases of adenocarcinoma of the gastrointestinal tract accompanying Paget's disease have also been reported. Thus, once a diagnosis of Paget's disease of the vulva is made, it is important for the gynecologist to rule out the presence of malignancy at other sites, including the breast. If no primary malignancy is uncovered,a total vulvectomy is usually performed. It is important to remove the full thickness of the skin to the subcutaneous fat to be certain that all of the skin adnexal structures are excised, as they may have a subclinical malignancy. Insofar as the disease may recur resulting in multiple surgical procedures, some experts have advocated less extensive initial therapy. Those women who have been treated for Paget's disease of the vulva should have, as part of the routine follow-up, annual examination of the breast, cytologic evaluation of the cervix and vulva, and screening for gastrointestinal disease, at least by testing for occult blood in the stool.
25. **B,** (1, 2), Pages 1013-1014; Fig. 30-20. Melanoma is the most frequent non-squamous cell malignancy of the vulva, comprising about 5% of primary cancers of this area. Although the diagnosis may be established by excisional biopsy, the treatment should be provided by radical vulvectomy and bilateral inguinal-femoral lymphadenectomy. Pelvic node dissection is reserved for those patients who have positive inguinal-femoral nodes. Melanomas may arise from either junctional or compound nevi. Although previously thought to bypass the inguinal-femoral nodes and progress directly to the deep pelvic nodes, recent series have not demonstrated pelvic node involvement without inguinal node involvement.
26. **E** (3 only), Page 991. In the past, a number of ambiguous terms have been used to describe gross lesions of the vulva. Terms

such as leukoplakia and leukoplakic vulvitis have been discarded since they imply, without biopsy confirmation, both precancerous lesions as well as inflammation. Under the new classification scheme used by the International Society for the Study of Vulvar Diseases and adopted by the International Society for Gynecologic Pathology these gross lesions should be referred to as vulvar atypia with biopsy confirmation needed to make the final diagnosis. The histologic architecture of these lesions defines whether or not surgical or medical therapy should be offered.

27. **C** (2, 3), Pages 996-997. Certain diagnostic aids may be useful in the initial evaluation of a patient with suspected vulvar atypia in preparation for biopsy. Lugol's solution as a cytoplasmicstain is not particularly helpful because of the numerous false positive areas as well as the fact that it does not penetrate the hyperkeratosis associated with many of these disorders. Toluidine blue, which is a nuclear stain, may assist in delineating vulvar atypia when positive since the superficial keratin layers of the vulvar do not normally contain nuclei. It should be remembered however that ulcerations and fissures in the skin also retain this dye. Acetic acid is used in patients who have suspected vulvar atypia in preparation for colposcopic (vulvoscopic) exam of the vulva. The magnification of the colposcope is practical in following patients with intraepithelial neoplasia of the vulva. Using this instrument, directed biopsy are obtained. The colposcope is not used for routine vulvar examination, but is primarily employed for those who are being evaluated or followed for vulvar atypia or intraepithelial neoplasia.

28. **A** (1, 2, 3), Page 1000. Progression of vulvar intraepithelial neoplasia (VIN) to invasive carcinoma is rare and has been estimated to occur in approximately 6% of all cases. Moreover, a comparable proportion of VIN cases spontaneously regress. The risk of progression to invasive cancer is higher for those who are older as well as for those who are immunosuppressed. Further, the risk of invasion is higher in women who have raised lesions with irregular surface patterns. Thus, patients who are older and those with irregular raised lesions have the greatest risk of unrecognized invasive cancer.

29. **A** (1, 2, 3), Page 1005. Although it is well known that regional lymph node involvement is an important prognostic factor, other observations are also important in determining therapy and survival. Numerous studies indicate that tumor stage, location on the vulva, microscopic differentiation, presence or absence of vascular space involvement, and tumor thickness are also important prognostic factors. In a large study done by the Gynecology Oncology Group (GOG) it was noted that labial lesions were associated with 7.4% positive nodes while clitoral lesions were associated with 27.4% positive nodes. Lesion size is also a factor with studies suggesting that lesions under 1 cm in diameter have limited metastatic potential to the regional nodes whilelesions over 4 cm in diameter may have regional node involvement in up to half of the cases.

CHAPTER 31 Premalignant and Malignant Diseases of the Vagina

DIRECTIONS for questions 1 - 12: Select the one best answer or completion.

1. Recurrences of squamous cell carcinoma of the vagina are most likely to occur as
   A. local recurrence
   B. bone metastases
   C. liver metastases
   D. lung metastases
   E. brain metastases
2. Of the following treatment modalities, the most frequently used in the treatment of squamous cell carcinoma of the vagina is
   A. laser ablation
   B. wide local excision
   C. radical surgery
   D. radiation therapy
   E. chemotherapy
3. The current recommendation for the initial evaluation of girls exposed to diethylstilbestrol in utero is to examine them
   A. following the menarche
   B. following the menarche or by age 14, whichever is first
   C. starting at age 18
   D. starting when they are sexually active
   E. starting at age 11
4. A "field defect" in gynecology denotes
   A. a blind spot in the visual field as a result of metastatic genital cancer
   B. the propensity of the squamous epithelium of the lower genital tract to undergo premalignant change
   C. herniation of fatty tissue through the inguinal canal
   D. adenosis of the vagina as a result of in utero exposure to diethylstilbestrol
   E. an area not affected by radiation therapy
5. A stage II vaginal cancer indicates that
   A. there is ureteric involvement
   B. the lesion extends to the pelvic wall
   C. the lesion is limited to the vaginal wall
   D. the lesion involves subvaginal tissue but does not extend to the pelvic wall
   E. the lesion involves the rectal mucosa
6. An 80 year-old woman who is in good health has a routine gynecologic examination. She had a total abdominal hysterectomy at age 45 for benign disease. The pap smear is reported as showing severe atrophy with inflammatory changes and a few atypical cells. The appropriate management is to
   A. prescribe topical 5-fluorouracil
   B. repeat the pap smear in one year
   C. prescribe a course of estrogen followed by a repeat pap smear in three months
   D. perform colposcopy
   E. perform a vaginectomy
7. A patient with primary squamous cell carcinoma of the vagina is found to have hydronephrosis. The tumor seems to be filling the pelvis, but the bladder and rectum appear to be free of disease. The remainder of her evaluation does not reveal distant disease. The appropriate stage to be assigned to this patient is
   A. 0
   B. I
   C. II
   D. III
   E. IV
8. A 60 year-old gravida 6 has recently experienced vaginal bleeding. Until this event, she was healthy and was not receiving any medications. On examination, a fungating, ulcerative lesion is found on the left lateral wall of the vagina near the fornix. The next step in her medical care is to
   A. perform a pap smear
   B. look at the lesion with a colposcope
   C. biopsy the lesion
   D. perform vaginectomy
   E. order radiation therapy
9. A 41 year-old patient underwent a total abdominal hysterectomy for moderate dysplasia of the cervix and uterine myomata. This patient should be advised that she
   A. does not need to have vaginal cytology
   B. needs a pap smear every 4-5 years
   C. needs a pap smear every 2-3 years
   D. needs a pap smear annually

E. should be followed with yearly colposcopic examinations

10. In vaginal carcinoma in situ (VAIN-3), abnormal cells are
    A. confined to the outer 1/3 of the epithelium
    B. confined to the inner 2/3 of the epithelium
    C. throughout the entire thickness of the epithelium
    D. invade the basement membrane
    E. invade sub-epithelial tissues
11. A 2 year-old is seen after passing a "grape-like" structure from the vagina. Otherwise the child is asymptomatic. One should
    A. obtain vaginal secretions for culture and sensitivity
    B. admit the child for observation in the hospital
    C. empirically treat the child with penicillin
    D. warn the parents about the problem of children inserting foreign objects into the vagina
    E. perform vaginoscopy under anesthesia
12. A 40 year-old patient, who is five years status post vaginal hysterectomy for carcinoma in situ of the cervix, is found to have diffuse multicentric vaginal intraepithelial neoplasia (VAIN). The most appropriate treatment is
    A. surgical excision
    B. laser ablation
    C. 5-fluorouracil cream
    D. radiation therapy
    E. systemic chemotherapy

DIRECTIONS For each numbered item 13 - 21, indicate whether it is associated with
A only (A)
B only (B)
C both (A) and (B)
D neither (A) nor (B)

13-15. Match the appropriate treatment option with the lesion
(A) radical hysterectomy and vaginectomy
(B) radiation therapy
(C) both
(D) neither

13. appropriate treatment for vaginal intraepithelial neoplasia
14. appropriate treatment for Stage II clear cell adenocarcinoma of the vagina
15. appropriate treatment for Stage III squamous cell carcinoma of the vagina

16-18. Match the lesion with the question
(A) clear cell carcinoma of the vagina
(B) squamous cell carcinoma of the vagina
(C) both
(D) neither

16. histologically demonstrates hobnail cells
17. in utero exposure to diethylstilbestrol
18. chemotherapy is first line of treatment

19-21. Characteristic of the neoplasia
(A) vaginal intraepithelial neoplasia (VAIN)-I
(B) cervical intraepithelial neoplasia (CIN)-I
(C) both
(D) neither

19. associated with herpes simplex virus infection
20. requires radiation therapy
21. characterized by abnormal maturation of the epithelium

DIRECTIONS for questions 22 - 31: For each of the questions below, ONE or MORE of the responses is correct. Select the best answer based on the following
A if 1, 2, and 3 are correct
B if only 1 and 2 are correct
C if only 2 and 3 are correct
D if only 1 is correct
E if only 3 is correct

22. A malignant melanoma of the vagina
    1. invades deeply into the tissues
    2. usually affects older patients
    3. rarely metastasizes
23. The diagnosis of sarcoma botryoides has been established in a 2 year-old. Management of this patient should include
    1. chemotherapy
    2. surgery
    3. radiation therapy
24. Symptoms commonly associated with vaginal cancer encompass
    1. urinary frequency
    2. vaginal discharge
    3. abnormal vaginal bleeding
25. The presence of an abnormal vaginal epithelium can be detected using
    1. Lugol's stain
    2. Colposcopy
    3. vaginal cytology
26. Appropriate therapy for vaginal intraepithelial neoplasia (VAIN) includes
    1. cryotherapy
    2. laser ablation
    3. 5-fluorouracil cream
27. Appropriate modalities used in the treatment of carcinoma in situ of the vagina include
    1. radiation therapy
    2. laser ablation
    3. 5-fluorouracil cream

28. The interpretation of routine pap smears is adversely affected by
    1. a vaginal infection
    2. menopausal changes
    3. menstruation
29. Factors affecting the prognosis of patients with clear cell adenocarcinoma of the vagina embody the
    1. age of the patient
    2. size of the tumor
    3. depth of invasion
30. The initial treatment of a patient with a malignant melanoma of the vagina may include
    1. radical surgery
    2. radiation therapy
    3. systemic chemotherapy
31. Alpha fetoprotein is secreted by
    1. an endodermal sinus tumor of the vagina
    2. a vaginal squamous cell carcinoma
    3. sarcoma botryoides

ANSWERS

1. **A,** Page 1027. Initially squamous cell carcinoma of the vagina recurs locally, just as squamous cell carcinoma of the cervix and vulva do. Although distant metastases occur, most patients will present with local recurrences. Since an effective chemotherapy program for recurrent vaginal carcinoma has not been developed, in patients who have only localized recurrence, an exenterative procedure should be considered if the tumor was initially treated with radiation.
2. **D,** Page 1026. In recent years, radiation therapy has been the most frequent mode of treatment for squamous cell carcinoma of the vagina. External radiation therapy with megavoltage equipment is utilized initially to shrink the tumor. This is then followed by a local cesium or radium implant placed interstitially with needles or by intracavitary radiation using a tandem similar to the delivery systems used for cervical carcinoma.
3. **B,** Page 1019. The current recommendations for the initial evaluation of girls exposed to diethylstilbestrol in utero are to examine them if there is bleeding or a lesion. If they are asymptomatic, the initial evaluation should occur shortly after menarche, or at age 14, whichever comes first. Because of the association of in utero exposure to diethylstilbestrol with both malignant and benign conditions, it is imperative to identify and appropriately evaluate all such patients. Refer to Chapter 14 for a complete discussion of diethylstilbestrol exposure. Because diethylstilbestrol was no longer available after the early 1970's, a patient less than 14 years of age is not likely to be seen in contemporary practice.
4. **B,** Page 1023. A "field defect" describes the propensity of squamous epithelium of the lower genital tract (cervix, vagina and vulva) to undergo premalignant changes. The epithelium of the lower genital tract is derived from a common embryonic origin. Since these structures are subjected to similar environmental stimulants, e.g. human papillomavirus and herpes simplex virus type II, similar premalignant changes might be anticipated. Areas of such neoplastic changes need not be contiguous and in fact, may arise in multiple sites throughout the genital tract. The recognition of field defect phenomenon is important since patients with cervical intraepithelial neoplasia are more likely to also develop vaginal intraepithelial neoplasia and vulvar intraepithelial neoplasia.
5. **D,** Page 1025; Table 31-1. The staging of vaginal cancer according to FIGO is done following clinical evaluation which includes examination under anesthesia, cystoscopy, sigmoidoscopy, and imaging studies (i.e. intravenous pyelogram, barium enema). Stage II involves the subvaginal tissue but does not extend to the pelvic wall.
6. **C,** Page 1023. An abnormal pap smear requires further evaluation. Since estrogen deficient state may adversely affect the interpretation of a pap smear, it should be repeated after the patient is given estrogen replacement therapy. Colposcopic

TABLE 31-1. International Federation of Gynecology and Obstetrics (FIGO) Staging Classification for Vaginal Cancer

Stage	Characteristics
0	Carcinoma in situ
I	Carcinoma limited to vaginal wall
II	Carcinoma involves subvaginal tissue but has not extended to pelvic wall
III	Carcinoma extends to pelvic wall
IV	Carcinoma extends beyond true pelvis or involves mucosa of bladder or rectum (bullous edema as such does not assign a patient to stage IV)

evaluation of the atrophic vaginal epithelium may be difficult due to the chronic inflammatory changes. If the repeat pap smear following estrogen replacement therapy is abnormal, colposcopic evaluation and biopsies will be necessary at that time. A vaginectomy without a histologic diagnosis may constitute either over or under treatment.

7. **D,** Page 1025; Table 31-2. The lesion extends into the pelvis and obstructs a ureter, indicating that the lesion has extended to the pelvic wall. The appropriate stage to be assigned according to the FIGO classification is stage III.
8. **C,** Page 1025. A large fungating, ulcerative lesion in this age group is likely to be a neoplasm. A biopsy of this or any significant lesion is a rapid and accurate way of making a definitive diagnosis; it should be performed at the initial visit. Treatment should not be undertaken until a diagnosis is made. This diagnosis must be based on a biopsy, not on pap smear or colposcopy results.
9. **D,** Pages 1023-1024. Considering the concept of a field defect, this patient with premalignant changes of the cervix is more likely to develop premalignant changes of the vagina. If left undetected, this may later progress to invasive cancer. A patient who has had moderate cervical dysplasia is at an increased risk of developing a vaginal or vulvar malignancy. As a screening tool vaginal cytology rather than colposcopy remains most cost-effective.
10. **C,** Page 1021; Figure 31-1, *C*. Vaginal carcinoma in situ (VAIN-3) denotes an intraepithelial neoplasm not invading the basement membrane or involving the subepithelial tissues, but in which dysplastic cells extend throughout the entire epithelial layer.
11. **E,** Page 1030. Although children sometimes insert foreign bodies into the vagina, passing a "grape-like" structure by a two year-old is extremely suspicious of the presence of a sarcoma botryoides. Since the prognosis for the child is directly related to the rapidity in which the diagnosis is established, one should perform vaginoscopy under anesthesia and biopsy all suspicious lesions as soon as possible.
12. **C,** Page 1024. 5-Fluorouracil cream is most appropriate for diffuse, multicentric lesions, while surgical excision is reserved for apical lesions, commonly found after hysterectomy. Laser is generally used for discrete lesions.

13-15. 13, **D;** 14, **A;** 15, **B;** Pages 1024, 1026-1027. In a patient with intraepithelial neoplasia (VAIN), local excision or laser ablation of the epithelium is the procedure of choice. In young patients with clear cell adenocarcinoma, an attempt should be made to preserve ovarian function and coital function. Thus, radical hysterectomy with partial or complete vaginectomy, pelvic lymphadenectomy and vaginal reconstruction is most often performed. When the tumor is extremely small, the use of local irradiation may be sufficient to ablate the tumor and preserve fertility. A Stage II lesion would not fall into this category. Radiation therapy is most often utilized for treatment of patients with extensive vaginal carcinoma. Patients with Stage III squamous cell carcinoma of the vagina would normally receive radiation therapy.

16-18. 16, **A;** 17, **A;** 18, **D;** Pages 1027-1029; Figure 31-4. The characteristic of the tubulocystic pattern of clear cell adenocarcinoma is hobnail cells extruding into the lumina of tubular structures. Clear cell adenocarcinoma may have other patterns as well, such as solid or papillary. It affects young women usually with a history of in utero exposure to diethylstilbestrol. The tumor is rarely found in patients who do not have a history of diethylstilbestrol exposure. Chemotherapy is reserved for patients with systemic disease or patients who failed other modalities of therapy.

19-21. 19, **C;** 20, **D;** 21, **C;** Pages 1023-1024; Figure 31-1, *A*. VAIN is the abbreviation used to describe intraepithelial neoplasms of the vagina, while CIN is used to describe cervical intraepithelial neoplasms. Both conditions are a result of a faulty maturation process in the surface epithelium. Risk factors include: previous venereal disease, herpes virus type II infection, human papilloma virus infection, and sexual activity at an early age with multiple sexual partners. Both lesions result in the exfoliation of abnormal cells into the vagina which can be detected on a routine pap smear collected from the cervix and the posterior vaginal pool. Both are treated surgically. Although vaginal intraepithelial neoplasia (VAIN) is most often in the upper 1/3 of the vagina, it is often multifocal, requiring examination of the vagina in its entirety.

22. **B** (1, 2), Page 1030. A malignant melanoma of the vagina is a rare neoplasm with only about 100 cases reported to date. It affects older women (mean age 60). The lesion invades deeply into the sub-vaginal tissue and metastasizes extensively. Pigmented lesions of the lower genital tract are more likely than pigmented lesions elsewhere in the body to undergo malignant transformation. If there is any question regarding a pigmented lesion, it should be excised and submitted for histologic evaluation.
23. **A** (1, 2, 3), Page 1031. Although exenterative procedures were performed in the past in the treatment of children with embryonal rhabdomyosarcoma (sarcoma botryoides), effective control with less radical surgery appears to have been achieved with a multimodality approach consisting of chemotherapy (Vincristine, Actinomycin D and Cyclophosphamide) combined usually with surgery. Radiation therapy has also been utilized. Such a combined approach appears to result in effective treatment with less mutilating surgery.
24. **C** (2, 3), Page 1025. The most common symptoms of vaginal cancer are abnormal vaginal bleeding and vaginal discharge. Urinary frequency is sometimes noted in patients with a large anterior lesion while tenesmus is noted in patients with a large posterior lesion. These symptoms appear only when the lesions are large and therefore are late in the course of disease. Similarly, pain is usually a symptom of an advanced tumor which has invaded into the deep tissues.
25. **A** (1, 2, 3), Page 1023. The presence of dysplastic vaginal epithelium is most frequently detected initially on pap smear. The abnormal area can be delineated by colposcopy or Lugol's stain. It should be biopsied for histologic evaluation.
26. **A** (1, 2 3), Pages 1024. The premalignant changes of vaginal intraepithelial neoplasia (VAIN) are localized to that epithelial layer alone. Ablation of the epithelium results in eradication of the disease. Cryotherapy, laser ablation, 5-fluorouracil cream application, and surgical excision of small lesions are all acceptable methods of treating these lesions.
27. **C** (2, 3), Page 1024. While both vaginectomy and radiation therapy would ablate carcinoma in situ of the vagina, this would be considered over treatment. The lesion is limited to the epithelial area only and thus removal of the epithelial layer either with laser therapy or the application of 5-fluorouracil cream is sufficient. In either instance, follow-up is required to assure elimination of all abnormal areas. Like all patients with lower genital tract malignancies, the patient is at a higher risk of developing similar neoplasms along the lower genital tract. Therefore, close gynecological surveillance is necessary for the remainder of the patient's life.
28. **A** (1, 2, 3), Pages 1023-1024. Inflammatory changes and estrogen deficiency affect the appearance of the exfoliating cells and thus make interpretation of cytologic smears more difficult. It is recommended that an infection be treated and cleared, and patients with severe atrophic changes be given hormonal replacement treatment. The cytologic smears should be repeated following completion of therapy. Menstrual blood creates technical difficulties by obscuring the sample.
29. **A** (1, 2, 3), Page 1028. Factors favorable in the survival of patients with clear cell adenocarcinoma of the vagina include:
    1. low stage
    2. older age
    3. tubulocystic pattern
    4. small tumor diameter
    5. reduced depth of invasion
    6. no lymph node involvement
30. **A** (1, 2, 3), Page 1030. Treatment of patients with malignant melanoma of the vagina consists of radical surgery with wide excision of the vagina, uterus and dissection of the retroperitoneal nodes (pelvic and inguinal). Lower vaginal lesions require treatment similar to vulvar carcinoma while upper vaginal lesions require treatment similar to cervical carcinoma. Adjunctive radiation therapy and chemotherapy also have been used. Despite all this, the five year survival is dismal. Local recurrence is common and the disease is usually fatal.
31. **D** (1 only), Page 1030. An endodermal sinus tumor (adenocarcinoma) is a rare vaginal tumor. It affects very young girls, usually under age 2 years. The tumor is aggressive, with an unfavorable prognosis since the tumor is usually fatal. It produces α-fetoprotein, which can be detected in the serum and can serve as a tumor marker.

CHAPTER 32

Malignant Disease of the Fallopian Tube

DIRECTIONS for questions 1 - 14: Select the one best answer or completion.

1. The least common primary female genital tract malignancy originates in the
   A. ovary
   B. fallopian tube
   C. uterus
   D. vagina
   E. vulva
2. Pain is the most frequent presenting symptom in cancer of the
   A. ovary
   B. fallopian tube
   C. endometrium
   D. cervix
   E. none of the above
3. The diagnosis of primary tubal carcinoma is most commonly made by
   A. history
   B. physical examination
   C. ultrasound
   D. CT scan
   E. surgical exploration
4. A 62 year old patient has persistent uterine bleeding despite two dilatation and curettages and two trials on conjugated equine estrogens-progestin therapy. No endometrial pathology has been found and the pelvic examination is unremarkable. The next step should be
   A. vaginal hysterectomy
   B. abdominal hysterectomy
   C. laparoscopy/laparotomy
   D. irradiation of the pelvis
   E. hysteroscopy/laser ablation of the endometrium
5. A 57 year old patient complains of vaginal bleeding, a profuse, intermittent watery discharge, and lower abdominal pain. On pelvic examination, a 5 cm right adnexal mass is palpated. These findings are most typical of
   A. a functional ovarian cyst
   B. ovarian carcinoma
   C. endometrial carcinoma
   D. a fallopian tube carcinoma
   E. a leiomyosarcoma
6. The percentage of patients with fallopian tube carcinoma who have positive vaginal cytology is
   A. <1%
   B. 2-5%
   C. 10-20%
   D. 50-60%
   E. >70%
7. At the time of exploratory laparotomy for a right adnexal mass in a 60 year old patient, a dilated right fallopian tube is discovered. When opened, it is filled with tumor. No other tumors are noted but the peritoneal fluid is found to be positive for malignant cells. The "unofficial stage" of the tubal carcinoma is
   A. Ia
   B. Ib
   C. Ic
   D. II
   E. III
8. The most frequent site of metastatic spread of tubal carcinoma is
   A. liver
   B. lung
   C. bone
   D. peritoneum
   E. retroperitoneal nodes
9. At the time of exploratory laparotomy, a 30 year old gravida 1 para 1 is found to have a primary tubal carcinoma confined to the right tube. The appropriate operation is
   A. right salpingectomy
   B. right salpingo-oophorectomy
   C. bilateral salpingectomy
   D. bilateral salpingo-oophorectomy
   E. total abdominal hysterectomy with bilateral salpingo-oophorectomy
10. In performing an exploratory laparotomy for a suspected tubal carcinoma, the first step upon entering the abdominal cavity should be:
    A. ligation of the distal and proximal ends of the affected tube
    B. palpation of the liver
    C. palpation of the para-aortic nodes
    D. obtaining peritoneal cytology

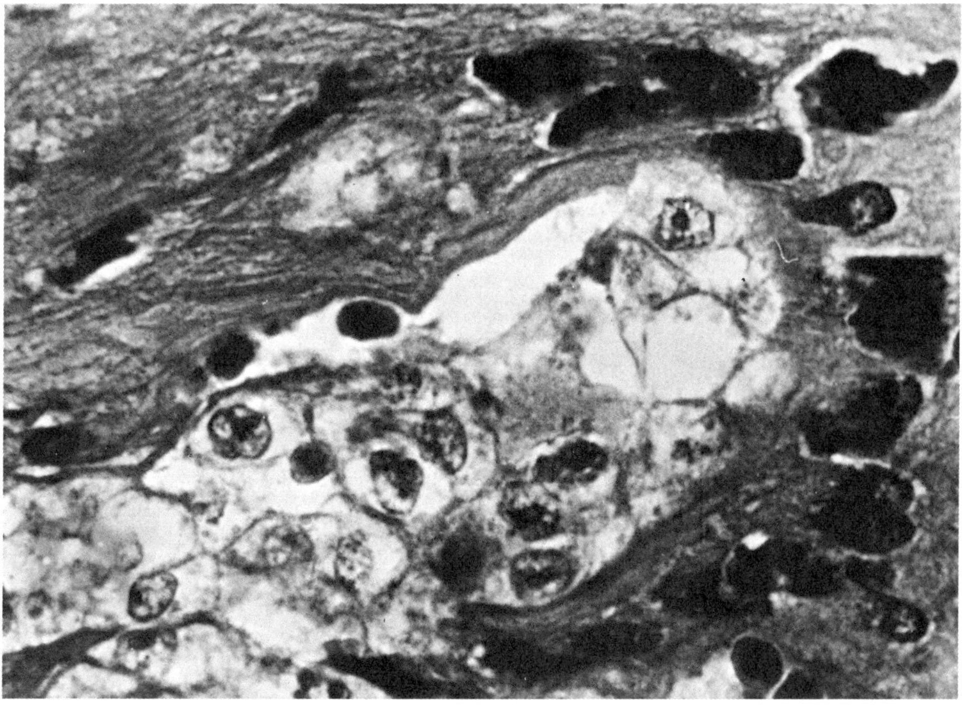

FIGURE 32-1.

E. palpation of the omentum

11. Figure 32-1 is a high-powered microscopic view of a section through a tumor of the fallopian tube. It is a
    A. papillary adenocarcinoma
    B. medullary adenocarcinoma
    C. carcinosarcoma
    D. mixed mesodermal tumor
    E. choriocarcinoma
12. The family of a patient with tubal carcinoma confined to the tube (Stage I) asks about the prognosis. It would be accurate to inform them that five year survival is
    A. <5%
    B. 10-20%
    C. 30-40%
    D. 50-60%
    E. 70-80%
13. In a postmenopausal woman, the classic symptoms suggestive of tubal carcinoma are included in the triad of
    A. pain, watery discharge, anorexia
    B. bleeding, watery discharge, adnexal mass
    C. bleeding, pain, adnexal mass
    D. anorexia, watery discharge, bleeding
    E. anorexia, pain, adnexal mass
14. Adenocarcinoma of the fallopian tube occurs most commonly in patients who are
    A. 40-49 years old
    B. 50-59 years old
    C. 60-69 years old
    D. 70-79 years old
    E. 80-89 years old

DIRECTIONS: For each numbered item 15 - 17, indicate whether it is associated with

A only (A)
B only (B)
C both (A) and (B)
D neither (A) nor (B)

15-17. Characteristic of
(A) primary tubal carcinoma
(B) primary ovarian carcinoma
(C) both
(D) neither

15. commonly spreads to para-aortic nodes
16. overall five year survival exceeds 50%
17. less common than metastatic disease

DIRECTIONS for questions 18 - 26: For each of the questions below, ONE or MORE of the responses is correct. Select the best answer based on the following

A if 1, 2, and 3 are correct
B if only 1 and 2 are correct
C if only 2 and 3 are correct
D if only 1 is correct
E if only 3 is correct

18. The criteria used to diagnose primary tubal carcinoma include
    1. the tumor is primarily within the lumen of the tube

2. the mucosa of the tube is involved with the tumor
3. a transition can be demonstrated between the malignant and nonmalignant tubal epithelium.

19. True statements concerning the staging of tubal carcinoma include that it
    1. was officially adopted by FIGO in 1986
    2. is based on clinical findings, histologic grade, depth of invasion
    3. is based on the system used for primary ovarian carcinoma
20. A 52 year old patient is found to have a Stage Ia carcinoma of the fallopian tube. Proper therapy should include
    1. total abdominal hysterectomy, bilateral salpingo-oophorectomy, para-aortic node biopsy, omentectomy
    2. intraperitoneal ^{32}P
    3. cyclophosphamide (Cytoxan) and megestrol acetate (Megace)
21. A 58 year old asymptomatic patient is seen for a routine office visit. A pap smear is performed. It is reported as "cells consistent with adenocarcinoma". The differential diagnosis should include adenocarcinoma of the
    1. endometrium
    2. ovary
    3. fallopian tube
22. A 48 year old patient undergoes surgery for a left adnexal mass. While exploring the pelvis, you note a tumor of the left fallopian tube. If you suspect metastatic cancer to the tube, you should pay particular attention to the
    1. ovaries
    2. intestines
    3. uterus
23. Abnormal uterine bleeding is the most common complaint associated with malignancies of the
    1. uterus
    2. fallopian tube
    3. ovary
24. The term "hydrops tubae profluens" is associated with
    1. vaginal discharge
    2. a disappearing pelvic mass
    3. pelvic pain
25. The prognosis for patients with tubal carcinoma is related to
    1. stage
    2. vessel invasion
    3. depth of tubal wall invasion
26. Initial adjunctive chemotherapy with a cisplatinum based regimen has been shown to improve survival in patients with advanced carcinoma of the
    1. endometrium
    2. fallopian tubes
    3. ovaries

ANSWERS

1. **B,** Page 1035. Fallopian tube carcinoma comprises approximately 0.3% to 1.1% of gynecologic malignancies. Up to 90% are metastatic from other sites, usually the ovary or uterus. Metastatic fallopian tumors are ten times more frequent than primary tumors.
2. **E,** Page 1035. In none of the malignancies of the female genital tract does pain represent the most frequent presenting symptom. In the case of tubal carcinoma, pain may occur, but is less frequent a presenting symptom than abnormal or excessive vaginal bleeding or discharge.
3. **E,** Pages 1035, 1039. Although tubal carcinoma may present with excessive bleeding or discharge, and although an adnexal mass is occasionally found, history and physical examination do not usually lead one to the correct diagnosis. Similarly, imaging studies are not pathognomonic. The diagnosis is most frequently made after surgical exploration for other diagnoses.
4. **C,** Page 1036. In a patient with postmenopausal uterine bleeding for whom two dilatation and curettages fail to reveal the cause of bleeding, the possibility of tubal carcinoma must be considered. Laparoscopy can aid in establishing this diagnosis. Hysterectomy would not necessarily address the possibility of adnexal pathology although an abdominal approach would allow thorough inspection of tubes and ovaries. Irradiation of the pelvis for bleeding of unknown etiology is inappropriate. Hysteroscopy with laser ablation of the endometrium would not rule out an adnexal etiology for the bleeding.
5. **D,** Pages 1035, 1036. The triad of bleeding, watery discharge and adnexal mass (hydrops tubae profluens) in a postmenopausal woman is considered highly suggestive of tubal carcinoma. These findings, however, only rarely occur together. The diagnosis is usually made postoperatively, as the physician's index of suspicion is low. An adnexal mass in a postmenopausal patient must not be considered functional. The diagnosis of ovarian carcinoma is less likely because of the watery vaginal discharge. Postmenopausal bleeding should be considered endometrial carcinoma un-

til proven otherwise, but the watery discharge and an adnexal mass suggest a different primary process. Leiomyosarcoma would present as a uterine mass rather than an adnexal mass and without the watery discharge.

6. **C,** Page 1036; Benedet JL, White GW, Fairey RN, Boyes DA: Adenocarcinoma of the fallopian tube. Obstet Gynecol 50: 654, 1977; Hirai Y, Kaku S, Teshima H, et al: Clinical study of primary carcinoma of the fallopian tube: Experience with 15 cases. Gynecol Oncol 34:20, 1989. Only 10% of the patients with tubal carcinoma in the series by Benedet have positive vaginal cytology while Hiraiet al have reported positive preoperative cytology in 6 of 15 cases (40%). Therefore, the pap smear is not a reliable screening tool, and a negative smear does not rule out the possibility of tubal carcinoma.
7. **C,** Page 1039; Table 32-1. Although there is no official FIGO staging system for primary tubal carcinoma, the suggested system places a tumor confined to one tube with positive washings at Ic. Had the washings been negative, the stage would be Ia. If confined to both tubes with negative washings, the stage would be Ib. Stage IIa is a tumor involving one or both tubes and spread to either the ovary or the uterus. In stage IIb the tumor has extended to other pelvic tissues. A stage III tumor involves one or both tubes with intraperitoneal spread including retroperitoneal nodes. Finally, a Stage IV lesion involves one or both tubes with metastases outside the peritoneum or to the parenchyma of the liver. If pleural fluid contains malignant cells the tumor is considered Stage IV.
8. **D,** Page 1038. The peritoneum is the most frequent site of metastatic spread of tubal carcinoma. Retroperitoneal nodes are also a common site. Hepatic and lung metastases are less common and denote stage IV disease when they occur.
9. **E,** Page 1039. Although the patient described is young (30 years old) and of low gravidity and parity, the appropriate operation is total abdominal hysterectomy with bilateral salpingo-oophorectomy. If no intraperitoneal spread is apparent, para-aortic node biopsy should be performed. An omentectomy should also be done.
10. **D,** Pages 1036, 1039. In carrying out operative staging for presumed tubal or ovarian cancer, the first surgical procedure performed once in the peritoneal cavity should be peritoneal cytology. It is done by lavage using 200-300 ml of normal saline mixed with 5000 units of heparin. If any other manipulations are carried out prior to obtaining appropriate cytology, one runs the risk of shedding tumor cells into the peritoneal cavity, thus altering the staging evaluation.
11. **E,** Page 1040. The photomicrograph depicted in Figure 32-1 (from Bigelow B: Gestational trophoblast disease. In Blaustein A, ed: Pathology of the female genital tract, 2nd ed. New York, Springer-Verlag, 1982) is a high-power view of a choriocarcinoma. Central pale cytotrophoblasts are surrounded by syncytiotrophoblasts. These tumors tend to be hemorrhagic and necrotic. No villi are seen. Choriocarcinoma of the tube is thought to result from trophoblastic disease associated with ectopic pregnancy.
12. **E,** Page 1040. The overall five year survival for all stages of tubal carcinoma combined is 38%. Patients with disease confined to the tube have the best prognosis, expecting a 70-80% five year survival.
13. **B,** Page 1035. The classic description of tubal carcinoma is the triad of abnormal uterine bleeding, adnexal mass and watery discharge in a postmenopausal woman. Pain is reported, but less frequently. Anorexia is not typically associated with tubal carcinoma.
14. **B,** Figure 32-2; Page 1036. The average age of women with adenocarcinoma of the fallopian tube is 54.9 years. The decade in which most cases occur is 50-59 years.

15-17. 15, **C;** 16, **D;** 17, **A;** Pages 1038-1039; 1040; 1035. Richardson GS, Scully RE, Nikrui N, et al: Common epithelial cancer of the ovary, N Engl J of Med 312:415, 1985. Both ovarian and tubal carcinoma commonly spread to the para-aortic nodes. This is of particular importance when the primary tumor appears to be confined to the ovary or tube. Para-aortic nodes should be palpated and sampled. The overall five year survival for both malignancies is below 50%. In cases of tubal carcinoma, survival is approximately 38%. Richardson, et al, reported ovarian cancer survival to be 30.6%. Whereas metastatic tumors comprise only a small portion of tumors in the ovary, 90% of tubal cancers are metastatic, mostly from ovary, uterus or the gastrointestinal tract.

18. **A** (1, 2, 3), Pages 1036, 1038; Hu CY, Tay-

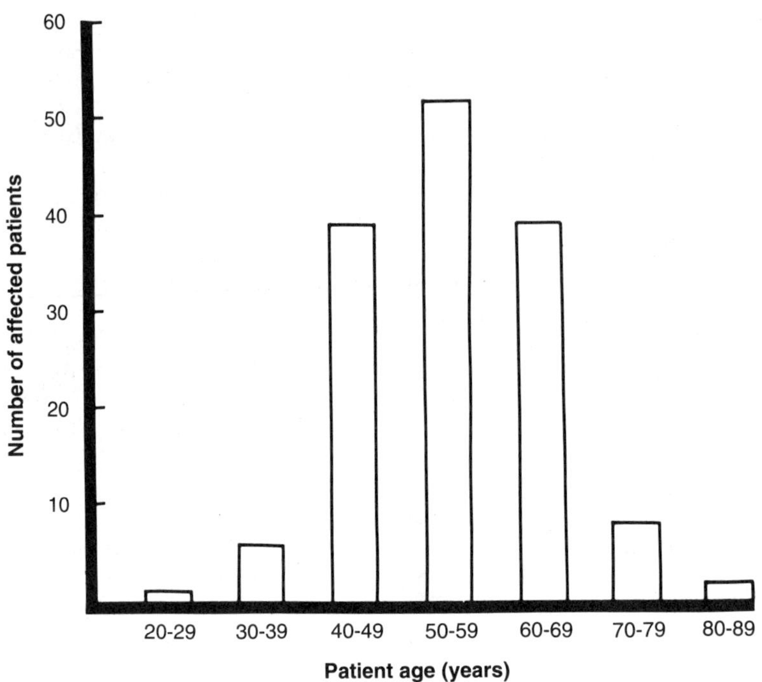

FIGURE 32-2.
Histogram illustrating age distribution of patients with tubal carcinomas.
(From Podczaski D, Herbst AL: Cancer of the vagina and fallopian tube. In Knapp RC. Berkowitz RS, eds: Gynecologic oncology. New York, Macmillan Publishing Co. 1983.)

mor ML, Hertig AT: Primary carcinoma of the fallopian tube. Am J Obstet Gynecol 59:58, 1950. The criteria used in the diagnosis of primary tubal carcinoma were suggested by Hu, et al. They include:

1. The primary tumor is grossly within the lumen of the tube.
2. The mucosa of the tube is involved with the tumor, which displays a papillary or medullary pattern.
3. A transition can be demonstrated between the malignant and nonmalignant tubal epithelium if the tubal wall is involved to a great extent.

19. **E** (3 only), Page 1038. A staging system for primary tubal carcinoma has not been officially adopted by FIGO. Since the spread of the disease is similar to that of epithelial carcinoma of the ovary, many authors have suggested a staging system similar to the one for ovarian cancer. The suggested staging system is accomplished clinically, at the time of surgery. The histologic grade and depth of invasion are considerations in determining the staging of endometrial, not tubal adenocarcinoma.
20. **D** (1 only), Page 1039. Therapy for Stage Ia, tubal carcinoma confined to the lumen with negative cytology, usually consists of primary surgery only (total abdominal hysterectomy, bilateral salpingo-oophorectomy, para-aortic node biopsy and omentectomy). If peritoneal cytology is positive, intraperitoneal 32P or whole abdominal radiation is also used. Chemotherapy is reserved for widespread intraperitoneal disease or for recurrent metastatic carcinoma.
21. **A** (1, 2, 3), Pages 1035-1036. Vaginal cytology has been reported to be positive in 10-40% of fallopian tube carcinomas. Ruling out endometrial carcinoma must be the primary consideration; however, the diagnoses of tubal carcinoma, as well as endocervical or ovarian carcinoma, should be considered in patients with vaginal cytology positive for adenocarcinoma in whom endometrial carcinoma has been excluded.
22. **A** (1, 2, 3), Page 1035. Since 90% of tubal cancers are metastatic, it behooves the clinician to know the likely primary sites, i.e. the ovary, uterus or intestines.
23. **B** (1, 2), Pages 1035-1036. Abnormal or excessive vaginal bleeding is the most commonly associated sign of cancers of the

uterus, fallopian tubes and cervix. Cervical cancer is classically associated with contact bleeding (post coital or post douche). Ovarian cancer tends to present as vague swelling of the abdomen caused by ascites unless the ovarian neoplasm is the relatively rare granulosa cell tumor.

24. **A** (1, 2, 3), Page 1035. Hydrops tubae profluens, sometimes associated with tubal carcinoma, refers to a symptom complex of abnormal vaginal discharge and pelvic pain associated with a pelvic mass. This mass may disappear after the discharge is noted. This symptomatology is presumably explained by blockage of the distal part of the tube, peristalsis of the tube resulting in vaginal discharge and disappearance of the mass as the dilated tube is emptied.
25. **A** (1, 2, 3), Page 1039. Asmussen M, Kaern J, Kjoerstad K, et al: Primary adenocarcinoma localized to the fallopian tubes: Report on 33 cases. Gynecol Oncol 30:183, 1988; Peters WA, Andersen WA, Hopkins MP, Kumar NB, Morley GW: Prognostic features of carcinoma of the fallopian tube. Obstet Gynecol 71:757,1988. Although the "staging" of tubal carcinoma is not officially accepted by FIGO, it is commonly used. Prognosis in cases of tubal carcinoma is related to this unofficial staging. Asmussen found that vessel invasion was a poor prognostic factor in a series of 33 cases. Peters reported that depth of invasion of the tubal wall was also a negative factor in those cases in which the tumor was confined to the tube.
26. **C** (2, 3), Pages 1039 and 1040; Peters WA, Andersen WA, Hopkins MP, Kumar NB, Morley GW: Prognostic features of carcinoma of the fallopian tube. Obstet Gynecol 71:757,1988. Combination chemotherapy with cis-platinum appears to be superior to other chemotherapy for the treatment of both ovarian carcinoma (see Chapter 29) as well as disseminated fallopian tube carcinoma. This was demonstrated in a multicenter analysis reported by Peters et al, in which combination chemotherapy included platinum, Cytoxan, and Adriamycin. At this time cis-platinum is not a standard adjunctive chemotherapeutic agent for advanced endometrial carcinoma.

CHAPTER

33 Gestational Trophoblastic Disease

DIRECTIONS for questions 1-8: Select the one best answer or completion.

1. A 37-year-old gravida 5, para 4 is referred with a confirmed diagnosis of a hydatidiform mole. This was not a planned pregnancy; the patient felt that she had completed her childbearing. During the evaluation of this patient, it is noted that the uterus is greater than expected by dates and that she has bilateral ovarian cysts approximately 10 cm in diameter. Which of the following is the best therapy?
   A. sharp curettage
   B. chemotherapy
   C. hysterotomy
   D. hysterectomy
   E. hysterectomy with bilateral oophorectomy
2. Which is the most common site of metastasis for gestational trophoblastic tumor (GTT)?
   A. brain
   B. lung
   C. liver
   D. ovary
   E. vagina
3. A 30-year-old gravida 3, para 2 delivered a normal 3000g male infant. On the first postpartum day she had a bilateral tubal ligation. She developed excessive bleeding 3 ½ weeks postpartum. A D&C was performed 4 weeks postpartum. The tissue is pictured in Figure 33-1. What is this?
   A. a hydatidiform mole
   B. a partial mole
   C. a choriocarcinoma
   D. evidence of retained secundines
   E. a normal finding
4. A 22-year-old gravida 2, para 1 delivered a 3600g female infant by cesarean section. Bleeding could not be controlled and a hysterectomy was performed. The tissue is pictured in Figure 33-2. What is this?
   A. a hydatidiform mole
   B. a partial mole
   C. a choriocarcinoma
   D. evidence of retained secundines
   E. a normal finding
5. Choriocarcinoma is most likely to develop after
   A. a normal pregnancy
   B. a partial mole
   C. a hydatidiform mole
   D. an ectopic pregnancy
   E. an incomplete abortion
6. The risk of developing a hydatidiform mole is highest if pregnancy occurs in women who are
   A. less than 20 years of age
   B. 20 to 29
   C. 30 to 39
   D. 40 to 49
   E. over 50 years of age
7. A 20-year-old gravida 1, para 0 is seen at 21 weeks of pregnancy by menstrual dates. The uterus is the size of a 25-week gestation. Having made the diagnosis of a hydatidiform mole, you would
   A. start oxytocin immediately
   B. evacuate by hysterotomy
   C. give prophylactic chemotherapy
   D. perform a suction curettage
   E. perform a hysterectomy
8. Signs and symptoms of a complete hydatidiform mole include all of the following **EXCEPT**
   A. abdominal pain
   B. ovarian enlargement
   C. hyperemesis gravidarum
   D. fetal heart tones
   E. uterus small for dates

DIRECTIONS for questions 9-10: For each numbered item, select the one heading most closely associated with it. Each lettered heading may be used once, more than once, or not at all.

Blood Types

	Wife	Husband
A.	A	A
B.	A	0
C.	B	A
D.	AB	0

E. The couple's blood type has not been shown to be a risk factor

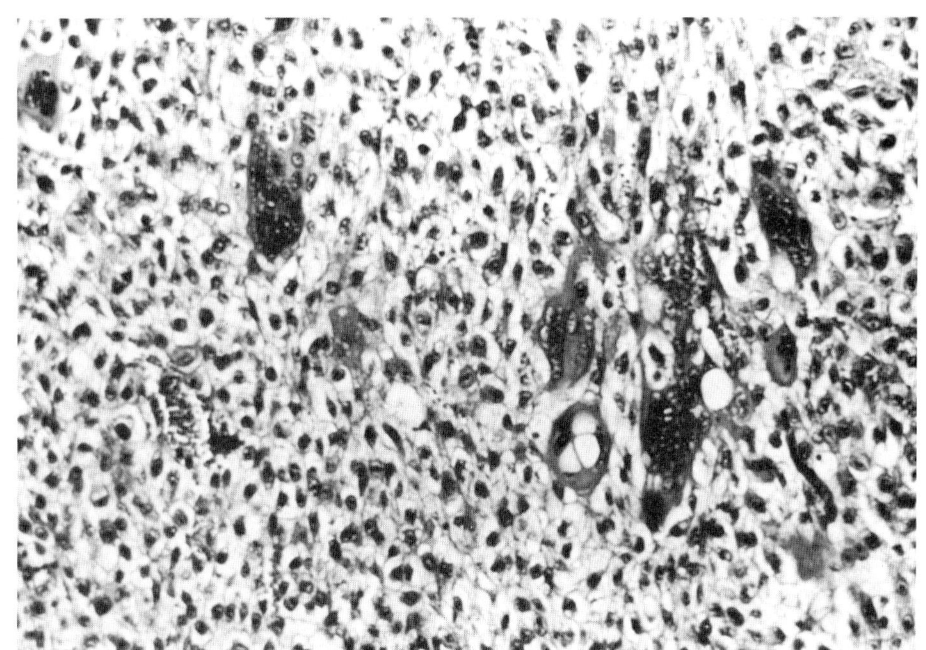

FIGURE 33-1.
(Courtesy of Robert C. Maier, MD, Medical College of Georgia.)

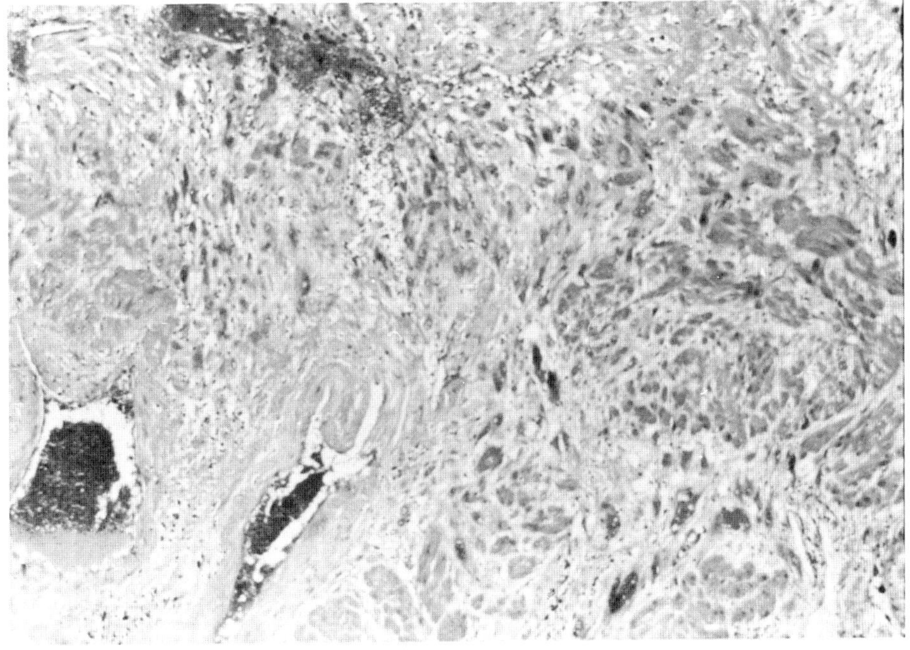

FIGURE 33-2.
(Courtesy of Robert C. Maier, MD, Medical College of Georgia.)

9. A woman at a higher risk for developing a hydatidiform mole
10. A woman at a higher risk for developing a choriocarcinoma

DIRECTIONS for questions 11-13: For each numbered item, select the one heading most closely associated with it. Each lettered heading may be used *only once.*

(A) Androgenesis
(B) Partial mole
(C) Complete mole
(D) Gestational trophoblastic tumor
(E) Placental-site trophoblastic tumor

11. A condition with some normal and some swollen villi plus fetal or cord or amniotic membrane elements associated with polyploidy.
12. A placental abnormality involving swollen placental villi and trophoblastic hyperplasia with loss of fetal blood vessels.
13. A tumor that consists of excessive groups of mononucleate and multinucleate trophoblastic cells in the area of implantation which is accompanied by an inflammatory cell reaction.

DIRECTIONS for questions 14-23: For each numbered item, indicate whether it is associated with

A only (A)
B only (B)
C both (A) and (B)
D neither (A) nor (B)

Questions 14-20

(A) Partial Mole
(B) Complete Mole
(C) Both
(D) Neither

14. Hyperplasia of the syncytiotrophoblast
15. Hyperplasia of the cytotrophoblast
16. Usually a 47, XY karyotype
17. Both maternal and paternal origin
18. Immediate evacuation of a 26-week-sized uterus
19. Weekly serum β-HCG determinations until 2 normal values have been obtained
20. Nuclear DNA is completely paternal and mitochondrial DNA is maternal

Questions 21-23

A. Low-risk gestational trophoblastic tumor GTT
B. High-risk gestational trophoblastic tumor GTT
C. Both
D. Neither

21. Recurrence rate is less than 30%
22. Patients treated with chemotherapy should not get pregnant until they have gone at least one year without evidence of recurrence
23. A score of 8 using the World Health Organization scoring system based on prognostic factors

DIRECTIONS for questions 24-34: For each of the questions below, ONE or MORE of the responses are correct. Select the best answer based on the following

A if 1, 2, and 3 are correct
B if only 1 and 2 are correct
C if only 2 and 3 are correct
D if only 1 is correct
E if only 3 is correct

Questions 24-25

24. Each of three patients has had a hydatidiform mole evacuated from her uterus. After consulting the graph in Figure 33-3, indicate those patient(s) who should be treated for gestational trophoblastic tumor.
   1. Patient 1

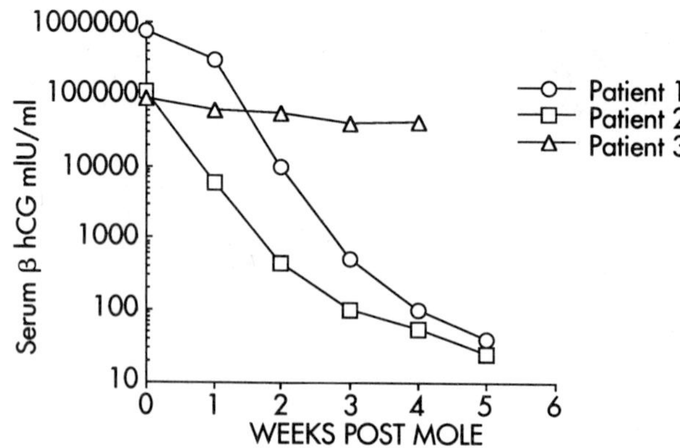

FIGURE 33-3.

2. Patient 2
3. Patient 3

25. All three patients whose β-HCG is depicted in Figure 33-3 are in their late twenties, multigravidas, and had their last menstrual period 14 weeks ago. Their uteri are consistent with a 14-week pregnancy and their ovaries are not palpable. Management of the patient(s) *with* gestational trophoblastic neoplasia identified in the previous question, assuming all additional relevant studies are normal, should include
    1. a chest x-ray
    2. single agent chemotherapy
    3. a sensitive test, specific for β-HCG every 2 weeks for 1 year
26. Appropriate treatment regimens for low risk (metastatic) gestational trophoblastic tumor (GTT) include
    1. one additional course of chemotherapy after a negative β-HCG has been obtained
    2. Actinomycin D
    3. VP-16 (etoposide)
27. Malignant sequelae following a hydatidiform mole appear to be more common when the signs and symptoms include
    1. hyperemesis gravidarum
    2. a uterus large for dates
    3. ovarian enlargement
28. A 32-year-old gravida 5, para 4 is now 20 weeks pregnant by her menstrual dates. The uterus is felt to be the size of a 16-week gestation. An ultrasound is obtained and is pictured in Figure 33-4. The β-HCG is markedly elevated for 20 weeks. In discussing the possible outcomes, you would tell this patient that
    1. the fetus has a life expectancy of less than 1 month
    2. she will need to have serial β-HCG levels obtained postpartum
    3. there is a 20% risk of malignant sequelae
29. It is established that individuals more likely to develop a hydatidiform mole include a woman with a history of
    1. a prior hydatidiform mole
    2. recurrent abortions

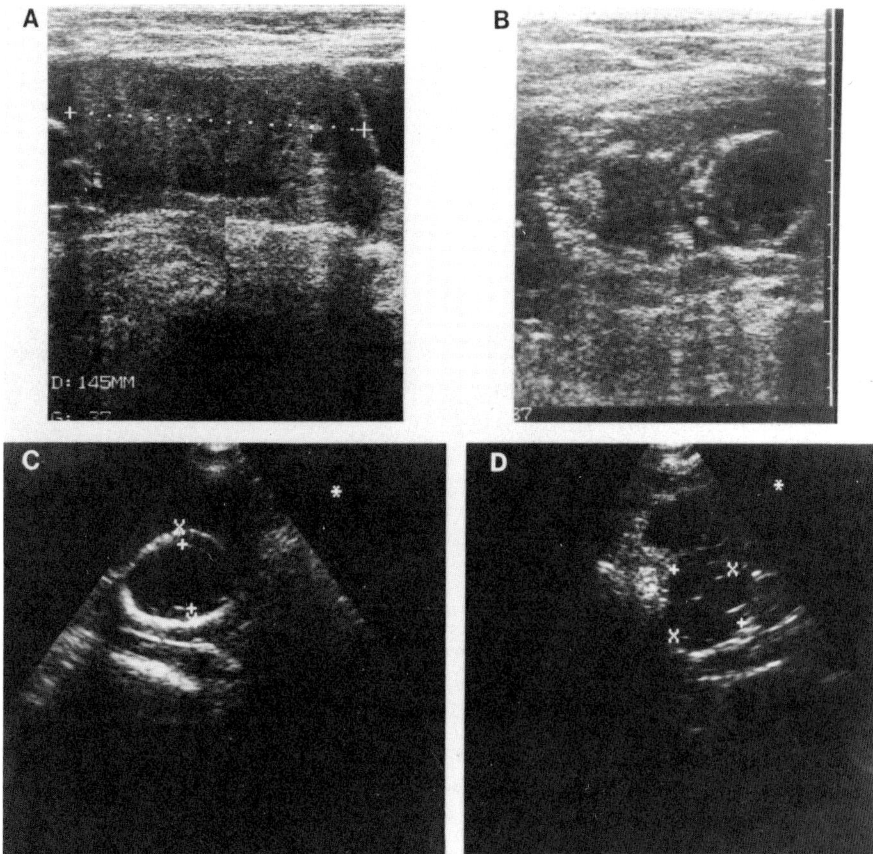

FIGURE 33-4.

3. poor nutrition

30. True statements about gestational trophoblastic tumor (GTT) include:
    1. one third arise after a molar pregnancy
    2. one third arise after a normal pregnancy
    3. Given a complete mole, approximately 20% will develop into GTT
31. Normal trophoblastic tissue
    1. metastasizes
    2. invades locally
    3. contains multinucleated cells
32. Which tests currently are used in the diagnosis and management of a complete or partial mole?
    1. an arteriogram
    2. a serum β-HCG
    3. ultrasound

Questions 33-34

33. A patient's uterus is symmetrically large for dates. The referring physician ordered a β-HCG. The result is charted on the laboratory's report shown in Figure 33-5. Your differential diagnosis includes
    1. twins
    2. a complete mole
    3. incorrect dates
34. Having established the differential diagnosis in question 33, you order an ultrasound. The image is reproduced in Figure 33-6. Given the most likely diagnosis, abnormal laboratory tests sometimes reported with this problem include
    1. elevated serum thyroxine
    2. x-ray evidence of a pulmonary lesion
    3. polycythemia

ANSWERS

1. **D,** Pages 1051-1052. If the patient has completed childbearing, hysterectomy, "D", should strongly be considered if the patient is older with an enlarged uterus or theca lutein cysts. The ovarian lutein cysts regress after termination of the pregnancy, and oophorectomy should not be performed unless there is other ovarian pathology or there is an acute episode such as rupture. Older patients or those with risk factors for ovarian carcinoma may wish to consider elective removal.
2. **B,** Page 1054. The most frequent site of metastatic GTN is the lungs (80 to 90% of cases), and less frequently the liver, brain, ovary, and vagina. However, metastatic disease can occur at any site. Given the diagnosis of GTN, a careful survey for metastatic disease should be initiated using CT examination of the brain and the abdomen. Tests of renal and liver chemistries should also be performed in addition to a hematologic profile.
3. **C,** Pages 1047-1048. The photomicrograph depicted in Figure 33-1 is a high-power view of a choriocarcinoma. Both pale cytotrophoblasts and syncytiotrophoblasts can be seen. These tumors tend to be hemorrhagic and necrotic. No villi are seen. With a complete or partial hydatidiform mole, the villi are edematous and lack fetal blood cells. One would expect to see villi rather than hemorrhage or necrosis with retained secundines. Choriocarcinoma may develop after a normal pregnancy. Trophoblastic tissue regresses within 2 to 3 weeks after normal delivery. The finding of trophoblastic cells in the uterus more than 3 weeks after delivery

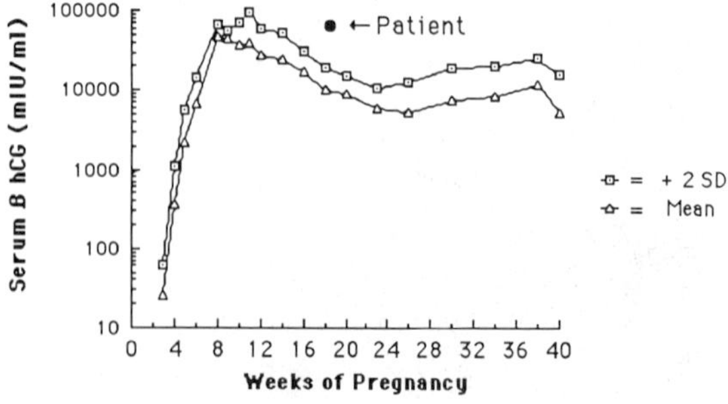

FIGURE 33-5.

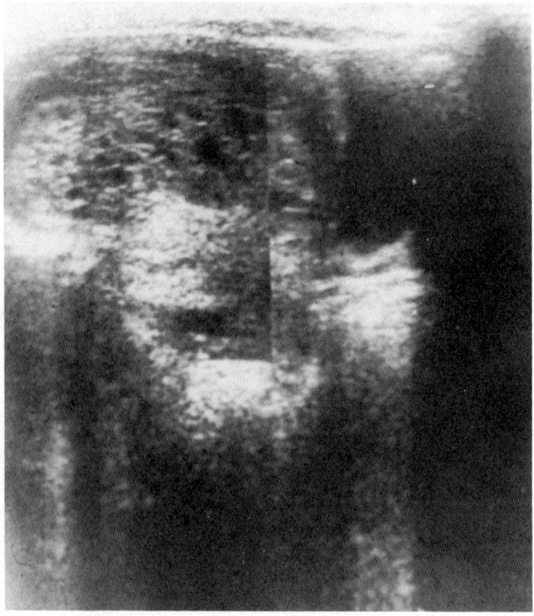

FIGURE 33-6.

should lead one to consider the possibility of choriocarcinoma. This scenario is indeed rare as the incidence of choriocarcinoma following a normal term pregnancy is 1 in 40,000 in the United States.

4. **D.** This photomicrograph depicts decidua and syncytiotrophoblasts within the myometrium. One should remember that trophoblasts invade the myometrium in a normal pregnancy. This is *not* indicative of gestational trophoblastic neoplasia. In all probability this patient will have no further difficulties. She does not require β-HCG monitoring.
5. **C,** Pages 1047, 1054. Although most choriocarcinomas occur after complete molar pregnancies, occurrences have been reported after incomplete moles and rare choriocarcinomas have developed after a normal pregnancy (1 per 40,000 term pregnancies). The disease also follows incomplete abortion and ectopic pregnancy.
6. **E,** Page 1048; Table 33-1. The risk of developing a hydatidiform mole in women who are pregnant is lowest in the 25-29 year age bracket. If the risk assigned to this group is 1, the risk in a woman under 20 years of age is 1.53 and in women over 50 it is 80.76, this being the highest risk group. Since not many women who are 50 years of age become pregnant, numerically few hydatidiform moles are seen in this age group.
7. **D,** Pages 1051 and 1052. Intravenous oxytocic agents are used during the evacuation and immediately postoperatively to aid in uterine contraction and to help reduce blood loss. However, it is not advisable to use oxytocic drugs before evacuation of the molar pregnancy because of the risk of disseminating abnormal trophoblastic cells. Suction curettage has proven to be safe and effective even with a larger uterus. After evacuation by suction curettage is complete, a gentle sharp curettage should be performed to ensure completion of the procedure. There is no need to do a hysterotomy. Prophylactic chemotherapy has not gained widespread acceptance because giving chemotherapy at the time of evacuation of the mole exposes the patient to toxic and dangerous drugs, and 80% of patients with a complete mole do not require further treatment. Since this patient is a 20 year-old and a gravida 1, it should be assumed that she has not completed childbearing. Therefore, she is not a candidate for a hysterectomy.
8. **D,** Pages 1049 and 1050 (box). Signs and symptoms associated with a hydatidiform mole include abnormal bleeding in early pregnancy, lower abdominal pain, preeclampsia before 24 weeks of gestation, hyperemesis gravidarum, a uterus large for dates, a uterus small for dates, enlargement of the ovaries, absent fetal heart tones and fetal parts, expulsion of swollen villi, and rarely hyperthyroidism. With an incomplete, not a complete, hydatidiform mole a fetus is usually present.

9-10. 9, **E;** 10, **B;** Page 1049; 1048. No differential in the risk for *hydatidiform mole* for ABO blood groups has been demonstrated. However, studies have shown that women with type A blood married to men with type O and vice versa are at higher risk for *choriocarcinoma* in comparison to matings of other blood groups.

11-13. 11, **B;** 12, **C;** 13, **E;** Pages 1044 and 1048. A hydatidiform mole is a placental abnormality involving swollen placental villi and trophoblastic hyperplasia with loss of fetal blood vessels. There are two types, partial and complete. A partial mole is a molar pregnancy with some normal and some swollen villi plus some fetal or cord or amniotic membrane elements associated with polyploidy. A complete mole is the most common type of gestational trophoblastic disease (GTD), occurring in the United States in 0.75 per 1000 pregnancies. The term placental-site trophoblastic tumor (trophoblastic pseudotumor) has been used to describe a rare variety of tumor that consists of excessive groups of mononucleate and multinucleate trophoblastic cells at the implantation site which is accompanied by an inflammatory cell reaction. These tumors tend to stain more for lactogen than for HCG, and both HCG and HPL should be monitored.

14-20. 14, **C;** 15, **B;** 16, **D;** 17, **A;** 18, **C;** 19, **C;** 20, **B;** Pages 1044, 1050-1051, 1052. The three morphologic characteristics of a complete mole are: (1) a mass of distended villi that appear as large grape-like dilations, (2) a loss of fetal blood vessels in the villi, and (3) hyperplasia of the syncytiotrophoblast and cytotrophoblast. With a partial mole, in addition to the presence of a fetus, there is hyperplasia of the syncytiotrophoblast *only*. In complete mole, only paternal chromosomes are believed to be present; there are 46 chromosomes and they are nearly always 46, XX, although a few moles with 46, XY karyotype have been reported. This is the result of a process known as androgenesis, which is the impregnation of an inactive egg by a paternal haploid sperm that duplicates its chromosomes to provide a diploid complement (See Figure 33-2, page 1046). The nuclear genome is entirely paternal, whereas mitochondrial genome is maternal per usual. This anomaly is due to a fertilization error occurring at the time of Maternal Meiosis II.

Incomplete or partial moles are triploid and have 69 chromosomes of both maternal and paternal origin (See Figure 33-3, page 1046). The most common mechanism for the origin of partial mole is a haploid egg being fertilized by two sperm, resulting in three sets of chromosomes. In all cases mitochondrial DNA is maternal. Not all triploidic concepti demonstrate molar degeneration since duplication of paternal DNA plays some unknown role. Consequently a 69, XXY fetus in which 2 of 3 haploid sets are maternal (e.g. Maternal Meiotic I error) would have a normal placenta. The ultimate severity of the triploidic phenotype depends on this imprinting mechanism.

Immediate evacuation of a 26-week-sized uterus may be an ethical and legal problem, if the uterus contains a partial rather than a complete mole, but triploidy is incompatible with *sustained* life.

The malignant potential of a partial mole is lower than that for a complete mole. In spite of rare subsequent malignancy, patients with partial moles need the same follow-up as those with a complete mole. Following the evacuation of a mole weekly serum β-HCG determinations should be obtained until 2 values are normal.

21-23. 21, **C**; 22, **C**; 23, **B**; Pages 1056-1057; Table 33-4. The recurrence rate for low-risk metastatic GTT is approximately 5%. The recurrence rate for non-metastatic GTT is 1% to 2%. As many as 20% of patients with metastatic high-risk GTT who attain a negative β-HCG titer have a recurrence. Non-metastatic GTT and metastatic low-risk GTT are almost 100% curable by chemotherapy. After 1 year of negative follow-up the patient may again attempt pregnancy whether she is high or low-risk. Using the World Health Organization scoring system based on prognostic factors, a total score less than or equal to 4 is considered low risk, a total score of 5-7 is considered middle risk, and a total score of 8 or higher is considered high risk. The most frequent site of metastatic GTT is the lungs (80% to 90% of cases), and less frequently the liver, brain, ovary, and vagina are involved

24. **E** (3 only), Pages 1052-1054. Usually, there is a gradual decline of β-HCG after evacuation of a hydatidiform mole, reaching a normal range of 3 to 5 mIU/ml by the 14th week after evacuation. There may be an abnormal regression curve after evacuation of a mole, as shown in patient 3, and in such instances the patient requires therapy for a gestational trophoblastic tumor. A rise in titer or a plateau in titer (failure to decrease over a 3-week interval) indicates the presence of postmolar trophoblastic neoplasia.

25. **B** (1, 2), Pages 1053 and 1054. Management of a patient with a hydatidiform mole includes
    1. A chest x-ray initially and repeated if abnormal or if the β-HCG plateaus or rises.
    2. Contraception for 1 year.
    3. A pelvic examination every 2 weeks until normal, then every 3 months
    4. Weekly serum determinations of β-HCG until normal for two values, then monthly for 1 year.

    In this question the option was to monitor β-HCG every 2 weeks and not weekly. Single agent therapy is sufficient because with the information given patient 3 has non-metastatic disease. Before chemotherapy is initiated, however, a CT of the brain and the liver should obtained, as well as a pelvic ultrasound, renal and liver chemistries, and a hematologic profile.

26. **A** (All), Pages 1055 and 1056. There are several different regimens that employ either methotrexate or actinomycin D for low risk GTN therapy. VP-16 (etoposide) has also been effectively used as single-agent therapy. One additional course of the agent being used should be given after a negative β-HCG has been obtained.

27. **C** (2, 3), Pages 1044, 1049-1050, and 1052. Malignant sequelae following a hydatidiform mole appear to be more common among those with an enlarged uterus. Enlargement of the ovaries is associated with a higher frequency of future malignant sequelae (approximately 50%) as compared to less than 15% for those without ovarian enlargement.

28. **B** (1, 2), Pages 1050, 1052. The ultrasound depicted in Figure 33-4 reveals placenta tissue suggestive of a hydatidiform mole (A), oligohydramnios (B), hydrocephaly (C), and a cystic structure (D) which in this patient is a theca lutein cyst. This is a case of a partial mole associated with an abnormal fetus. Survival of such an infant beyond the early neonatal period has not been reported. Partial moles are rarely associated with the subsequent development of malignant trophoblastic disease. In spite of this fact, patients with partial moles need the same follow-up as those with complete moles including serial β-HCG determinations.
29. **B** (1, 2), Page 1048. A history of prior hydatidiform mole increases the risk of a subsequent mole by 20 to 40 times. Recurrent spontaneous abortion is also a risk factor. The increased frequency of moles in lower socioeconomic groups and in underdeveloped areas has led to the suggestion that poor nutrition is a factor in the development of the disease. The evidence is conflicting, and a dietary etiology is not supported by current data.
30. **E** (3 only), Page 1052. GTT develops after approximately 20% of complete hydatidiform moles. Conversely, about half the cases of GTT arise after molar pregnancy while one fourth occur after normal pregnancy and one fourth after abortion or ectopic pregnancy.
31. **A** (All), Page 1044. Trophoblastic tissue is unusual insofar as it shares certain characteristics with malignancies, such as the ability to divide rapidly, to invade locally, and occasionally to metastasize to distant sites such as the lung. The syncytiotrophoblast is a multinucleated cell layer.
32. **C** (2 3), Pages 1050, 1052, 1054. The most valuable aid in the diagnosis of a hydatidiform mole is ultrasound. Other diagnostic tests, such as amniograms and arteriograms, were previously used. HCG is important in the diagnosis and follow-up of a molar pregnancy, but one should use a sensitive immunoassay (radioimmunoassay [RIA] or enzymatic immunoassay [EIA]) specific for the subunit. Always know the specificity and sensitivity of the test you are using. A single elevated β-HCG is not diagnostic because the patient may have twins or her dates may be in error. One should have a baseline β-HCG before beginning treatment.
33. **A** (All), Pages 1049-1050. Levels of β-HCG can appear elevated in a twin pregnancy. This patient's value would fall into an acceptable range if she were really 12, not 18 weeks. Patients with a complete mole usually have an elevated β-HCG. A single β-HCG is often not diagnostic, especially if the level is not elevated. In 30 to 50% of cases, the uterus will be large for dates. Patients with an incomplete mole tend to have lower levels of β-HCG.
34. **B** (1, 2), Pages 1050-1051. Occasionally a patient with a mole will manifest hyperthyroidism, disseminated intravascular coagulation, or trophoblastic disease in the lungs. These patients can develop pulmonary insufficiency. These patients are not polycythemic. If anything, they are anemic due to blood loss.

PART FIVE

ENDOCRINOLOGY AND INFERTILITY

Dysmenorrhea and Premenstrual Syndrome

DIRECTIONS for questions 1 - 4: Select the one best answer or completion.

1. A 36 year-old gravida 3, para 3, who underwent a tubal ligation eight years ago is under treatment for premenstrual syndrome (PMS). She has responded well to ovarian suppression with danazol. No other previous therapy has been beneficial and she now seeks a more permanent solution. She should be offered
   A. hysterectomy
   B. hysterectomy with bilateral oophorectomy
   C. endometrial ablation
   D. dilatation and curettage
   E. presacral neurectomy

Questions 2-3

2. A 32 year-old woman has been arrested and charged with the murder of her husband. In her defense, she has entered a plea of temporary insanity by virtue of the premenstrual syndrome. You have been subpoenaed to testify. On the witness stand, the prosecuting attorney asks you to define the "premenstrual syndrome". Your testimony should indicate that the symptoms of PMS
   A. occur no more than 14 days prior to menstruation
   B. occur no more than 5 days prior to menstruation
   C. occur in a severe form in more than 10% of patients
   D. are sometimes absent immediately after menstruation
   E. are primarily emotional, not physical
3. The woman's defense attorney (question 2) has entered into evidence a graph of the defendant's "symptoms" over the past two months. You are asked to review Defendant's Exhibit A (Figure 34.1) Based on this graph, you might reasonably testify that the accused
   A. has "PMS"
   B. is a manic-depressive
   C. was insane at the time of the murder
   D. has severe dysmenorrhea
   E. none of the above
4. A 20 year-old nulligravida complains of severe lower abdominal cramping pain, nausea, vomiting and diarrhea, which occur approximately eight hours after the onset of menstruation and lasts for one to two days. The patient's periods take place regularly every 26 to 28 days and last five days. She is not sexually active, uses no birth control, and normally takes Extra Strength Tylenol(acetaminophen) with little relief. Her physical, including pelvic examination, is unremarkable. The cause of these symptoms is most likely
   A. adenomyosis
   B. endometriosis
   C. cervical stenosis
   D. excess prostaglandin
   E. leiomyomata

DIRECTIONS For each numbered item 5 - 16, indicate whether it is associated with
A only (A)
B only (B)
C both (A) and (B)
D neither (A) nor (B)

5-9. Match the complaint, cause, or response
(A) premenstrual syndrome
(B) dysmenorrhea (primary or secondary)
(C) both
(D) neither

5. lower abdominal pain solely prior to menstruation
6. pelvic heaviness and bloating
7. prostaglandin mediated
8. may respond to non-steroidal anti-inflammatory drug (NSAID) therapy
9. approximately 15% of sufferers have severe symptoms

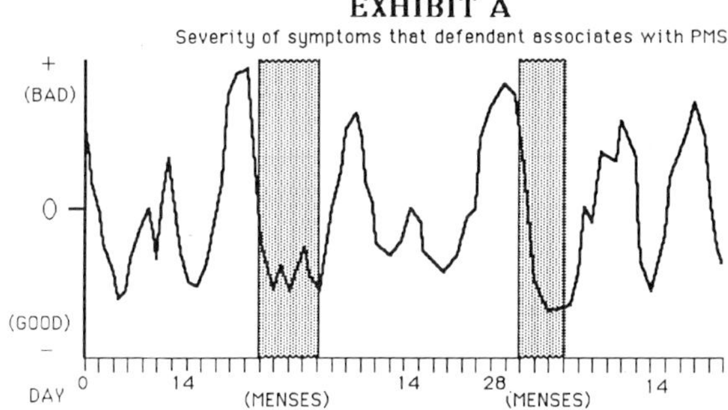

FIGURE 34-1.

10-16. Differences and commonalities between primary and secondary dysmenorrhea
   (A) primary dysmenorrhea
   (B) secondary dysmenorrhea
   (C) both
   (D) neither

10. likely to improve with mild to moderate strength analgesics
11. probable diagnosis for menstrual discomfort in a 42 year-old multipara
12. generally associated with a normal pelvic examination
13. likely to have a familial pattern
14. major cause of school absences
15. associated with throbbing abdominal pain and a sense of pelvic heaviness
16. symptoms start 3 to 4 days prior to menses

DIRECTIONS for questions 17 - 32: For each of the questions below, ONE or MORE of the responses is correct. Select the best answer based on the following

A if 1, 2, and 3 are correct
B if only 1 and 2 are correct
C if only 2 and 3 are correct
D if only 1 is correct
E if only 3 is correct

17. A 19 year-old nulligravid college student requests contraception. Her only significant history is that of dysmenorrhea for six years. Her examination is normal. Recommended contraceptive choices for her should include
   1. oral contraceptives
   2. a diaphragm
   3. an intrauterine contraceptive device
18. It is currently thought that cause or causes of the premenstrual syndrome (PMS) include
   1. estrogen excess
   2. endorphin imbalance
   3. serotonin deficiency
19. A 17 year-old nulligravida requests treatment of her primary dysmenorrhea. Contraindications to the use of nonsteroidal anti-inflammatory agents in this patient would encompass
   1. aspirin sensitive asthma
   2. a history or diarrhea with menstruation
   3. premenstrual irritability and bloating
20. Which of the following would be useful in making the diagnosis of premenstrual syndrome?
   1. a clinical trial of 200 mg per day of Vitamin B_6
   2. a serum estrogen level
   3. a diary of symptoms over a 2 to 3 month period
21. A 32 year-old desires treatment for the premenstrual syndrome (PMS). She has previously taken bromocriptine and asks about taking it again. She should be told that it
   1. is appropriate when breast tenderness is the major symptom
   2. causes a greater improvement in mood than does placebo treatment
   3. reduces the elevated level of prolactin found in these patients
22. Prostaglandin $F_{2\alpha}$ has been implicated as a possible cause of primary dysmenorrhea because
   1. it is found in higher amounts in women with dysmenorrhea
   2. it is capable of stimulating the smooth muscle of the uterus
   3. inhibition of its production through the use of nonsteroidal anti-inflammatory drugs results in the relief of symptoms
23. The role of progesterone in the treatment of premenstrual syndrome (PMS) is based on
   1. the observation that PMS symptoms are absent during pregnancy
   2. large open uncontrolled trials
   3. the reduced levels of progesterone in patients with PMS
24. Appropriate initial therapy for premenstrual symptoms in a 29 year-old gravida 3, para 2, abortus 1, female who has had her "tubes tied" includes
   1. reassurance
   2. a balanced diet
   3. vitamin B_6 100 mg p.o. b.i.d
25. In a 19 year-old nulligravida with the clinical diagnosis of primary dysmenorrhea, appropriate therapy consists of two tablets at the onset of pain and then one tablet t.i.d. PRN of
   1. Anaprox 275 mg
   2. Ponstel 250 mg
   3. Motrin 800 mg

26. A 30 year-old patient is referred for cyclic fluid retention as a primary focus of the premenstrual syndrome (PMS). She should be told that fluid retention has been implicated in PMS because symptomatology is associated with
    1. an increase in total body weight
    2. an increase in abdominal girth
    3. a perception of swelling
27. A 36 year-old gravida 3, para 3, health food store owner asks your opinion about using vitamin B_6 in a dosage of 650 mg twice a day for the treatment of premenstrual syndrome (PMS). You can respond that this regimen
    1. will help to slow the metabolism of estrogen
    2. is potentially dangerous
    3. has not been proven effective

Questions 28-29

28. A 34 year-old gravida 1, para 1, using an intrauterine device (IUD) for contraception complains of heavy, crampy periods since the birth of her child one year ago. She had experienced menstrual pain during most of her periods prior to her last pregnancy. This discomfort had responded to therapy with Motrin (ibuprofen). Her current discomfort is somewhat worse than it was previously. She has tried an over-the-counter ibuprofen medication without success. This patient's physical examination, including pelvic examination, is normal and her IUD string is visible. Possible diagnoses include
    1. primary dysmenorrhea
    2. secondary dysmenorrhea
    3. premenstrual syndrome
29. In an effort to help the patient depicted in Question 28, you might reasonably recommend
    1. surgical sterilization
    2. a nonsteroidal anti-inflammatory agent
    3. removal of the IUD
30. A 16 year-old has disabling primary dysmenorrhea. Her history is otherwise negative and her physical examination is normal. Initial therapeutic options include
    1. oral contraceptives
    2. prostaglandin synthetase inhibitors (NSAID's)
    3. analgesics
31. Factors which affect the severity of premenstrual syndrome symptoms include
    1. age
    2. number of children
    3. evidence of clinical depression
32. A 38 year-old gravida 4, para 4, has a two year history of emotional lability, irritability and difficulty with fellow workers. She admits to episodes of inexplicable crying and feels that sometimes people are "out to get her." She has not sought help for this, but believes that it may be the premenstrual syndrome (PMS). In addition to PMS, a differential diagnosis for this patient should include
    1. anxiety
    2. depression
    3. psychosis

ANSWERS

1. **B,** Page 1075. As reported recently, some patients who respond to ovarian suppressing doses of medication may be candidates for hysterectomy and bilateral salpingo-oophorectomy as the definitive treatment for the premenstrual syndrome (PMS). Removing the uterus alone will not alter the symptoms as it only removes the source of bleeding and not the source of other premenstrual symptoms. Endometrial ablation would also only reduce or eliminate menstrual bleeding while not addressing the symptoms. Dilatation and curettage as well as presacral neurectomy have no role in the treatment of premenstrual syndrome (PMS). Hysterectomy with bilateral oophorectomy should only be employed in the unusual case where other therapies have failed and in a patient who clearly responds to ovarian suppression. In addition to danazol, GnRH agonists have been used successfully to treat PMS. Patients who undergo surgical castration can be given estrogen replacement therapy without symptoms recurring.
2. **A,** Page 1074, Premenstrual syndrome and dysmenorrhea, Dawood MY, McGuire JL and Demers LM (eds), Urban & Schwarzenberg, Baltimore, 1985. Probably the best working definition of the premenstrual syndrome is one that restricts the recurrence of significant, distressing emotional and physical symptoms to no more than 14 days before menses. These symptoms must recur episodically and predictably and do not have to occur every month, although they usually do so. In addition, the symptoms must spontaneously and completely disappear with, or soon after, the onset of menstrual flow. While the premenstrual syndrome (PMS) is thought to affect anywhere from 5% to 95% of women, only about 2% to 3% have severe symptoms.

3. **E,** Page 1069. The pattern of symptoms illustrated in Figure 34-1 is typical of patients who have complaints that become linked or entrained with the recurrent rhythm of the period, not true premenstrual syndrome (PMS). Note that there is a true "symptom-free" period following each menstrual flow. No mention of menstrual pain has been made to support the diagnosis of dysmenorrhea. As a gynecologist, you are not in a position to diagnose what that disorder is nor to make legal assessments regarding her guilt or accountability.
4. **D,** Pages 1063-1065. Primary dysmenorrhea is caused by an excess of prostaglandin F2α. This prostaglandin excess also is responsible for the presence of nausea, vomiting and diarrhea which are not seen with adenomyosis or cervical stenosis. The pain associated with endometriosis generally precedes the onset of menstrual flow and improves after flow is established.

5-9. 5, **A;** 6, **C;** 7, **B;** 8, **C;** 9, **B;** Pages 1069; 1074; 1063; 1064; 1075. While the most commonly recognized symptoms of premenstrual syndrome are emotional, many somatic pre-period symptoms may be present. When these symptoms exist solely in the premenstrual period, they may correctly be termed a part of "premenstrual syndrome". These same somatic symptoms may also be present in primary or secondary dysmenorrhea and the differentiation between these and premenstrual syndrome (PMS) is based on the timing of the complaints. Even though both premenstrual syndrome (PMS) and dysmenorrhea may respond to non-steroidal anti-inflammatory drug (NSAID) therapy, there is no evidence currently available that prostaglandins play a significant role in the development of PMS. Severe symptoms are found in 2-3% of "PMS" patients and 10 to 15% of women with dysmenorrhea.

10-16. 10, **C;** 11, **B;** 12, **A;** 13, **A;** 14, **A;** 15, **B;** 16, **D;** Pages 1064-1068. The best therapy for secondary dysmenorrhea is ultimately directed toward the cause, but both primary and secondary dysmenorrhea may be treated successfully with analgesics. The distinction between primary and secondary is most often made on the basis of a normal pelvic examination associated with primary dysmenorrhea. The peak age of incidence for primary and secondary dysmenorrhea is very different. Primary dysmenorrhea is much more likely in younger women. Thus, it accounts for a significant number of school absences. In older women, secondary dysmenorrhea is more apt to be the correct diagnosis even though primary dysmenorrhea is still possible. While causes of secondary dysmenorrhea such as myomata may have a familial pattern, it is primary dysmenorrhea that is most closely associated with a familial tendency. The symptoms of pelvic heaviness and throbbing pain are more common with secondary dysmenorrhea. The pain of primary dysmenorrhea is usually described as sharp or "labor-like" in character. In neither primary nor secondary dysmenorrhea do the symptoms start appreciably before the onset of menstrual flow.

17. **B** (1, 2), Pages 1065-1066. Because primary dysmenorrhea is associated with ovulatory cycles, suppression of ovulation with oral contraceptives will often provide at least some measure of relief. A diaphragm would be an acceptable barrier form of contraception if the patient were sufficiently motivated to use it correctly. Her dysmenorrhea would then have to be treated with a nonsteroidal anti-inflammatory agent. While some studies indicate no effect of intrauterine device (IUD) use on the incidence of dysmenorrhea, many authors feel that it may contribute to menstrual pain and classify it as a cause of secondary dysmenorrhea. Progesterone containing IUD's are less like to be associated with dysmenorrhea. The patient is, however, a nulligravida. Therefore, the potential adverse effect on fertility must be weighed and the IUD should be avoided.
18. **C** (2, 3), Pages 1070-1073. While many possible causes for premenstrual syndrome (PMS) have been advanced over the years, all remain unproven. Currently, the best that can be said is that PMS isa multifactorial psychoendocrine disorder. There is growing evidence that serotonin and endorphins may have a central role in PMS.
19. **D** (1 only), Page 1065. Aspirin sensitive asthma, inflammatory bowel disease and a gastric ulcer are contraindications for most nonsteroidal anti-inflammatory drugs (NSAIDs). While there is an incidence of from 3 to 10% of diarrhea with the use of NSAIDs, many studies have indicated that

there is a reduction in the incidence of period related diarrhea with these drugs. Premenstrual syndrome (PMS) is not a contraindication to the use of these drugs and indeed, patients may respond favorably to their use.

20. **E** (3 only), Page 1069. The most useful tool for making the diagnosis of premenstrual syndrome is a diary of symptoms. There is no evidence that changes in estrogen levels would be helpful in making the diagnosis. Since the value of Vitamin B_6 therapy is debatable, any response noted would be non diagnostic because of the possibility of a placebo effect.
21. **D** (1 only), Page 1071. Studies have been unable to demonstrate an abnormal level of prolactin in women with premenstrual syndrome (PMS). In controlled studies of bromocriptine use in the treatment of the premenstrual syndrome (PMS), only breast tenderness responded, and only in doses above 5 mg per day.
22. **A** (1, 2, 3), Page 1064, Ylikorkala O, Dawood MY, New concepts in dysmenorrhea. Amer J Obstet Gynecol 130:833-847, 1978. Prostaglandin $F_{2\alpha}$ has been found in levels of 5 to 10 times the usual amount in women with primary dysmenorrhea. It is a potent stimulator of smooth muscle both in the uterus and in the gastrointestinal tract. In the uterus, this prostaglandin $F_{2'}$ action may be responsible for intrauterine pressures in excess of 400 mmHg. (During contractions of the uterus during menstruation, the uterine pressure is 60-80 mmHg). In the gastrointestinal tract, the increased motility caused by the stimulatory effects of prostaglandin $F_{2'}$ may account for the frequent observation of nausea, vomiting and diarrhea in patients with primary dysmenorrhea. While the success of NSAID therapy supports the role of prostaglandins in primary dysmenorrhea, it does not by itself conclusively establish a cause and effect relationship.
23. **B** (1, 2), Page 1072-1074. The use of progesterone therapy in the treatment of premenstrual syndrome (PMS) has been most vocally championed by Dr. Katharina Dalton of England. She observed that PMS symptoms were absent in her own pregnancy and in her patients during pregnancy. This has led to the use of progesterone in uncontrolled open trials of more than 30,000 patients world-wide. Despite this experience, no controlled blind study has been able to confirm a superiority over placebo. No study of any kind has been able to confirm any consistent alteration of progesterone levels.
24. **A** (1, 2, 3), Page 1074. Though unproven by double blind trials, reassurance, a good diet and a exercise program are always appropriate. Exercise may help induce endogenous endorphin production. A substantial number of patients will benefit from just undergoing the process of investigation and the identification of a diagnostic condition. Supplementation with small doses of vitamin B_6, which is a coenzyme in the production of serotonin, is probably very reasonable therapy in almost any patient with premenstrual syndrome (PMS).
25. **A** (1, 2, 3), Page 1065 (Table 34-2). Anaprox (naproxen sodium), Ponstel (mefenamic acid), and Motrin (ibuprofen) are all approved for the treatment of dysmenorrhea and would be appropriate in the absence of contraindications. Because of evidence of receptor site activity by the fenamates (Ponstel and Meclomen) there may be some theoretical advantage favoring these agents. In practice, this may be reflected in a slightly faster onset of action. For most patients, however, these differences are probably of little consequence.
26. **E** (3 only), Page 1072. Controlled studies have been unable to demonstrate any changes in abdominal measurements or in total body weight, even in those patients who complain of swelling and bloating. These patients do believe that during the period of symptomatology, they are bloated and swollen.
27. **C** (2, 3), Page 1074, Hagen I, Neshem BI, Tamtland T. Acta Obstet Gynecol Scand 64:667-670, 1985. The rationale for using B_6 as therapy for premenstrual syndrome (PMS) comes from the fact that it is a coenzyme in the production of serotonin in the brain. Because reduced levels of serotonin have been found in patients with depression, some authors have postulated that replacing B_6 may favorably affect the emotional symptoms of PMS. Vitamin B_6 therapy for premenstrual syndrome PMS has not been adequately studied to make any case for efficacy. While some patients may experience improvement, there are no blinded studies to suggest a response greater than seen with placebo. Peripheral nerve damage has been reported in dosages above 200 mg per day. Dosage in the magnitude suggested for this patient should not be used.

28. **B** (1, 2), Pages 1063-1068; Dysmenorrhea, Dawood MY (ed), Williams and Wilkins, Baltimore, 1981. Chan WY, Dawood MY, Fuchs F. Relief of dysmenorrhea with the prostaglandin synthetase inhibitor ibuprofen: effect on prostaglandin levels in menstrual fluid. Am J Obstet Gynecol 135:102, 1979. While the most likely diagnosis for this patient is dysmenorrhea secondary to an intrauterine device (IUD), continuing primary dysmenorrhea is still a possibility. The patient's history is not typical for the premenstrual syndrome (PMS). It does suggests that she may have had primary dysmenorrhea before her pregnancy. Studies reported by Dawood indicate that pregnancy and delivery do not relieve dysmenorrhea. As many as 20% of women with dysmenorrhea will experience a return of symptoms with the return of ovulation. The lack of response of the patient's symptoms to over-the-counter strengths of ibuprofen most likely reflects inadequate dosage rather than an indication of a non-prostaglandin mediated etiology.
29. **C** (2, 3), Pages 1064-1066, Premenstrual syndrome and dysmenorrhea, Dawood MY, McGuire JL, Demers LM(eds), Urban & Schwarzenberg, Baltimore, 1985. When intrauterine device (IUD) use was more common, it represented a not uncommon cause for secondary, though iatrogenic, dysmenorrhea. It has been postulated that the increased prostaglandins related to IUD use not only may have been partially responsible for the contraceptive effect, but also may have been the cause of the accompanying menstrual pain. This association is supported by studies that indicate moderate success in treating these women with therapeutic doses of prostaglandin inhibitors. To attempt to differentiate between secondary dysmenorrhea from her IUD and primary dysmenorrhea, it may be necessary to advise the removal of the IUD. If this is done, an alternative contraceptive should be provided. Sterilization would not be appropriate as it does not address the complaint of dysmenorrhea.
30. **A** (1, 2, 3), Pages 1064-1065. Oral contraceptives relieve the symptoms of primary dysmenorrhea in 90% of patients. This may be due to a modulating effect on the hypothalamus or because of a reduction in the amount of endometrium. Prostaglandin synthetase inhibitors are a logical alternative. Analgesics can be used as back-up drugs if the other two options are ineffective. Narcotics are to be avoided!
31. **A** (1, 2, 3), Pages 1069-1070. It is known that environmental stressors do affect the severity of the symptoms of the premenstrual syndrome (PMS). In one study, 34% of symptom severity was attributable to PMS in the patient's mother, a low level of exercise, a younger age, and a larger number of children. In another study, PMS patients were shown to have episodes of "luteal phase depression" when compared to controls, but that these episodes were different from those suffered by patients with "endogenous depression."
32. **A** (1, 2, 3), Pages 1069-1070. Premenstrual syndrome (PMS) must be differentiated from other psychiatric disorders such as depression, anxiety reactions, and psychosis. A critical point in making the diagnosis of PMS is that PMS symptoms only occur during the luteal phase. A prospective symptom diary over severalmonths will help to identify this pattern. Although continuous use of psychoactive drugs such as tricyclics and lithium have not yielded good PMS symptom relief, alprazolam or fluoxetine hydrochloride given on days 20-28 of the cycle have significantly relieved the severity of premenstrual nervous tension, mood swings, irritability, anxiety, depression, fatigue, forgetfulness, crying, cravings for sweets, abdominal bloating, cramps, and headaches. Fluoxetine hydrochloride should not be given to patients with bipolar depression. These newer drugs seem to hold promise for relieving PMS symptoms when properly used and seem to be required in small doses only.

CHAPTER

35 Abnormal Uterine Bleeding

DIRECTIONS for questions 1 - 18: Select the one best answer or completion.

1. A woman complaining of menorrhagia has flow lasting a total of ten days. The majority of her menstrual blood loss most likely occurs
   A. within the first 3 days of menstruation
   B. during the 4th, 5th, and 6th day of menstruation
   C. during the last 3 days of menstruation
   D. at a different time each month
2. A 38 year-old gravida 3, para 3 presents with a history of progressive menorrhagia over the past eight months. This has never happened previously. The patient weighs 170 pounds and is 5 feet 2 inches tall. She has no rash, but her skin is dry. An office endometrial aspirate at her initial visit 1 month ago revealed proliferative endometrium. Her hemoglobin was 10.8 gm. The systemic disease ***most likely*** to be associated with these findings is
   A. systemic lupus erythematosis (SLE)
   B. idiopathic thrombocytopenic purpura (ITP)
   C. von Willebrands disease
   D. hypothyroidism
   E. diabetes mellitus
3. The mechanisms that normally stop menstrual blood loss include all of the following **EXCEPT**
   A. localized vasoconstriction
   B. formation of a platelet plug
   C. vascular fibrin deposition
   D. fibrinolysis
   E. myometrial contraction
4. Anovulatory patients have heavier bleeding than ovulatory patients because anovulatory patients appear to have a deficiency in
   A. prostaglandin $F_{2\alpha}$
   B. prostaglandin E_2
   C. thromboxane
   D. prostacycline
   E. arachidonic acid
5. A 28 year-old gravida 1, para 1 with menorrhagia over the past six months had her endometrium sampled on day 22 of her cycle. The report states: "secretory endometrial fragments." Since the biopsy, menstrual flow has been heavier and longer. A work-up for other potential causes for this bleeding is unrevealing. The next step in her management should be
   A. a repeat office endometrial aspiration
   B. a dilatation and curettage
   C. a vaginal probe ultrasound
   D. hysteroscopy
   E. a midluteal progesterone level
6. In treating patients with severe menorrhagia secondary to anovulation, a theoretic advantage of high dose conjugated equine estrogens over a high dose combination oral contraceptive is that estrogen alone
   A. promotes rapid endometrial growth
   B. increases spiral artery recoil
   C. increases platelet aggregation
   D. promotes synthesis prostaglandin F_2,
   E. can be given intravenously
7. A thirteen year-old virgin complains of a three month history of menometrorrhagia. The rectal abdominal exam is normal. An office urine pregnancy test is negative. The hemoglobin and hematocrit are 9.8 gm and 29% respectively. The treatment of choice for this patient is
   A. combination oral contraceptives
   B. cyclic progestin therapy for ten days every month
   C. dilatation and curettage
   D. outpatient hysteroscopy
   E. daily high dose conjugated oral estrogen
8. An 18 year-old gives a 2 month history of intermittent, irregular bleeding. Her last normal menstrual period was 3 months ago. Prior to that, her cycle was regular at 28 days. A pelvic examination is normal. The next step in management should be
   A. endometrial aspiration
   B. pelvic ultrasound
   C. a pregnancy test
   D. laparoscopy
   E. hysteroscopy

9. A 45 year-old gravida 3, para 3, who has had menorrhagia for 6 months underwent a dilation and curettage 4 weeks ago. The uterus was normal in size. The cavity felt smooth, and the pathologist reported that the endometrium was secretory. The preferred management is
   A. cyclic medroxyprogesterone acetate
   B. continuous medroxyprogesterone acetate
   C. continuous conjugated estrogens
   D. cyclic danazol
   E. combination oral contraceptives
10. An 18 year-old has had one extremely heavy period for which she was prescribed conjugated estrogen, 10 mg in divided doses. Assuming that the bleeding is markedly diminished within 24 hours, the next step in the treatment of this patient should be
   A. conjugated estrogen, 10 mg per day in divided doses plus medroxyprogesterone acetate 10 mg per day for 2 weeks
   B. conjugated estrogen, 20 mg per day in divided doses for 2 weeks
   C. a cycle of oral contraceptives containing 30-35 mcg of ethinyl estradiol
   D. vitamin E for 30 days
   E. office endometrial aspiration
11. The mean volume of blood lost during normal menstruation is
   A. 15 ml
   B. 35 ml
   C. 55 ml
   D. 75 ml
   E. 95 ml
12. A 38 year-old gravida 4, para 3, abortus 1 states that she has had heavy vaginal bleeding for 9 days. Her pulse is 110, blood pressure 80/60, and pelvic examination is normal. A βhCG is negative, the hemoglobin 10 gm and the hematocrit 30%. The most efficacious treatment is
   A. parenteral high dose conjugated estrogen for 10 days
   B. dilation and curettage
   C. medroxyprogesterone acetate 20 mg per day for 10 days
   D. danazol 400 mg per day for 10 days
   E. oral contraceptive tablets four per day for 10 days
13. A 14 year-old comes to the emergency department with a 3 day history of excessive menstrual flow. Her hemoglobin is 8.2 gm and her hematocrit is 23%. A pregnancy test is negative. The blood pressure is 80/40 and the pulse 120. The most likely diagnosis is
   A. von Willebrand's disease
   B. a prothrombin deficiency
   C. leukemia
   D. anovulation
   E. an endometrial polyp
14. A 28 year-old woman, 3 or 4 times per year for the past 2 years, has been about 7 days late for her period. The flow eventually starts with spotting. A βhCG is negative at the time of her office visit. An endometrial biopsy done on the fourth day of her "late flow" reveals mixed proliferative and secretory endometrium. These findings are indicative of
   A. an inadequate corpus luteum
   B. anovulation
   C. repetitive subclinical abortions
   D. a chronic ectopic pregnancy
   E. a persistent corpus luteum (Halban's syndrome)
15. A 38 year-old, 5 feet 4 inch, 135 pound gravida 2, para 2 woman presents with a 4 month history of irregular menstruation. She has very heavy flow every 60 to 120 days. A βhCG is negative. The pelvic examination is normal. The next step in management should be
   A. office hysteroscopy
   B. office endometrial aspiration
   C. serum clotting studies
   D. hysterosalpingogram
   E. pelvic ultrasound
16. After successful treatment of an acute episode of anovulatory bleeding in a 13 year-old, long-term treatment is best accomplished by
   A. dilation and curettage
   B. cyclic oral contraceptives
   C. cyclic conjugated estrogens
   D. cyclic medroxyprogesterone acetate
   E. cyclic danazol
17. A 42 year-old woman with Class III valvular heart disease has a history of progressive menorrhagia over the past 8 months. Previous attempts to decrease the bleeding using medroxyprogesterone acetate have failed. An endometrial aspiration is reported to be proliferative endometrium without inflammation. The hemoglobin is 10.8 gm. At this point you would
   A. start cyclic oral contraceptives
   B. start nonsteroidal anti-inflammatory drugs
   C. start antibiotic therapy
   D. perform an endometrial ablation procedure such as laser vaporization
   E. perform a dilatation and curettage
18. The rationale for the therapeutic use of

conjugated estrogen for the immediate treatment of dysfunctional uterine bleeding is based on the fact that it
A. stabilizes endogenous serum clotting factors
B. causes a decrease in platelet adhesiveness
C. causes decidualization of the endometrium
D. leads to rapid proliferation of the endometrium
E. is followed by a uniform endometrial slough upon withdrawal

DIRECTIONS for questions 19 - 21: For each numbered item, select the one heading most closely associated with it. Each lettered heading may be used once, more than once, or not at all.

Appropriate therapeutic

(A) danazol
(B) ergot alkaloid
(C) epsilon amniocaproic acid
(D) medroxyprogesterone acetate

19. inhibitor of fibrinolysis; associated with a 60% reduction in menstrual blood loss in patients with menorrhagia
20. does not reduce menstrual blood loss in patients treated for menorrhagia
21. enhances activity of 17-α-dehydrogenase to favor conversion of estradiol to estrone

DIRECTIONS for questions 22 - 30: For each of the questions below, ONE or MORE of the responses is correct. Select the best answer based on the following

A if 1, 2, and 3 are correct
B if only 1 and 2 are correct
C if only 2 and 3 are correct
D if only 1 is correct
E if only 3 is correct

22. In assessing the quantity of blood loss during a patient's subjective report of "heavy" blood flow during menstruation, the most reliable feature obtained by history is the
 1. number of pads used
 2. patient's description of passage of blood clots
 3. number of days of flow
23. The histologic appearance of the endometrium of a patient who is anovulatory is likely to show
 1. proliferation of the endometrium
 2. areas of necrosis of the endometrium
 3. an eosinophilic infiltrate
24. True statements regarding menstruation include
 1. the normal mean cycle is 28 days
 2. the normal mean duration of flow is 4 days
 3. the number of sanitary pads used by a patient is an accurate indicator of the amount of flow
25. The pharmacologic actions of nonsteroidal anti-inflammatory drugs used in treating menorrhagia are
 1. the inhibition of platelet aggregation
 2. interference in the conversion of arachidonic acid to prostaglandins
 3. blocking formation of prostacyclin
26. The hematologic profile of a group of women who lose more than 80 ml of blood each menstrual cycle would include a
 1. reduced serum iron level
 2. lower mean hemoglobin
 3. lower mean hematocrit
27. Medroxyprogesterone acetate
 1. reduces vascularity in the basalis layer of the endometrium
 2. inhibits estrogen receptor replenishment in the cytosol
 3. activates 17-hydroxysteroid dehydrogenase
28. Theraupetics efficacious in reducing mean menstrual blood loss include
 1. cyclic synthetic progestins
 2. nonsteroidal anti-inflammatory drugs
 3. progestin releasing intrauterine devices (IUDs)
29. The advantages of "roller ball" electrocautery endometrial ablation over laser ablation of the endometrium include
 1. hormonal "pretreatment" is not necessary
 2. fewer long term complications
 3. less expense
30. A 20 year-old, gravida 0, complains of "heavy menstruation," which is now in its seventh day. The pelvic examination is normal except for the presence of clotted blood filling the posterior fornix. A βhCG is negative and an office hematocrit is 35%. The recognized standard management options include
 1. high dose conjugated estrogen therapy (10 mg/day in divided doses) until bleeding stops
 2. medroxyprogesterone acetate, 10 mg/day for 10 days
 3. dilatation and currettage

ANSWERS

1. **A,** Page 1080. Menorrhagia has been reported to occur in up to 14% of healthy woman participating in studies of measurement of menstrual blood loss. In women complaining of menorrhagia, just as with women who have normal menstruation, 70% of the blood is lost within the

first two days of menstruation and 92% is passed by the end of the third day. There seems to be no relation between the number of days of menstrual bleeding and total menstrual blood loss. The majority of patients with menorrhagia did not have increased duration of flow, but rather had a marked increase in amount of menstrual flow for the first few days of menstruation.

2. **D,** Page 1082; Wilanksy DL and Greisman B: Early hypothyroidism in patients with menorrhagia, Am J Obstet Gynecol 160:663, 1989. Hypothyroidism is frequently associated with menorrhagia as well as intermenstral bleeding. Thyroid stimulating hormone (TSH) should be measured in women with menorrhagia of undetermined etiology. In a study by Wilansky and Greisman 15 of 67 women had early hypothroidism which was detected by an abnormal thyrotropin releasing hormone (TRH) stimulation test. Following treatment the TSH levels in the affected women returned to normal and the menorrhagia disappearedwithin three to six months. Although this study awaits corroboration, hypothyroidism should be kept in mind in patients with otherwise unexplained menorrhagia. The history given in this question is not typical for diabetes mellitus, systemic lupus erythematosis, idiopathic thrombocytopenic purpura, and von Willebrands disease.
3. **E,** Page 1083. The mechanism for hemostasis in reaction to vascular injury is similar in the endometrium as in other injured tissues of the body. There are five basic actions including: 1) localized vasoconstriction; 2) platelet adhesion; 2) formation of the platelet plug; 4) reinforcement of the platelet plug with fibrin and 5) removal of the coagulated material by fibrinolysis. This process is slightly altered in the endometrial vessels when compared to vessel damage elsewhere in that the hemostatic plugs in the endometrium are smaller, have a different morphology, and persist for a shorter time than those in other tissues.
4. **A,** Page 1084. Smith SK, Abel MH, Kelly RW, and Baird DT: The synthesis of prostaglandins from persistent proliferative endometrium, J Clin Endocrinol Metab 55:284, 1982. Smith, et al found that the levels of prostaglandin $F_{2\alpha}$ were lower in women with anovulatory abnormal uterine bleeding with a persistently proliferative endometrium than were the levels in woman with a normal secretory endometrium. Prostaglandin $F_{2\alpha}$ is known to promote vasoconstriction in the spiral arterioles of the endometrium. It has been shown that prostaglandin $F_{2\alpha}$ binds to receptors in the spiral arteries in the late secretory phase to cause vasoconstriction and presumably help control menstrual flow. Prostaglandin E_2 is a vasodilator and thromboxane promotes platelet aggregation while prostacycline inhibits this process. Arachidonic acid is the precursor for both prostaglandin $F_{2\alpha}$ and prostaglandin E_2.
5. **D,** Page 1085; Gimpelson RJ and Rappold HO: A comparative study between panoramic hysteroscopy with directed biopsies and dilatation and curettage, Am J Obstet Gynecol 158:489, 1988; March CM: The endometrium in the menstrual cycle. In Mishell DR Jr, Davajan V, and Lobo RA, editors: Infertility, contraception and reproductiveendocrinology, Cambridge, Mass, 1991, Blackwell Scientific Publications. In those patients who are ovulating and have menorrhagia, it is important to rule out the presence of a uterine lesion such as an endometrial polyp, submucous myoma, or carcinoma. Although a number of tests, including vaginal probe ultrasonography, might reveal the source of the problem, many authors prefer hysteroscopy which can be performed in the office under local anesthesia. It has been estimated that a dilatation and curettage misses the diagnosis in 10%-25% of patients. Gimpelson and Rappold found that hysteroscopy permitted the accurate diagnosis in 60 of 342 patients in whom the diagnosis was not made by dilatation and curettage. March has reported that one fourth of patients with a presumptive diagnosis of dysfunctional bleeding were found to have a uterine lesion at the time of hysteroscopy.
6. **A,** Page 1086. To control an acute bleeding episode, after organic causes have been ruled out, the use of oral conjugated estrogen in very high doses (10 mg in four divided doses) is a therapeutic regimen that many authors feel is clinically useful. Although high dose combination oral contraceptives have been found to be effective, some studies suggest that this is not as efficacious as high doses of conjugated estrogen alone. The difference might be due to the fact that the combined use of estrogen and progestin will not afford as rapid an endometrial growth as estrogen alone. The progestin decreases the syn-

thesis of estrogen receptors and increases estradiol dehydrogenase in the endometrial cell inhibiting the growth promoting action of estrogen. Other mechanisms such as estrogen's effect on spiral artery recoil, platelet function or prostaglandin synthesis seem to be unrelated.

A great deal of controversy surrounds the issue of what constitutes the best treatment. As evidenced by the ENT literature, estrogen may have a direct effect on blood vessels. Those authors who prefer a combination of estrogen and progestin point out that the progestin in a combination oral contraceptive acts more slowly and thus doesn't initially counter the estrogen effects on endometrial growth.

7. **B,** Page 1087. This question ignores the possibility of a blood dyscrasia and that possibility should always be considered, especially in a teenager. Adolescent anovulatory patients represent an ideal model for the use of progestins in the treatment of dysfunctional uterine bleeding. Since these patients exhibit immaturity of the hypothalamic pituitary axis, this treatment is preferred over oral contraceptives because the therapy does not prolong hypothalamic pituitary inhibition and may, according to the older literature, delay the maturation of this axis. In the young virginal patient with these findings, dilatation and curettage and hysteroscopy are not necessary. Treating the patient with estrogen alone will not help since her problem is primarily that of unopposed estrogen secretion.
8. **C,** Page 1082. The most common cause of vaginal bleeding during the reproductive age are accidents of pregnancy such as a threatened, incomplete, or missed abortion, or an ectopic pregnancy. This warrants performance of a sensitive βhCG test, either by serum or urine as part of the immediate diagnostic evaluation. Endometrial aspiration and hysteroscopy are contraindicated in this patient until a diagnosis of pregnancy is ruled out. After the results of the pregnancy test are available, one might perform a pelvic ultrasound or laparoscopy in this patient with a normal pelvic exam if one were concerned about a pregnancy abnormality.
9. **A,** Pages 1083-1084, 1086. After dilatation and curettage is used to treat acute bleeding in a woman in her late reproductive years, further therapy is indicated if the histology shows secretory endometrium. This is best accomplished by using cyclic medroxyprogesterone acetate to effect an orderly withdrawal bleeding each month. Continuous medroxyprogesterone acetate will be associated with degrees of endometrial atrophy from which the patient is likely to bleed again. Both cyclic and continuous conjugated estrogens are contraindicated since they will cause excessive endometrial proliferation which may cause futher irregular, heavy bleeding. Cyclic danazol is not indicated and is a less cost effective measure to control bleeding in the patient. Since this woman is 45, and thus in a perimenopausal age group, she should be treated even though the endometrium is secretory. At this time it is possible that she isnot ovulating each month. Oral contraceptives are a less safe choice in this patient.
10. **A,** Page 1086. When high dose conjugated estrogen therapy has been successful in reducing the amount of uterine bleeding within the first 24 hours, immediate progestin support of the endometrium is also required. Therefore conjugated estrogen therapy is continued at the same dosage and a progestin, usually medroxyprogesterone acetate, 10 mg per day is added. Both hormones are continued for 2 weeks, after which treatment is stopped to allow withdrawal bleeding. Doubling the conjugated estrogen dose for 2 weeks is likely to cause abnormal hyperplasia of the endometrium and more bleeding. Initiation of oral contraceptives at this point is another option in this patient, but there is no compelling reason to switch to another regimen, a combination estrogen-progestin oral contraceptive four times a day for seven days. Vitamin E has not been scientifically proven to be of benefit. Since this patient has responded to high dose conjugated estrogen therapy, office endometrial aspiration is unnecessary at this point. If the patient were not to respond to the above outlined therapy, endometrial sampling would be indicated.
11. **B.** Page 1080. There are two reliable objective methods that can be used to quantify menstrual blood loss. One involves radioisotope tagging of a patient's red cells; the other involves photometric measurement to quantify the amount of hematin collected on sanitary napkins. Using these techniques, it has been found in several studies that the mean amount of menstrual blood loss in normal women

(women with normal hemoglobin, hematocrit, and plasma iron) is about 35 ml.

12. **B,** Pages 1092-1093. A dilatation and curettage should be used to stop the acute bleeding episode in patients over the age of 35, since the incidence of anatomical problems and pathologic findings is increased in this age group. The performance of a dilatation and curettage can be both diagnostic and therapeutic. A dilatation and curettage is the quickest way to stop acute bleeding and is indicated in patients with severe menorrhagia who may be hypovolemic. It should be remembered that, although the dilatation and curettage is effective for the treatment for acute bleeding, long-termcures are unusual since the underlying pathophysiology is unchanged.
13. **D,** Page 1083. Certain systemic diseases, especially disorders of blood coagulation such as von Willebrand's disease and prothrombin deficiency, may often present as abnormal uterine bleeding. Other disorders that produce platelet deficiencies, such as leukemia, occasionally present in this fashion. Coagulation disorders are found in about 20% of adolescent females who require hospitalization for abnormal uterine bleeding.
14. **E,** Page 1083. Certain disorders that may cause dysfunctional uterine bleeding relate to the life span of the corpus luteum. Prolonged life of the corpus luteum has been reported as a cause for abnormal bleeding similar to that presented by this patient (Halban's syndrome or a persistent corpus luteum). The etiology is uncertain and the treatment is expectant. This entity must be differentiated from early pregnancy loss by obtaining a sensitive serum or urine pregnancy test. Since this disorder is associated with a normal appearing secretory endometrium, the diagnosis is made when a biopsy obtained on the fourth day of the patient's flow is both proliferative and secretory, and the βhCG assay is negative.
15. **B,** Page 1082-1084. In this age group, having ruled out pregnancy and given a normal pelvic examination, one must rule out malignancy even though it is unlikely. A cost effective method is to perform an office endometrial aspiration. An endometrial biopsy is ideally obtained at the onset of the bleeding episode to help determine whether or not ovulation has occurred. This knowledge will help determine therapy. Office hysteroscopy is not indicated until the endometrial histology is known. A hysterosalpingogram and pelvic ultrasound are unnecessary at this time. Serum clotting studies are largely unrevealing in a patient in this age group with a short history of a bleeding abnormality.
16. **D,** Pages 1086-1087. Anovulatory, adolescent patients represent an ideal model for the use of progestins in the treatment of dysfunctional uterine bleeding. Because these teenagers are likely to have animmature hypothalamic-pituitary axis, progestin therapy for 10 days each month is a reasonable mode of treatment to produce regular cyclic bleeding until maturity of the postitive feedback system is achieved. Although **controversial**, it is probably best that oral contraceptives not be used in these patients, unless there is a need for contraception, since this therapy prolongs hypothalamic-pituitary inhibition. Dilatation and curettage is not indicated in this patient, whose acute bleeding episode has been controlled. Cyclic conjugated estrogens and cyclic danazol therapy are not valid choices. Danazol is expensive and carries with it the risk of undesirable side effects.
17. **D,** Pages 1093-1095; Goldrath MH, Fuller, FA, Segal S: Laser Photo Vaporization of Endometrium for the Treatment of Menorrhagia, Am J of Obstet Gynecol 140:14; 1981. Laser photovaporization of the endometrium for treatment of menorrhagia has been recently advocated by some investigators. This procedure for endometrial ablation may be used as an alternative to hysterectomy in patients where other modalities have failed or are contraindicated. This technique has been reported by Goldrath et al., who showed that it was curative in 160 of 180 patients. The efficacy of this approach awaits conformation by other investigators. Cyclic oral contraceptives are contraindicated in this patient and the effectiveness of nonsteroidal anti-inflammatory drugs and antifibrinolytics in patients with systemic disease is poor, but some would argue for a trial before attempting an operative procedure, such as an ablation or dilatation and curettage. The latter may only afford temporary relief.
18. **D,** Page 1086. The rationale for the therapeutic use of estrogen for the immediate treatment of abnormal uterine bleed is based on the fact that estrogen in pharma-

cologic doses causes rapid growth of the endometrium. Thus, bleeding that results from most causes of dysfunctional bleeding will respond to such therapy because a rapid growth of endometrial tissue occurs over the denuded and raw epithelial surface. Acute bleeding from most causes is usually controlled by this method. Appreciable changes in either systemic or local clotting factors or changes in platelet adhesiveness have not been well documented. Decidualization of the endometrium does not occur in the absence of progestin therapy. Likewise, uniform endometrial slough after estrogen withdrawal does not occur unless the estrogen treatment has been followed by adequate doses of progestins. As suggested in the answer to question #6, there are many respected physicians who would opt to use a combination oral contraceptive.

19-21. 19, **C**; 20, **B**; 21, **D**; Pages 1089; 1091; 1087-1088. Nilsson L and Rybo G: Treatment for Menorrhagia, Am J Obstet Gynecol 110:713, 1971. Episilon-amniocaproic acid is one of a number of potent inhibitors of fibrinolysis and therefore has been used in the treatment of various hemorrhagic conditions including menorrhagia. It is associated with a significant reduction of blood loss in these patients. The blood loss reduction was most in those patients who originally exhibited the greatest loss. Ergot derivatives are not recommended. They are rarely effective and have a high incidence of side effects including nausea, vertigo, and abdominal cramps. One study demonstrated no reduction in blood loss in 82 women with menorrhagia treated with ergot alkaloid preparations. This therapeutic is not effective at the cellular level. It is efficacious postpartum because myometrial contractions are important in reducing blood loss. One mechanism of action of medroxyprogesterone acetate is to enhance the converison of a potent estrogen, estradiol, to the less potent estrogen, estrone. This effectively reduces the cellular proliferation of the endometrium and reduces menstrual flow in patients with menorrhagia.

22. **B** (1, 2), Pages 1079-1080. There is a poor coorelation between a woman's perception of menstrual blood loss and the actual amount lost. Determining the number of sanitary pads used is a moderately unreliable indication of menstrual blood loss except when a patient is **soaking** a large number of pads. Asking the patient to estimate the amount of blood loss is also unreliable and it has been shown that 40% of women with a blood loss greater than 80 ml consider their menstrual flow to be small or moderate in amount. The patient's age alone does not correlate with menstrual blood loss unless concomitant pelvic pathology such as myomata are found. Likewise, the number of days of flow has not correlated in patients who bleed seven days or less. Queries about the passage of blood clots or the degree of inconvenience caused by the bleeding are most helpful in the assessment of the amount blood loss during menses.

23. **B** (1, 2), Page 1083. In most patients with dysfunctional uterine bleeding, ovulation fails to occur. There is continuous estradiol production without corpus luteum formation and progesterone secretion. This leads to a continually proliferating endometrium and the formation of areas of necrosis which occur as the endometrium outgrows its blood supply. In contrast to normal menstruation, a uniform slough of the endometrium to the basalis layer does ***not*** occur and there is excessive uterine blood flow. Acute inflammation or eosinophilic infiltration typically is ***not*** part of the histology of the endometrium of patients with dysfunctional uterine bleeding. Chronic endometrial inflammation may contribute to irregular bleeding patterns. It is discussed in Chapter 22.

24. **B** (1, 2), Page 1079. To define abnormal uterine bleeding, it is necessary first to recognize the characteristics of normal menstrual flow. The mean cycle interval is 28 days q 7 days and the mean duration of flow is 4 days. Bleeding for for more than 7 days is abnormally prolonged and termed menorrhagia. Subjective assessments of menstrual blood loss are poorly correlated with objective measurements of menstrual blood loss. One study suggests that 40% of women with blood loss greater than 80 ml considered their menstrual flow to be small or moderate in amount. Determining the number of sanitary pads used is an unreliable indication of menstrual blood loss. There is a great variability in the absorption of blood with different types of sanitary pads as well as marked variations in the fastidiousness among patients in their need to change sanitary products.

25. **A** (1, 2, 3), Page 1088-1089. Nonsteroidal

anti-inflammatory drugs are prostaglandin synthetase inhibitors. They inhibit the biosynthesis of cyclic endoperoxides which catalyze the conversion of arachidonic acid to prostaglandins. In addition, these agents may block the action of prostaglandins by interferring directly at their receptor sites. All nonsteroidal antiinflammatory drug are cyclooxygenaseinhibitors and thus block the formation of both thromboxane and the prostacyclins. Thromboxane increases platelet aggregation. A number of agents are available including mefenamic acid, meclofenamate, and naproxyn sodium. These drugs are usually given for the first three days of menses or throughout the bleeding episode. They appear to have similar levels of effectiveness.

26. **A** (1, 2, 3), Page 1080. Hallberg L. and Nilsson L.: Determination of Menstrual Blood Loss, Scan J. Clin Lab Invest 16:244, 1964. Using quantitative methods, Hallberg et al. found that individuals with a monthly menstrual blood loss of greater than 80 ml have a significant lower mean hemoglobin, hematocrit, and serum iron levels. Therefore, a menstrual blood loss greater than 80 ml should be regarded as hypermenorrhea. The anemia demonstrated in these patients is secondary to blood loss and is not related to abnormal clotting factors or platelet aggregation abnormalities. Abnormalities of these factors may contribute to excessive blood loss in a smaller select group of patients.
27. **C** (2, 3), Page 1088. Medroxyprogesterone acetate, given to patients with adequate amounts of endogenous estrogen, produces regular withdrawal bleeding. When used as maintenance therapy over longer periods of time, medroxyprogesterone acetate is usually prescribed in a dose of 10 mg daily for 10 to 13 days each month. Progestins act as antiestrogens. They diminish the effect of estrogen on the target cells by inhibiting estrogen receptor replenishment in the cytosol and influence the activation of 17-dehydroxysteroid dehydrogenase, which converts estradiol to the less active estrone. These findings account for the antimitotic, antigrowth effect of progestins. Natural progesterone stimulates secretory activity which does not occur with long term use of medroxyprogesterone acetate. There is no evidence suggesting that endometrial vascularity is reduced by the use of medroxyprogesterone acetate.
28. **A** (1, 2, 3), Pages 1087 and 1088. All of the listed treatments may be efficacious in reducing menstrual blood loss. Progestins not only stop endometrial growth, but support and organize the endometrium in such a way that an organized slough occurs after its withdrawal. This organized slough to the basalis layer allows a rapid cessation of bleeding. In addition progestins stimulate arachidonic acid formation in the endometrium increasing the prostaglandin $F_{2\alpha}$/prostaglandin E ratio. The progesterone releasing intrauterine device (IUD) has also been found to be effective in the treatment of women with ovulatory abnormal uterine bleeding. In various studies after one year, between a 60% and 80% reduction in menstrual blood loss has occured after the introduction a progestin releasing intrauterine device. Several nonsteroidal anti-inflammatory drugs have been administered during menstruation to groups of women with menorrhagia and ovulatory abnormal uterine bleeding. They have reduced mean menstrual blood loss by about 20-50%.
29. **E** (3 only), Pages 1093 and 1095. Both laser ablation and electrocautery of the endometrium can be applied successfully to treat patients with heavy menstrual flow. It is suggested that with both methods, patients be pretreated for approximately 1-2 months with a hormonal agent to effect endometrial atrophy. This renders the laser or cautery ablations more effective. High dose progestins or danazol may be used in this capacity. The long-term effects of all techniques of endometrial ablation are not yet known. The clinician should be aware that a certain percentage of patients will return with continued menstrual flow and that the patient may need to have a second treatment with these techniques. In addition, the long-term effect on the rates of potentially serious endometrial pathology, such as endometrial carcinoma, are not known. The time needed to learn the roller ball technique is shorter than that for laser and the equipment is considerably less expensive.
30. **B** (1, 2), Pages 1086-1087. There are several approaches to the treatment of acute "endocrinologic" uterine bleeding. Each has its advocates. In this 20 year-old patient, acute bleeding is usually controlled

adequately by administration of oral conjugated estrogens in a dose of 10 mg/day in divided doses until the bleeding markedly slows or stops or by medroxyprogesterone acetate,10 mg/day for 10 days. According to some authors medroxyprogesterone acetate is less effective in providing immediate relief from the bleeding. Oral contraceptive agents containing 50 mcg of estrogen have been used in the immediate treatment of this problem. In this age group, it is important to have ruled out pregnancy. Judging from the amount of bleeding and the age of the patient, the bleeding is likely to be secondary to anovulation. Endometrial sampling is not indicated in this patient with a low risk for neoplastic disease. This procedure will not remove the underlying cause for her bleeding. Dilatation and curettage is not necessary unless there is a poor clinical response to estrogen therapy.

CHAPTER

36 Amenorrhea

DIRECTIONS for questions 1 - 13: Select the one best answer or completion.

1. Normal pubertal development is the result of
   A. adrenal maturation
   B. increased sensitivity of the hypothalamic-pituitary-gonadal axis to circulating estrogen
   C. decreased REM sleep
   D. maturation of the hypothalamic-pituitary-gonadal axis
   E. weight loss
2. A 17-year-old states she has never had a period. On examination, the findings are as shown in Figure 36-1. The most likely diagnosis is
   A. pregnancy
   B. androgen insensitivity
   C. gonadal dysgenesis
   D. imperforate hymen
   E. Rokitansky-Kuster-Hauser syndrome
3. Given the probable diagnosis in Question 36-2, the most useful initial diagnostic test would be a
   A. buccal smear
   B. FSH determination
   C. serum estrogen determination
   D. GnRH (LH-RH) stimulation test
   E. x-ray to determine the patient's bone age
4. Eight months after the delivery of her second child, a patient complains that she has not had a period. The patient did not breast-feed because she could not produce milk. A pregnancy test and progestin withdrawal test are negative. The most likely diagnosis is
   A. Sheehan's syndrome
   B. hyperprolactinemia
   C. polycystic ovarian disease
   D. androgen insensitivity
   E. Rokitansky-Kuster-Hauser syndrome
5. Anorexia nervosa is characterized by all the following **EXCEPT**
   A. dry skin
   B. hypotension
   C. tachycardia
   D. hypothermia
   E. constipation
6. A 14-year-old with normal secondary sexual development is seen in the emergency department complaining of abdominal pain. She has never menstruated. On examination, you palpate a large central abdominopelvic mass which extends to the umbilicus and feels like an enlarged uterus. Fetal heart tones are not heard. The most likely diagnosis is
   A. Rokitansky-Kuster-Hauser syndrome
   B. androgen insensitivity
   C. a complete transverse vaginal septum
   D. pregnancy
   E. gonadal dysgenesis
7. Of the following conditions, the most common cause of secondary amenorrhea in an adolescent woman is
   A. polycystic ovarian syndrome
   B. anorexia nervosa
   C. hyperprolactinemia
   D. Rokitansky-Kuster-Hauser syndrome
   E. gonadal dysgenesis
8. A 27-year-old marathon athlete asks for your advice regarding her menstrual cycles. In the past 4 1/2 years she has menstruated only once. The examination is within normal limits. Appropriate advice would be to ask the woman to
   A. reduce physical activity to a minimum
   B. increase caloric intake and gain weight
   C. take oral contraceptive pills
   D. await the results of a progestin withdrawal test
   E. obtain a psychiatric evaluation
9. A 17-year-old who has had regular periods every 28 to 30 days since she was 12 is now 2 weeks late for her period. Her past medical history is negative, and the physical exam is within normal limits. Which of the following tests is indicated?
   A. serum prolactin
   B. FSH
   C. β-HCG
   D. serum estradiol
   E. karyotype

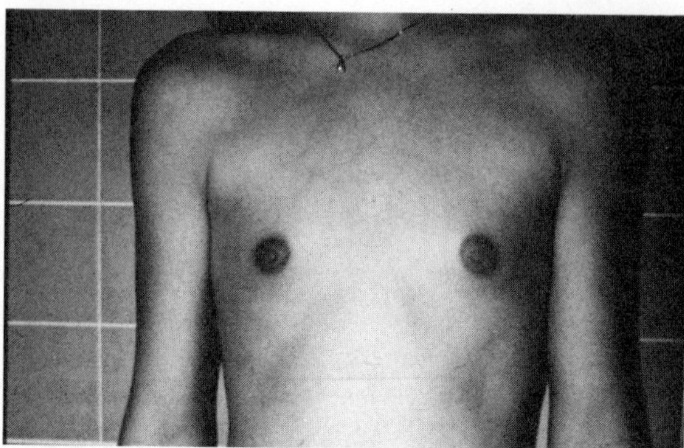

FIGURE 36-1.

10. A 16-year-old woman tells her doctor that she is 4 weeks late for her period. She is sexually active. The past medical history is negative, and the physical exam is within normal limits. The pregnancy test is negative. The most likely diagnosis is
    A. ectopic pregnancy
    B. anovulation
    C. gonadal failure
    D. hypothyroidism
    E. anorexia nervosa
11. The appropriate therapeutic modality for an anovulatory adolescent is
    A. clomiphene citrate
    B. progestin withdrawal
    C. Pergonal (menotropins)
    D. GnRH agonist
    E. Premarin (conjugated estrogens)
12. A 14-year-old high school student is referred for evaluation of primary amenorrhea. She is an excellent athlete and runs almost 5 miles daily. On examination it is noted that her breasts are Tanner stage 1, and pubic hair development is graded as Tanner stage 2. The remainder of the examination is within normal limits. The first step in her evaluation should include a
    A. pregnancy test
    B. serum LH
    C. serum FSH
    D. karyotype
    E. serum testosterone
13. A 27 year old woman has had no menstrual periods for 6 months. She feels well, exercises moderately, and has no other symptoms or complaints. She does not have a history of a uterine infection. Her general physical evaluation is normal. This woman does not have withdrawal bleeding after progesterone. Her laboratory tests include a normal CBC, a prolactin of 10 ng, a LH of 15 mIU/ml, a FSH of 10 mIU/ml, and an estradiol which was 44 pg/ml. The most likely diagnosis is
    A. polycystic ovary syndrome
    B. premature ovarian failure
    C. hypothalamic failure
    D. gonadotrophin resistant ovary syndrome
    E. hypothalamic dysfunction

DIRECTIONS for questions 14 - 17: For each numbered item, select the one heading most closely associated with it. Each lettered heading may be used once, more than once, or not at all.

14-17. Match the hormonal level with syndrome or finding
    (A) low FSH
    (B) normal FSH
    (C) high FSH
    (D) high ACTH
14. Turner's syndrome
15. positive progestin withdrawal test
16. Kallman's syndrome
17. resistant ovary syndrome (Savage syndrome)

DIRECTIONS for questions 18 - 30: For each of the questions below, ONE or MORE of the responses is correct. Select the best answer based on the following
A if 1, 2, and 3 are correct
B if only 1 and 2 are correct
C if only 2 and 3 are correct
D if only 1 is correct
E if only 3 is correct

18. Typically patients with the Rokitansky-Kuster-Hauser syndrome are differentiated from patients with androgen insensitivity by
    1. progesterone withdrawal test results
    2. the presence of a short blind vagina
    3. karyotype
19. One would expect a patient with anorexia nervosa to have a
    1. low T 4
    2. low T 3
    3. low FSH
20. Which of the following karyotypes may be obtained from individuals with gonadal dysgenesis?
    1. 46,XX or 46,XY
    2. 45,X/46,XX
    3. 45,X/46,XY
21. Procedures appropriate in the management of patients with androgen insensitivity syndrome include
    1. gonadectomy
    2. vaginal dilation
    3. breast augmentation

22. Asherman's syndrome is associated with
    1. secondary amenorrhea
    2. dilation and curettage
    3. an elevated FSH
23. Gonadectomy should be performed on patients with
    1. androgen insensitivity
    2. pure gonadal dysgenesis
    3. Turner's syndrome
24. The somatic features of Turner's syndrome include
    1. short stature
    2. normal breast development
    3. cubitus varus
25. Ovarian failure may be caused by
    1. autoimmune disorder
    2. X-chromosome deletion
    3. autosomal recessive disorder in 46,XX individuals
26. In a 15-year-old presenting with primary amenorrhea and a large uterine mass the most plausible diagnoses are
    1. Rokitansky-Kuster-Hauser syndrome
    2. imperforate hymen
    3. pregnancy
27. The procedures useful in establishing the diagnosis of Asherman's syndrome are
    1. hysterogram
    2. hysteroscopy
    3. laparoscopy
28. Findings usually associated with anorexia nervosa include
    1. loss of at least 25% of original body weight
    2. onset before age 25
    3. a distorted attitude towards food
29. True statements regarding female athletes with exercise-induced amenorrhea include
    1. prolactin levels are extremely low
    2. exercise-induced amenorrhea causes high FSH levels
    3. a-endorphin levels are elevated during exercise
30. A non hirsute 28 year old female with secondary amenorrhea had withdrawal bleeding to progesterone. Further evaluation should include
    1. prolactin
    2. LH
    3. FSH

ANSWERS

1. **D,** Page 1105. Prior to puberty, gonadotrophin levels are low because the hypothalamic-pituitary-gonadal axis is extremely sensitive to the negative feedback of the low level of circulating estrogen. As the axis matures, this sensitivity diminishes and an episodic nocturnal rise in LH is observed. Next, pulses of FSH and LH are noted both at night and during the daytime. FSH and LH stimulate the gonad to produce estrogen which, in turn, affects secondary sexual development.
2. **C,** Pages 1106-1109. The combination of primary amenorrhea and absent breast development suggests failure of the gonads to produce estrogen. The only condition listed characterized by absent estrogen production is gonadal dysgenesis. In all other conditions, the amenorrhea is associated with adequate and appropriate breast development. The Rokitansky-Kuster-Hauser syndrome is characterized by an incomplete to atretic vagina and a rudimentary to bicornuate uterus. The tubes and ovaries are normal, and hence pubertal development is normal except for a lack of menstruation. The lower vagina usually consists of a short blind pouch. On rare occasions, a patient may have a functional endometrium and thus develop hematometra. Renal (50%) and skeletal malformations (10-15%) are moderately common.
3. **B,** Pages 1108-1109, 1112. Although all the tests listed have a place in the work-up of a patient with delayed puberty, a determination of the FSH serum concentration would be most valuable in this patient. A high FSH level will confirm gonadal failure, while a low FSH level will suggest constitutional delay or pituitary failure. A karyotype is important after the diagnosis of gonadal failure is established, since some of these patients will have a mosaic containing a Y chromosome. Because it contains a great deal more information, a karyotype is preferred over a buccal smear.
4. **A,** Page 1121. This postpartum patient was unable to produce milk which is the typical presentation of a patient whose pituitary gland was destroyed during pregnancy and delivery due to hemorrhage or thrombosis. This extremely rareconstellation of events is called Sheehan's syndrome. It is important to evaluate the function of other endocrine organs, particularly the thyroid and the adrenal glands, because "multi-gland" hormonal replacement therapy may be indicated. Androgen insensitivity is found in a genetic male while the Rokitansky-Kuster-Hauser syndrome includes an absent vagina. The clinical presentation is not typical of polycystic ovarian disease since a withdrawal bleed is expected in response to progestin therapy.

5. **C,** Page 1117. Patients with anorexia nervosa have bradycardia, not tachycardia. These patients may also have dry skin, hypotension, hypothermia, and constipation. If they gain weight their pattern of LH pulses go through the changes that usually occur in normal puberty. The ovaries do the same with increasing follicular size and development of a dominant follicle.
6. **C,** Pages 1102, 1110-1111. The large central mass is probably an enlarged uterus. The association of primary amenorrhea, an enlarged uterus, and pain suggest an obstruction of the outflow tract and retention of menstrual flow. The patient has normal sexual development indicating an active hypothalamic-pituitary-ovarian axis and adequate estrogen production, excluding the possibility of gonadal dysgenesis. If, in fact, the large abdominopelvic mass is a uterus, androgen insensitivity syndrome is excluded since a uterus is absent in these individuals. The absence of fetal heart tones makes pregnancy an unlikely possibility. Rokitansky-Kuster-Hauser syndrome with a uterus is very rare and is therefore far less likely than a complete transverse vaginal septum.
7. **B,** Page 1117. Any patient who presents with postpubertal amenorrhea should be considered to be pregnant until proven otherwise since pregnancy is the most common cause of amenorrhea in young females. Adolescents with anorexia nervosa, excessive stress, hyperprolactinemia, Rokitansky-Kuster-Hauser syndrome, and gonadal dysgenesis can all present with primary amenorrhea, but eating disorders are probably the most common cause of secondary amenorrhea in adolescents who are not pregnant. Polycystic ovarian syndrome may cause amenorrhea, but usually results in irregularuterine bleeding.
8. **D,** Pages 1123-1124. It is now believed that amenorrhea associated with strenuous exercise is also related to stress. While reducing physical activity to a minimum or increasing caloric intake to gain weight may alleviate the problem, most athletes refuse to do so. Amenorrhea by itself does the patient no harm. However, it reflects a hypoestrogenic state, which makes the patient susceptible to developing osteoporosis. Prior to the initiation of estrogen replacement therapy (ERT), a progestin withdrawal test is done. If positive (bleeding occurs), the patient is presumed to produce adequate amounts of estrogen, and ERT is not required. If negative, ERT is suggested to prevent the deleterious effects of estrogen deficiency on the bones.
9. **C,** Page 1123. The most common cause of secondary amenorrhea in young women is pregnancy. Although hyperprolactinemia, gonadal failure, and chromosome abnormalities may cause secondary amenorrhea, these are relatively rare. This patient has not met the criteria for secondary amenorrhea. Nevertheless, a pregnancy test should be performed. If the pregnancy test is negative, the patient can be reassured. It is most likely that she will resume normal menstruation. If she has 6 months of amenorrhea, a work-up should be initiated.
10. **B,** Pages 1123-1126. Anovulation is relatively common at both ends of the reproductive age group; that is, the young adolescent girls in the first 2 years after puberty and the perimenopausal women. Thus, anovulation is the most likely diagnosis in this patient whose hormonal and chromosomal studies are probably normal. If there is doubt, other laboratory tests such as a FSH, TSH, prolactin, estrogen, and karyotype can be performed.
11. **B,** Pages 1123-1125. Patients who suffer from chronic anovulation have unopposed estrogen production. Overgrowth of endometrium follows, and abnormal uterine bleeding occurs after a period of amenorrhea. Although the patient can be followed without treatment, progestin withdrawal would reassure the patient that there is no significant pathology as well as counteract the action of unopposed estrogen. Even though clomiphene citrate induces ovulation, and therefore can be used totreat chronic anovulation, the use of this medication should be reserved for patients who wish to become pregnant. Birth control pills should be used if the patient is sexually active.
12. **C,** Pages 1105, 1112, 1113, 1115-1116; Figure 36-7. Although exercise-induced amenorrhea is relatively common in this age group, this young woman has not begun her secondary sexual development. Therefore, as with all girls her age who have not commenced breast development, a complete evaluation is required. Breasts that are Tanner stage 1 signify a lack of estrogen production. A serum FSH would be most helpful in determining whether the estrogen deficiency is on the basis of gonadal dysgenesis or on the basis of a hy-

pothalamic-pituitary disorder. Elevated FSH levels (above 40 mIU/ml) would indicate gonadal failure, while a low FSH would suggest a hypothalamic disorder. A random LH is less helpful as episodic pulses may cause the results to be quite variable. A pregnancy test and a karyotype are not indicated at the present time. A serum testosterone is helpful when the patient is hirsute. In patients with a low FSH, consideration should be given to performing a GnRH stimulation test to determine the level of maturation of the hypothalamic pituitary ovarian axis.

13. **E,** Pages 1121, 1124. A woman with secondary amenorrhea, who does not withdraw to progesterone, generally has low estrogen. This may be due to a uterine, ovarian, or hypothalamic pituitary abnormality. Testing often reveals the most likely source. If the FSH and LH are high, ovarian failure is likely; if the FSH is normal and LH is high, polycystic ovary syndrome is likely; if the FSH and LH are normal or low and estrogen is normal or low, the disorder may be due to variations in GnRH pulses from the hypothalamus. In these cases, if the estradiol is above 40 pg/ml, the likely diagnosis is hypothalamic dysfunction, while if the estradiol is below 40 pg/ml, hypothalamic failure is more plausible.

14-17. 14, **C**; 15, **B**; 16, **A**; 17, **C**; Pages 1109-1111 . Normal levels of FSH suggest adequate estrogen production, and thus following progestin administration, withdrawal bleeding is expected. High levels of FSH indicate a hypoestrogenic state on the basis of gonadal failure or resistance (gonadal dysgenesis, Turner's syndrome, resistant ovary syndrome). Withdrawal-bleeding following progestin administration is not expected in these cases. Kallman's syndrome denotes individuals with hypo-gonadotrophic hypogonadism and anosmia. FSH levels are low as a result of inadequate production.

18. **E** (3 only). Pages 1110-1111 Patients with the Rokitansky-Kuster-Hauser syndrome and patients with androgen insensitivity have a short blind vagina and no uterus. Usually, they present to the physician complaining of primary amenorrhea. Because they have no outflow tract and Rokitansky syndrome often has no functioning uterus, a progestin withdrawal test is negative in both groups. The difference between these two groups of patients is the mechanism by which the müllerian duct fails to develop. In patients with androgen insensitivity, the müllerian inhibiting factor produced by the testes causes regression of the müllerian duct. Except for the karyotype, the findings are similar in both conditions. Patients with Rokitansky-Kuster-Hauser syndrome have a normal female karyotype (46,XX), while patients with androgen insensitivity syndrome possess a normal male karyotype (46,XY).

19. **C** (2, 3), Pages 1117-1118. Patients with anorexia nervosa have a hypothalamic disorder interfering with normal GnRH release. Thus, both FSH and estrogen levels are extremely low. In addition, the peripheral conversion of T 4 to T 3 is impaired, resulting in low levels of T 3, but T 4 levels are within the normal range.

20. **A** (1, 2, 3), Pages 1106-1107, 1109. Gonadal failure is usually the result of X chromosome deletion in all cells (45,X) or in some of the cells (a mosaic). A number of karyotypes have been found including, but not limited to, 45,X; 45,X/46,XX; and 45,X/46,XY. Some individuals may have a single gene defect resulting in gonadal dysgenesis (pure gonadal dysgenesis). These conditions are transmitted either as an autosomal recessive disorder in genetic females (46,XX) or as an X-linked recessive disorder in genetic males (46,XY).

21. **B** (1, 2), Pages 1110, 1112-1113. Patients with androgen insensitivity have normal testes located in the abdominal cavity or the inguinal canal. These gonads, if left in situ, are at increased risk of developing a malignancy, and so should be removed when pubertal development is complete. Estrogen replacement therapy should be given following castration. The vagina of these individuals is short and requires dilation and elongation. This can be achieved either by graduated dilation (Frank's method) or surgically (the McIndoe-Reed Procedure). Breast development is adequate, requiring no augmentation.

22. **B** (1, 2), Pages 1113-1114. Asherman's syndrome is characterized by intrauterine adhesions obliterating the endometrial cavity. The most frequent cause of Asherman's syndrome is a vigorous endometrial curettage, usually postpartum or postabortal; tuberculous endometritis is a rare cause. Patients with Asherman's syndrome have secondary amenorrhea, despite a normal FSH and serum estrogen.

23. **B** (1, 2), Pages 1110, 1113. Prophylactic gonadectomy should be performed on all patients with a Y chromosome complement. Thus, those patients with androgen

insensitivity, and with pure gonadal dysgenesis who have a 46,XY chromosome complement, require gonadectomy to eliminate the risk of developing a neoplasm (gonadoblastoma) in the gonad. Patients with Turner's syndrome, whose karyotype is 45,X, and patients with Rokitansky syndrome, who have a normal 46,XX karyotype, do not require gonadectomy. A word of caution—some patients with gonadal dysgenesis who seemingly have a 45,X karyotype may have mosaicism in which the 45,X cell line is mixed with a 46,XY cell line. These patients would also need a gonadectomy.

24. **D** (1 only), Page 1109. Patients with Turner's syndrome have gonadal dysgenesis and a karyotype of 45,X. In addition to primary amenorrhea and absent breast development, these individuals have other somatic abnormalities, the most prevalent being stature under five feet (the gene for stature being located on the short arm of the X chromosome). In addition, a web neck, short fourth metacarpals, a shield chest, widely spaced nipples, and cubitus valgus are some of the more prevalent somatic anomalies observed. Because of the short stature and these morphometric features, the diagnosis is usually made prior to puberty.
25. **A** (1, 2, 3), Pages 1121-1123. Ovarian failure may result from deletion of genetic material on the Xchromosome. When one X chromosome is missing in its entirety, Turner's syndrome results. However, various degrees of deletion have been described. If chromosome X material is missing, ovarian failure can occur. Individuals with premature ovarian failure may have antibodies to endocrine organs, suggesting an autoimmune etiology. In these cases the patients are usually less than 35-years-old and have elevated anti-nuclear and anti-thyroid antibodies. An infectious etiology such as mumps oophoritis has also been observed. Patients with a 46,XX karyotype may suffer from ovarian failure on the basis of an autosomal recessive disorder. Genetic males with 46,XY karyotype may present with "ovarian" failure on the basis of a X-linked recessive disorder. Because gonadal function is lost in utero, the external genitalia are not stimulated by androgens. As a result, the external genitalia appear female. These individuals are usually raised as girls. There is no secondary sexual development at the time of expected puberty. A karyotype should be obtained in patients under 25 years who have ovarian failure.
26. **C** (2, 3), Page 1102. A 15-year-old presenting with primary amenorrhea and a large abdominal mass may suffer from an outflow tract obstruction with the subsequent accumulation of menstrual flow behind the obstructing membrane. Thus, an imperforate hymen is a likely diagnosis. Although pregnancy is uncommon in patients who have not had a menstrual period, ovulation may occur in the first cycle, so pregnancy should always be considered. Patients with the Rokitansky-Kuster-Hauser syndrome usually have no uterus and therefore are not likely to have a uterine mass.
27. **B** (1, 2), Pages 1113-1114. Asherman's syndrome denotes intrauterine synechiae. These can be diagnosed by hysterogram or during hysteroscopy. On hysterogram, synechiae can be seen as filling defects, or there may be complete obliteration of the uterine cavity. During hysteroscopy intrauterine adhesions are seen directly and can be interrupted through an operating hysteroscope. Laparoscopy has no place in the diagnosis of intrauterine adhesions.
28. **A** (1, 2, 3), Page 1117. All the findings listed are helpful in making the diagnosis of anorexia nervosa. Usually there is absence of other medical or psychiatric disorders. In addition, at least two of the following manifestations are usually seen: 1) amenorrhea, 2) lanugo hair, 3) bradycardia, 4) periods of over activity, 5) episodes of spontaneous or self-induced vomiting after meals.
29. **E** (3 only), Page 1116. It is believed that amenorrhea associated with strenuous exercise is related to stress as well as to weight loss. Prolactin, β-endorphin, and catechol-estrogen levels are significantly higher and LH and FSH significantly lower in women who exercise strenuously.
30. **B** (1, 2), Page 1124. In women with secondary amenorrhea who withdraw from a progesterone challenge, FSH will be normal, but some will have a high LH and others will have a low LH. If the LH is greater than 25 mIU/ml polycystic ovarian syndrome should be suspected, even if the patient is not hirsute. Prolactin should be checked as a prolactin producing pituitary adenoma may be manifested only by amenorrhea.

CHAPTER 37

Hyperprolactinemia, Galactorrhea, and Pituitary Adenomas

DIRECTIONS for questions 1 - 22: Select the one best answer or completion.

1. A 37-year-old with galactorrhea has a prolactin of 40 ng/ml on two occasions. Her thyroid function studies are normal. Twenty minutes after a 500 μg IV bolus of thyrotropin-releasing hormone (TRH) the prolactin is 90 ng/ml. The next step would be to
   A. observe for 3 months
   B. obtain an anteroposterior and lateral coned-down views of the sella turcica
   C. obtain a MRI (magnetic resonance imaging) scan
   D. start bromocriptine
   E. refer for surgical resection
2. A patient who had been treated for a prolactin-secreting microadenoma has just delivered and wishes to breast feed. You would advise her
   A. not to breast feed
   B. to take bromocriptine while breast feeding
   C. to take bromocriptine for 2 to 3 weeks after breast feeding
   D. to have a serum prolactin determination before you decide what to advise
   E. to have a CT (computerized tomography) scan before you decide what to advise
3. All of the following can cause galactorrhea and hyperprolactinemia **EXCEPT**
   A. Cushing's disease
   B. low dose oral contraceptives
   C. chronic renal disease
   D. hyperthyroidism
   E. chest trauma
4. A 20-year-old gravida 0 complains of galactorrhea. She has no other complaints. Her periods are regular, occurring every 28 days. Her physical examination is normal except for her galactorrhea. A serum prolactin is reported to be 18 ng/ml. At this point you recommend a
   A. computerized tomography (CT) scan
   B. hypocycloidal tomography
   C. pneumoencephalography
   D. visual field examination
   E. follow-up in one year
5. "Big-big" prolactin
   A. is the principle form of prolactin measured in bioassays
   B. is the principal form of prolactin measured in immunoassays
   C. is a dimer of the small monomeric form
   D. has reduced binding to mammary tissue membranes in comparison to the monomeric form
   E. constitutes 50% of the secreted form
6. Select the patient in Figure 37-1 whose serum prolactin is most typical of the normal patient
   A. Patient A
   B. Patient B
   C. Patient C
   D. Patient D
   E. Patient E
7. In the normal patient lactation does not commence until after delivery because
   A. prolactin is not secreted until after delivery
   B. placental lactogen is only weakly lactogenic
   C. β-HCG blocks the action of prolactin on the breast
   D. the increase in cortisol associated with the delivery process is important in the initiation of lactation
   E. estrogen inhibits the action of prolactin on the breast
8. A 33-year-old, who is 5 feet 3 inches tall and weighs 180 pounds, has galactorrhea, oligomenorrhea, a serum prolactin of 18 ng/ml and a normal TSH. At this point you would
   A. do nothing for a year
   B. order an infusion of Thyrotropin-Releasing-Hormone (TRH) as a provocative stimulus of prolactin
   C. order a CT (computerized tomography) scan
   D. order a MRI (magnetic resonance imagery)

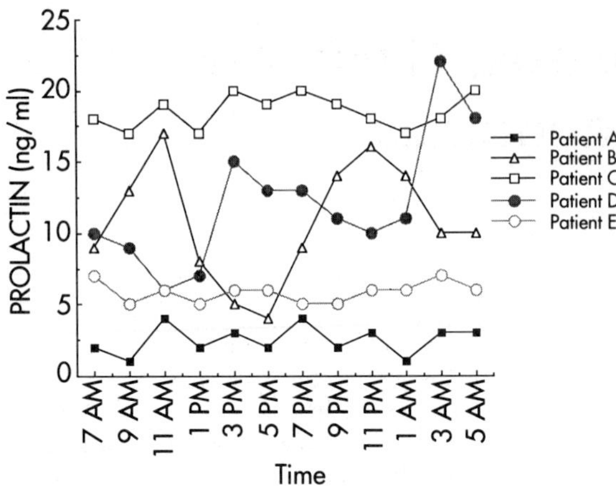

FIGURE 37-1.

E. order an anteroposterior and lateral coned-down views of the sella turcica

9. In which of the following patients with galactorrhea, all of whom might have an elevated serum prolactin, are you **most** likely to find that the prolactin actually is elevated?
   A. A 20-year-old with low estrogen and amenorrhea
   B. A 30-year-old, 8 months postpartum, breast feeding, and with amenorrhea, whose blood is drawn when the woman is in a basal state
   C. A 25-year-old with normal estrogen and oligomenorrhea
   D. A 30-year-old with normal estrogen and amenorrhea
   E. A 25-year-old with normal estrogen and normal menses
10. A woman who recently has developed trouble breast-feeding her 7-month-old infant has had a basal serum prolactin determination, which is reported to be 10 ng/ml. Having been asked for an opinion, you would state that
   A. this is too low a level for successful lactation
   B. that she is obviously under stress, and that if she relaxed, the prolactin would increase and she would be able to breast-feed
   C. the prolactin level is compatible with successful breast-feeding
   D. without knowing the conditions under which the result was obtained, you cannot offer an opinion
   E. the patient should be examined for Sheehan's syndrome
11. A 25-year-old single patient has oligomenorrhea, galactorrhea, and hyperprolactinemia (88 ng/ml). Thyroid function studies are normal. On MRI (magnetic resonance imagery) scan a 3 mm microadenoma was noted. The oligomenorrhea and galactorrhea are not of concern to the patient. Recommended therapy for this patient is
   A. bromocriptine
   B. external radiation therapy
   C. periodic progestin withdrawal
   D. surgical resection
   E. implantation of yttrium-90 rods
12. The major mechanism by which elevated levels of prolactin inhibit ovulation appears to be
   A. a direct action of big-big prolactin
   B. alterations in normal gonadotrophin-releasing hormone (GnRH) release
   C. direct inhibition of ovarian secretion of estradiol
   D. direct inhibition of ovarian secretion of progesterone
   E. interference with the positive estrogen effect on midcycle LH release
13. True statements about prolactin include all of the following **EXCEPT** it
   A. is synthesized in chromophobe cells located in the pituitary gland
   B. is stored in chromophobe cells located in the pituitary gland
   C. is synthesized in decidual tissue
   D. is synthesized in endometrial tissue
   E. has a half-life of 20 hours
14. Pituitary tumors that secrete mainly adrenocorticotropic hormone (ACTH) or growth hormone frequently secrete prolactin. Hyperprolactinemia has been reported to occur in approximately what percent of cases with

	Cushing's disease	**acromegaly**
A.	25%	10%
B.	10%	25%
C.	10%	10%
D.	25%	25%
E.	5%	10%

15. Findings commonly associated with patients who have hyperprolactinemia include all of the following **EXCEPT**
   A. galactorrhea
   B. amenorrhea
   C. anovulation
   D. oligomenorrhea
   E. polymenorrhea
16. Bromocriptine (2-Br-alpha-ergocryptine mesylate)
   A. is detectable in the circulation 24 hours after administration
   B. frequently (40-50% of the time) causes orthostatic hypotension

C. frequently (40-50% of the time) causes insomnia
D. is a dopamine receptor agonist
E. is ineffective when administered other than by mouth

17. A 19-year-old college student developed amenorrhea of 6 months duration. A work-up at Student Health revealed a normal physical, including a normal pelvic examination, a FSH in the low normal range, and an early morning serum prolactin of 70 ng/ml. At this point you would order a
A. quantitative β-HCG
B. thyroid-stimulating hormone (TSH)
C. repeat serum prolactin in the mid-afternoon
D. luteinizing hormone (LH)
E. MRI (magnetic resonance imagery)

18. A 28-year-old gravida 0 who consulted you because of infertility is found to have a prolactin microadenoma. In discussing bromocriptine treatment, you would tell this patient that
A. she will not get pregnant until her prolactin is less than 20 ng/ml
B. she should notify you immediately if she is late for a period so that you can stop the medication since there is evidence that it is teratogenic
C. even with a dose of bromocriptine of up to 20 mg/day (about three times the average), 40% of patients with a microadenoma fail to have prolactin levels return to normal
D. bromocriptine is not associated with an increase risk of spontaneous abortion
E. that if she stops bromocriptine during pregnancy, there is a 40% chance that she will develop visual field changes because of tumor growth

19. The patient is a 20-year-old white long-distance track star who consulted you because of amenorrhea. Initially, you felt the amenorrhea was due to her vigorous exercise. Then she developed galactorrhea, and you obtained a serum prolactin. Now, having made the diagnosis of a prolactin-secreting microadenoma, you would inform the patient that if she is not treated she is very likely to develop
A. primary empty sella syndrome
B. osteoporosis
C. visual problems
D. hypothyroidism
E. adrenal insufficiency

20. A 28-year-old patient with 6 months amenorrhea and a normal pelvic exam has been found to have a prolactin of 55 ng/ml. In discussing the diagnostic work-up to rule out a prolactinoma, you would suggest the following sequence in your evaluation.
A. (1) β-HCG, if negative; (2) CT (computerized tomography), if normal; (3) thyrotropin-releasing-hormone (TRH) test
B. (1) β-HCG, if negative; (2) thyrotropin-releasing-hormone (TRH) test, if response is 200%; (3) MRI (magnetic resonance imagery)
C. (1) TSH, if normal; (2) thyrotropin releasing-hormone (TRH) test, if response is <200%; (3) MRI (magnetic resonance imagery)
D. (1) TSH, if normal; (2) CT (computerized tomography), if normal; (3) MRI (magnetic resonance imagery
E. (1) TSH, if abnormal; (2) thyrotropin-releasing-hormone (TRH) test, if response is <200%; (3) MRI (magnetic resonance imagery)

21. The rationale for discontinuing bromocriptine in a woman who becomes pregnant and has a prolactin-secreting macroadenoma includes all of the following **EXCEPT**
A. it suppresses fetal prolactin
B. more than 50% of such patients have a decrease in visual fields during pregnancy
C. it crosses the placenta
D. prolactin levels increase during pregnancy
E. the long-term effects of bromocriptine on the newborn are unknown

22. A 40-year-old is found to have a prolactinoma. Her serum prolactin is 250 ng/ml, and she gives a history of 3 years of amenorrhea and galactorrhea. The patient has inquired about surgical correction. In discussing the possible outcomes following transsphenoidal microsurgical resection, it would be correct to tell this patient that
A. she will need to undergo radiation after surgery
B. the risk of permanent diabetes insipidus is greater than 40%
C. the risk of hypopituitarism is 25%
D. her age and the length of time she has had symptoms is unrelated to the likelihood of a cure
E. the basic defect in dopamine regulation of prolactin secretion persists after removal

DIRECTIONS for questions 23 - 27: For each numbered item, select the one heading most closely associated with it. Each lettered heading may be used once, more than once, or not at all.

23-24. Physiologic action
(A) dopamine
(B) epinephrine
(C) serotonin
(D) 2-Br-α-ergocryptine mesylate
(E) estradiol
23. prolactin-inhibiting factor (PIF)
24. prolactin-releasing factor (PRF)

25-27. Several pharmacologic agents are associated with galactorrhea and hyperprolactinemia. The pathophysiology depends upon the agent. Match the mechanism with the medication
(A) blocks dopamine uptake
(B) blocks hypothalamic dopamine receptors
(C) depletes catecholamines
(D) blocks the conversion of tyrosine to dopa
(E) blocks the conversion of tryptophan to serotonin
25. reserpine
26. haloperidol
27. tricyclic antidepressants

DIRECTIONS: For each numbered item 28-29, indicate whether it is associated with
A only (A)
B only (B)
C both (A) and (B)
D neither (A) nor (B)

28-29. Appropriate testing for
(A) prolactin-secreting macroadenoma
(B) prolactin-secreting microadenoma
(C) both
(D) neither
28. visual field testing
29. insulin tolerance test

DIRECTIONS for questions 30 - 33: For each of the questions below, ONE or MORE of the responses is correct. Select the best answer based on the following
A if 1, 2, and 3 are correct
B if only 1 and 2 are correct
C if only 2 and 3 are correct
D if only 1 is correct
E if only 3 is correct

30. Prolactin stimulates the
1. growth of mammary tissue
2. secretion of milk into the alveoli of breast glands
3. release of gonadotrophins

31. Bromocriptine has been advocated to treat a prolactin-secreting macroadenoma
1. prior to surgical resection in an effort to alter and shrink the tumor
2. after an irradiation failure
3. in a patient who has visual field impairment

32. Physiologic stimuli that increase prolactin release include
1. stress
2. exercise
3. sleep

33. An increase in serum prolactin is usually noted with
1. an infusion of thyrotropin-releasing-hormone (TRH)
2. a craniopharyngioma
3. the empty sella syndrome

ANSWERS

1. **C,** Page 1142. In cases with borderline elevations of prolactin (20 - 60 ng/ml) and an abnormal response to TRH (an increase of less than 200%), a MRI (magnetic resonance imaging) scan should be performed. Not all individuals with an abnormal TRH response will have radiologic evidence of a microadenoma, however.
2. **C,** Pages 1145-1146. Following delivery, breast feeding may be initiated without adverse effects on the tumor. Following completion of nursing, bromocriptine should be ingested for 2 to 3 weeks and then discontinued. At that time a serum prolactin measurement and a repeat MRI or CT scan should be performed so that the need for further treatment can be reassessed.
3. **D,** Page 1137. Pathologic causes of hyperprolactinemia, in addition to a prolactin-secreting pituitary adenoma, include other pituitary tumors that produce acromegaly and Cushing's disease. Additional causes are hypothalamic disease, various pharmacologic agents, *hypothyroidism* not hyperthyroidism, chronic renal disease, or any chronic type of breast nerve stimulation, such as may occur with a thoracic operation, herpes zoster, or chest trauma. Ingestion of oral contraceptive steroids can also increase prolactin levels, with a greater incidence of hyperprolactinemia occurring with higher estrogen formulations. Nevertheless, galactorrhea does not usually occur during oral contraceptive ingestion because the exogenous estrogen blocks the binding of prolactin to its receptors.
4. **E,** Pages 1137, 1142. In most laboratories a normal serum prolactin is under 22

ng/ml. Women with regular menses, galactorrhea, and normal prolactin levels do not have prolactinomas, and therefore radiologic studies do not need to be performed in such women. There would certainly not be a suspicion of a macroadenoma so visual fields would not be warranted. Since an 3-5% of patients with hyperprolactinemia will have hypothyroidism, a thyroid-stimulating hormone assay (TSH) is warranted at the time the prolactin is drawn. Since this patient does not have hyperprolactinemia, she should merely be followed.

5. **D,** Pages 1133-1134. Big-big prolactin (mol wt 100,000 daltons) may represent an aggregation of many monomeric molecules of prolactin (mol wt equals 22,000). The small form is biologically active, and about 80% of the hormone is secreted in the small form. The larger forms of prolactin, big and big-big, are immunoreactive, but most of the immunoassayable prolactin is in the small form. Big-big prolactin has reduced binding to mammary tissue membranes in comparison to the monomeric form and is thus inactive in some bioassays. Specific receptors for prolactin are present in the plasma membrane of mammary cells as well as in many other tissues.
6. **D,** Pages 1134-1135. Prolactin levels normally fluctuate throughout the day, with maximum levels observed during nighttime while asleep and a smaller increase occurring in the early afternoon.
7. **E,** Page 1134. During pregnancy the levels of prolactin increase, reaching about 200 ng/ml in the third trimester, and the rise is directly related to the increase in circulating levels of estrogen. Despite the elevated prolactin levels during pregnancy, lactation does not occur because estrogen inhibits the action of prolactin on the breast, most likely blocking prolactin's interaction with its receptor. A day or two following delivery of the placenta, both estrogen levels and prolactin levels decline rapidly and lactation is initiated. Prolactin levels reach basal levels in nonnursing women in 2 to 3 weeks.
8. **E,** Pages 1139-1140, 1142. A prolactinoma and hypothyroidism have been ruled out in this patient with oligomenorrhea, a normal prolactin, and normal TSH. Because a few patients with galactorrhea, abnormal menstrual function, and normal prolactin levels have been found to have the empty sella syndrome, anteroposterior and lateral coned-down views of the sella turcica should be obtained. If this X-ray is abnormal, the diagnosis should be confirmed by a CT (computerized tomography) or MRI (magnetic resonance imagery) scan.
9. **A,** Page 1137. Hyperprolactinemia has been reported to be present in 15% of all anovulatory women and 20% of women with amenorrhea of undetermined cause. The incidence of galactorrhea in women with hyperprolactinemia has been reported to range from 30% to 80%. The incidence of hyperprolactinemia is higher (88%) in those women with galactorrhea who have amenorrhea and low estrogen than in those with galactorrhea and normal menses, oligomenorrhea, or amenorrhea with normal estrogen levels (49%). Basal levels of circulating prolactin decline to the nonpregnant range about 6 months after parturition in nursing women.
10. **C,** Page 1134. Prolactin levels reach normal, nonpregnant concentrations in nonnursing women in 2 to 3 weeks. Although basal levels of circulating prolactin decline to the nonpregnant range about 6 months after parturition in nursing women, prolactin levels increase markedly following each act of sucking and stimulate milk production for the next feeding. A level of 10 ng/ml is in the normal range. Since the patient had established breast feeding, Sheehan's syndrome is not a consideration. Stress should increase, not decrease, the release of prolactin.
11. **C,** Pages 1135-1136, 1140, 1145. Bromocriptine therapy is used primarily in women with microadenomas who wish to conceive or who are disturbed by their symptoms. This patient is not married and did not indicate that conception was an objective. She is not bothered by either the galactorrhea or the oligomenorrhea. Since she has some menses, she is producing estrogen. Thus, she does not appear to be at increased risk for osteoporosis and should be treated with periodic progestin withdrawal (medroxyprogesterone acetate 10 mg per day for 10 days of treatment) to prevent endometrial hyperplasia. A barrier type of contraception is advisable. Surgical resection is an option for patients with larger tumors. Radiation is not a primary mode of treatment for this lesion. Results have been inconsistent and there is a delay of several months between treatment and resumption of ovulation.
12. **B,** Page 1135. The mechanism, which best

explains why elevated prolactin levels interfere with gonadotrophin release, has not been completely elucidated, but the major factor appears to be alterations in normal gonadotrophin-releasing hormone (GnRH) release. It has also been shown that elevated levels of prolactin directly inhibit basal as well as gonadotrophin-stimulated ovarian secretion of both estradiol and progesterone. However, this mechanism is probably not the primary cause of anovulation, because women with hyperprolactinemia can be stimulated to ovulate with various agents including pulsatile GnRH. Some patients with moderate hyperprolactinemia have a greater than normal proportion of the big-big form of prolactin. Because this form of prolactin has reduced bioactivity, these individuals can have normal pituitary and ovarian function.

13. **E,** Page 1134. Prolactin is synthesized and stored in the pituitary gland in chromophobe cells called lactotrophs, which are located mainly in the lateral areas of the gland. In addition, prolactin is synthesized in decidual and endometrial tissue. Prolactin circulates in an unbound form and has a 20 minute half-life.
14. **B,** Page 1139. Pituitary tumors that secrete mainly adrenocorticotropic hormone (ACTH) or growth hormone frequently secrete prolactin. Hyperprolactinemia has been reported to occur in about 10% of patients with Cushing's disease and 25% of patients with acromegaly.
15. **E,** Page 1135. Hyperprolactinemia is usually associated with galactorrhea and can produce disorders of menstrual function, including amenorrhea, oligomenorrhea, and anovulation. Polymenorrhea is not a finding associated with increased serum prolactin.
16. **D,** Page 1145. Bromocriptine directly stimulates dopamine receptors, and as a dopamine receptor agonist, it inhibits prolactin secretion both in vitro and in vivo. After ingestion, bromocriptine is rapidly absorbed, with peak blood levels reached 1 to 3 hours later. It is not detectable in the serum after 14 hours. For this reason the drug is usually given at least twice daily. The most frequent side effect is orthostatic hypotension, which occurs in about 15% of patients. To minimize the effects of orthostatic hypotension, the initial dose should be taken at bedtime with food. Less frequent adverse symptoms include headache, nasal congestion, fatigue (not insomnia), constipation and diarrhea. About 10% of women cannot tolerate oral bromocriptine because of severe side effects. Vermesh et al reported that the drug was very well absorbed vaginally without the presence of side effects. A long-acting injectable form of bromocriptine that is effective for 1 month has also been developed, but it is not yet available for clinical use.
17. **B,** Pages 1137-1138, 1142. About 3 to 5% of individuals with hyperprolactinemia have hypothyroidism. This is the result of the decreased negative feedback of thyroxine (T_4) on the hypothalamic-pituitary axis. The resulting increase in thyrotropin-releasing hormone (TRH) stimulates prolactin secretion as well as thyroid-stimulating hormone (TSH) secretion from the pituitary. Thus, a TSH assay should be obtained for all individuals with hyperprolactinemia. If the TSH level is elevated, triiodothyronine (T_3) and T_4 should be measured to confirm the diagnosis of primary hypothyroidism. This is necessary because occasionally the TSH will be elevated as a result of a TSH-secreting pituitary adenoma. In this patient, with a normal pelvic examination, a quantitative β-HCG is not indicated. One might have performed a qualitative β-HCG as an initial screening test. Measuring the level of luteinizing hormone (LH) would not be of any help in establishing a diagnosis. A serum prolactin obtained in mid-afternoon would be about the same or higher, not lower. A MRI is indicated if the TSH is normal.
18. **D,** Pages 1145-1147. The usual therapeutic dose of bromocriptine is 2.5 mg twice or three times a day. About 10% of patients with microadenomas fail to have prolactin levels return to normal despite administration of up to 20 mg per day. Nevertheless, despite the persistently elevated prolactin levels, many of these patients ovulate and conceive. There is no evidence that the drug is teratogenic or adversely affects pregnancy outcome. The incidence of spontaneous abortion and multiple pregnancy is not increased. Less than 1% of patients with microadenomas have changes in visual fields. About 20% of patients with macroprolactinomas develop adverse changes in visual fields and polytomographic or neurologic signs during pregnancy. Some of these patients re-

quire bromocriptine or operative treatment during pregnancy or shortly postpartum.

19. **B,** Pages 1144-1145. Several studies have demonstrated the benign course of untreated microadenomas. These tumors seldom enlarge. Therefore, treatment may not be necessary if the patient is not bothered by the amenorrhea or galactorrhea. In this case, this patient is at increased risk for osteoporosis because of the low estrogen associated with prolactin elevations and her long distance running. For this reason she should receive exogenous estrogen. Macroadenomas, not microadenoma are likely to enlarge and cause visual field distortion or disturbance of pituitary function. A cause, not a consequence of hyperprolactinemia, is the primary empty sella syndrome. This is a clinical situation in which an intrasellar extension of the subarachnoid space results in compression of the pituitary gland and an enlarged sella turcica.
20. **C,** Pages 1142, 1143; Figure 37-9. Also see Shangold GA, Kletzky OA, Marrs RP, et al: Obstet Gynecol 63:771, 1984. With 6 months of amenorrhea, a normal pelvic exam, and a moderately elevated prolactin, a β-HCG is not going to be cost effective. The elevated prolactin could be secondary to hypothyroidism. The first step in this work-up should be a TSH (thyroid-stimulating hormone) determination. Since this is normal, the next step is a thyrotropin-releasing-hormone (TRH) test. If prolactin is measured before and 20 minutes after administration of an intravenous bolus of 500 μg of TRH, normal individuals have at least a 200% increase (three times baselines) of prolactin. All patients with hyperprolactinemia above 20 ng/ml and CT evidence of tumor had less than a threefold increase in prolactin (Shangold et al). Since the response was less than 200%, a CT or MRI scan is indicated to rule out a prolactinoma.
21. **B,** Pages 1148-1149. Twenty percent, not 50% of patients with macroadenomas develop adverse changes in visual fields and polytomographic or neurologic signs during pregnancy. Bromocriptine crosses the placenta and does suppress fetal prolactin but does not suppress placental hormone production. Its long term effects on the newborn are unknown although the risk of congenital anomalies, spontaneous abortion, and multiple gestation does not appear to increase. Postnatal surveillance of more than 200 children born after their mothers had been on bromocriptine revealed no adverse effects to date. If stopped at the onset of pregnancy, it should be reinstated in those pregnant patients who develop visual impairment. During pregnancy women with a macroadenoma should have monthly visual fields and neurologic testing.
22. **E,** Pages 1115, 1134. Radiation therapy should be used only as adjunctive management following incomplete operative removal of large tumors. A prolactin of 250 ng/ml is high, but this alone doesn't mean that the lesion is so large that it cannot be completely removed at surgery. Transsphenoidal operations have a mortality of less than 0.5%. The risk of permanent diabetes insipidus and hypopituitarism is less than 2%. The initial cure rate for patients with a serum prolactin above 200 ng/ml is 35%. Operative treatment of tumors in patients older than 26 with amenorrhea for more than 6 months carries a poorer prognosis than tumors in younger patients with a shorter duration of amenorrhea. In patients with prolactinomas there is a defect in dopamine regulation of prolactin secretion that persists even after surgical removal of the adenoma. This loss of dopaminergic inhibition of prolactin that persists for years after tumor removal is thought to explain the high rate of recurrence of tumors in the long-term follow-up of patients.

23-24. 23, **A;** 24, **C;** Page 1134. Prolactin synthesis and release are controlled by central nervous system neurotransmitters. The major control mechanism is inhibition. It appears that the major physiologic inhibitor of prolactin release is the neurotransmitter dopamine, which acts directly on the pituitary gland. Dopamine appears to be the prolactin-inhibiting factor (PIF). Both serotonin and thyrotropin-releasing hormone (TRH) stimulate prolactin release. Since the latter stimulates prolactin release only minimally unless infused, it appears that serotonin is a prolactin-releasing factor (PRF). The rise in prolactin levels during sleep appears to be controlled by serotonin. Bromocriptine, 2-Br-alpha-ergocryptine mesylate, is a semisynthetic ergot alkaloid that is a dopamine receptor agonist and is used to treat hyperprolactinemia. Estrogen stimulates prolactin production and release and is especially important in this regard at the time of puberty and during pregnancy. It is not, however, considered a prolactin-releasing factor.

25-27. 25, **C**; 26, **B**; 27, **A**; Page 1137. One of the most frequent causes of galactorrhea and hyperprolactinemia is the ingestion of pharmacologic agents. The antihypertensive agent reserpine depletes catecholamines, and methyldopa blocks the conversion of tyrosine to dihydroxyphenylalanine (dopa). The tricyclic antidepressants block dopamine uptake, and haloperidol and phenothiazines block hypothalamic dopamine receptors. Amphetamines stimulate the serotoninergic system.

28-29. 28, **A**; 29, **A**; Pages 1140-1142. Visual field determination and tests of adrenocorticotropic hormone (ACTH) and thyroid function are not necessary in patients with microadenomas, as these small tumors do not interfere with overall pituitary function and do not extend beyond the sella. However, these evaluations should be performed in individuals with macroadenomas. An insulin tolerance test is a test of ACTH reserve.

30. **B** (1, 2), Page 1134. The main functions of prolactin are the stimulation of growth of mammary tissue and the production and secretion of milk into the alveoli. Prolactin interferes with gonadotrophin release. Women with hyperprolactinemia have abnormalities in the frequency and amplitude of luteinizing hormone (LH) pulsations, with a normal or increased gonadotrophin response following gonadotrophin-releasing hormone (GnRH) infusion.

31. **A** (1, 2, 3), Pages 1149-1150. Some authors advocate the use of bromocriptine in the management of all patients with macroadenomas. It shrinks 80-90% of all macroadenomas, and although recurrence after cessation of therapy is high, long-term therapy has been successful in some patients. This medication is expensive, however, and a number of women, especially those on higher doses, have unpleasant side effects so that there are patients who prefer surgical treatment. If given preoperatively to shrink the tumor, the drug should be continued until the time of operation because following withdrawal of the drug, the tumor size may increase just as rapidly as it shrank. Bromocriptine has been successfully used to treat patients with failure of, or recurrence after, operation or irradiation therapy. Visual field impairment has disappeared with bromocriptine treatment.

32. **A** (1, 2, 3), Page 1134. Nipple and breast stimulation increase prolactin levels in the nonpregnant female. Other stimuli include stress, exercise, and sleep.

33. **A** (1, 2, 3), Pages 1137-1138, 1139. Thyrotropin-releasing hormone (TRH) can cause the release of prolactin. The normal response to an infusion of 500 μg is greater than three times the baseline prolactin. A craniopharyngioma can produce hyperprolactinemia as can an infiltration of the hypothalamus by sarcoidosis, histiocytosis, leukemia, or carcinoma. The empty sella syndrome is a condition in which there is an intrasellar extension of the subarachnoid space resulting in compression of the pituitary gland and an enlarged sella turcica that may be associated with galactorrhea and hyperprolactinemia. Therefore, in patients with radiologic evidence of an enlarged sella, a CT (computerized tomography) or MRI (magnetic resonance imaging) scan should be obtained to establish or rule out the presence of empty sella syndrome.

CHAPTER

38 Hyperandrogenism

DIRECTIONS for questions 1 - 21: Select the one best answer or completion.

1. Typical clinical features of virilization include all of the following **EXCEPT**
   A. decreased breast size
   B. dryness of the vagina
   C. development over a relatively long time (more than 2 years)
   D. increase in muscle mass
   E. secondary amenorrhea
2. The majority of the peripheral clinical manifestations of hirsutism are caused by
   A. increased circulating levels of androstenedione
   B. increased circulating levels of dehydroepiandrosterone (DHEA)
   C. increased levels of 5α-reductase
   D. increased levels of free testosterone
   E. increased levels of sex hormone-binding globulin (SHBG)
3. In order to exert a biologic effect such as hirsutism, testosterone is metabolized peripherally in target tissues to
   A. 5α-dehydrotestosterone (DHT)
   B. dehydroepiandrosterone sulfate (DHEA-S)
   C. androstenedione
   D. free testosterone
   E. etiocholanolone
4. In the severe form of congenital adrenal hyperplasia with complete 21-hydroxylase deficiency, clinical manifestations become apparent in a female
   A. at the time of birth
   B. at the time of menarche
   C. sometime between childhood and adolescence
   D. in the late teens
   E. in the fourth decade and present as hirsutism
5. Biochemical characteristics of polycystic ovary syndrome include all of the following **EXCEPT**
   A. increased gonadotropin-releasing hormone (GnRH) pulse amplitude
   B. tonically elevated levels of luteinizing hormone (LH)
   C. decreased level of follicle stimulating hormone (FSH)
   D. increased levels of circulating ovarian androgens
   E. decreased levels of biologically active (non-SHBG bound) estradiol
6. A 26 year-old woman who is 5′3″ tall and weighs 100 kg has biochemically proven polycystic ovary syndrome. In addition she is most likely to have
   A. hypothyroidism
   B. congenital adrenal hyperplasia
   C. Addison's Disease
   D. impaired glucose tolerance
   E. primary hyperparathyroidism
7. Increased terminal hair growth in a patient is consistent with each of the following **EXCEPT**
   A. clinical hirsutism
   B. elevated levels of circulating androgen
   C. increased activity of 5α-reductase
   D. an increased amount of vellous hair
   E. a prolonged length of anagen
8. The major clinical difference between polycystic ovary syndrome and stromal hyperthecosis is a
   A. greater ovarian enlargement in stromal hyperthecosis
   B. thickened ovarian capsule in stromal hyperthecosis
   C. higher levels of circulating free estradiol in stromal hyperthecosis
   D. progressive androgen stigmata including virilization in stromal hyperthecosis
   E. anovulation in stromal hyperthecosis
9. A 28 year-old gravida 1, para 0 who is approximately 32 weeks pregnant has had an acute onset of progressive, bothersome hirsutism of the upper lip and chin. During this time she has developed acne. The most likely reason is that the patient
   A. has an increased rate of androgen conversion from placental progesterone
   B. has androgenic manifestations because of increased peripheral 5α-reductase activity
   C. has increased ovarian testosterone production

D. has increased maternal adrenal DHEA-S production
E. has increased peripheral conversion to 5α-dehydrotestosterone (DHT)

Questions 10-11

10. A 22 year-old, gravida 1 para 1, 125 pound woman is referred with bothersome central hirsutism. She has regular menstrual periods and the referring physician has obtained both serum testosterone and dehydroepiandrosterone sulfate (DHEA-S), which are normal. The most likely source of her problem is increased
A. free testosterone
B. androstenedione
C. androsterone
D. 5α-reductase activity
E. etiocholanolone

11. The best treatment for the patient in the above question, #10, is
A. Spironolactone
B. dexamethasone
C. conjugated estrogens
D. oral contraceptives
E. electrolysis

12. In evaluating a 30 year-old, oligomenorrheic, hirsute woman, a dehydroepiandrosterone sulfate (DHEA-S) of 4 ng/ml is found. (Normal = 0.8 to 3.4 ng/ml.) An ACTH stimulation test is performed to rule out primary adrenal disease, and the DHEA-S is found to triple. This is consistent with the diagnosis of
A. Cushing's disease
B. acromegaly
C. an adrenal carcinoma
D. polycystic ovarian syndrome
E. an androgen-secreting ovarian tumor

13. Symptoms of androgen excess in patients with congenital adrenal hyperplasia are the result of excessive
A. adrenal production of free testosterone
B. peripheral conversion of C_{19} steroids to testosterone
C. adrenal production of free dehydroepiandrosterone sulfate (DHEA-S)
D. adrenal production of free androstenedione
E. adrenal cortisol production

14. A 24 year-old, oligomenorrheic nulligravida is diagnosed as having polycystic ovarian syndrome. The patient is not anxious to get pregnant at this time. The best treatment is cyclic
A. medroxyprogesterone acetate
B. conjugated estrogens
C. norethindrone
D. levonorgestrel acetate
E. combination oral contraceptives

Questions 15-16

15. A 30 year-old, 5 feet 1 inch, 110 pound gravida 2 para 2 is referred to you for treatment of slowly progressive hirsutism. She has regular monthly menstrual periods. Her serum testosterone is 0.5 ng/ml (Normal = 0.2 to 0.8 ng/ml) and serum DHEA-S is 1.2 ng/ml (Normal = 0.8 to 3.4 ng/ml.). The most likely diagnosis is
A. Cushing's syndrome
B. idiopathic hirsutism
C. polycystic ovarian syndrome
D. congenital adrenal hyperplasia
E. stromal cell hyperthecosis

16. The best treatment of the patient in question #15 is
A. dexamethasone
B. combination oral contraceptives
C. conjugated estrogen
D. medroxyprogesterone acetate
E. Spironolactone

17. A 28 year-old, slender, athletic-looking, normotensive woman has an 18 month history of oligomenorrhea and 6 month history of progressive central hirsutism and clitoromegaly. Her serum testosterone is 0.8 mg/ml (Normal = 0.2 to 0.8 ng/ml). The DHEA-S is 10 mg/ml (Normal = 0.8 to 3.4 ng/ml.). The pelvic examination is normal. This patient should have
A. computerized tomography (CT) of the adrenal glands
B. an ACTH stimulation test
C. an overnight dexamethasone suppression test
D. complete dexamethasone suppression test (Liddle's test)
E. laparoscopic examination of the ovaries

18. The best laboratory test to confirm a suspected diagnosis of congenital adrenal hyperplasia is a
A. serum testosterone
B. serum DHEA-S
C. serum pregnanetriol
D. serum 17-hydroxyprogesterone
E. urinary 17-ketosteroids

19. A 26 year-old, infertile woman presents with oligomenorrhea. She is 5 feet 7 inches tall and weighs 160 pounds. The ovaries are bilaterally enlarged. She does *not* have hirsutism. Of the following, the most likely to be normal is
A. DHEA-S
B. 3α-diol-G
C. testosterone
D. androstenedione
E. LH

20. A 25 year-old woman delivers a 3200 gram

baby at term after an uncomplicated pregnancy. Newborn examination is normal except for the presence of ambiguous genitalia, including an enlarged clitoris, a vaginal dimple, and an incompletely developed scrotum. The most likely diagnosis is

A. congenital adrenal hyperplasia
B. androgen insensitivity syndrome (testicular feminization)
C. Cushing's syndrome
D. Turner's syndrome
E. adrenal carcinoma

21. A 26 year old woman is referred for evaluation of bothersome hirsutism. The referring physician has obtained a serum testosterone, which is 1.0 ng/ml (Normal = 0.2 to 0.8 ng/ml). Further information can be best gained by ordering a
    A. serum androstenedione
    B. serum androsterone
    C. serum etiocholanolone
    D. serum dehydroepiandrosterone sulfate (DHEA-S)
    E. urinary 17-ketosteroids

DIRECTIONS for questions 22 - 29: For each of the questions below, ONE or MORE of the responses is correct. Select the best answer based on the following

A if 1, 2, and 3 are correct
B if only 1 and 2 are correct
C if only 2 and 3 are correct
D if only 1 is correct
E if only 3 is correct

22. True statements regarding the genetic inheritance of late onset 21-hydroxylase deficiency include
    1. the phenotype is apparent after adolescence.
    2. it is highest in the Ashenazi Jewish population
    3. this is a homozygous condition with two severely defective alleles.
23. Late onset 21-hydroxylase deficiency is best differentiated from polycystic ovary syndrome by
    1. a basal serum 17-hydroxyprogesterone level
    2. an ACTH stimulation test
    3. urinary 17-ketosteroids
24. Historic features helpful in identifying the source of androgen in a 21 year-old woman complaining of progressive hirsutism for the past year include
    1. her menstrual history
    2. her prepubertal and pubertal linear growth history
    3. the age at which hair growth became noticeable
25. In treating hirsutism with various pharmacologic agents, patients should be told that
    1. they will need to continue therapy for the rest of their life
    2. a response may take at least three months to begin to be apparent
    3. approximately three quarters of patients will have a favorable response with one year of treatment
26. Biochemical characteristics associated with the ovarian histology shown in Figure 38-1 include
    1. increased pulsatility of GnRH
    2. tonically elevated LH
    3. increased total circulating estrogens
27. True statements concerning circulating testosterone include
    1. the majority is biologically inactive

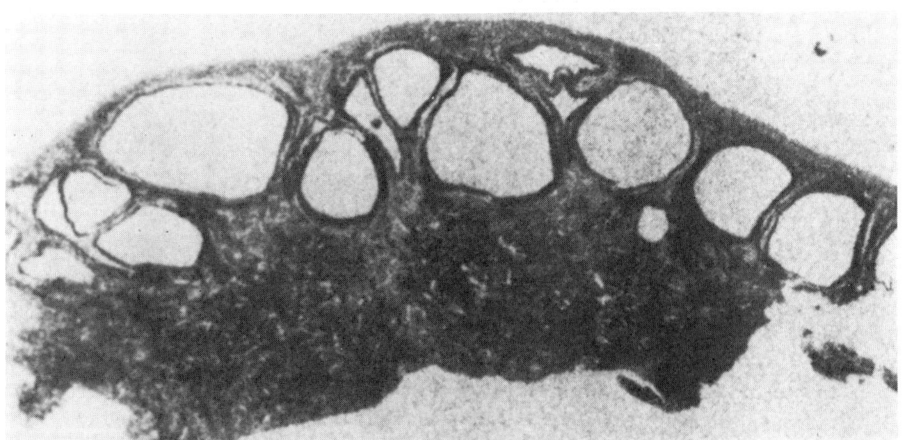

FIGURE 38-1.

2. it is metabolized in the periphery to 5α-dihydro-testosterone
3. the measurement reported when a serum testosterone is requested is the concentration of free hormone

28. True observations regarding the estrogen milieu in women with polycystic ovarian syndrome (polycystic ovary syndrome) include an increase in
    1. unbound circulating estradiol
    2. circulating estrone
    3. total estriol
29. The estrogen milieu in a patient with polycystic ovary syndrome as represented in Figure 38-2 encompass
    1. an increase in total circulating levels of estradiol
    2. an increase in biologically active estradiol
    3. an increase in total serum estrone

ANSWERS

1. **C,** Page 1158. Virilization is a relatively uncommon clinical finding and its presence is usually associated with markedly elevated levels of circulating testosterone (2 ng/ml or greater). In contrast to the gradual development of hirsutism, signs of virilization usually occur over a relatively short period of time. These signs are due to both the masculinizing and defeminizing action of testosterone and include temporal balding, clitoral hypertrophy, decreased breast size, dryness of the vagina, and increased muscle mass. Woman with virilization are nearly always amenorrheic and the presence of an androgen secreting neoplasm should always be suspected in this clinical situation.
2. **D,** Pages 1161-1162. Androstenedione and dehydroepiandrosterone (DHEA) do not have androgenic activity, but are peripherally converted at a slow rate to a biologically active androgen, testosterone. About two thirds of the daily testosterone produced in a woman originates from the ovaries. Thus, increased circulating levels of testosterone usually indicate abnormal ovarian androgen production. Most testosterone in the circulation (about 85%) is tightly bound to sex hormone binding globulin (SHBG) and is believed to be biologically inactive. An additional 10-15% is loosely bound to albumin with only about 1%-2% not bound by any protein (free testosterone). Both the free and albumin-bound fraction are biologically active. Serum testosterone can be measured as the total amount, the amount that is believed to be biologically active (non-SHBG bound), and as the free form.
3. **A,** Pages 1162, 1164 (Table 38-4). To exert a biologic effect, testosterone is metabolized peripherally in targeted tissues to the more androgenic 5α-dehydrotestosterone (DHT) by the enzyme 5α-reductase. Even with normal circulatory levels of androgen, increased 5a-reductase activity in the pilosebaceous unit will result in increased androgenic activity

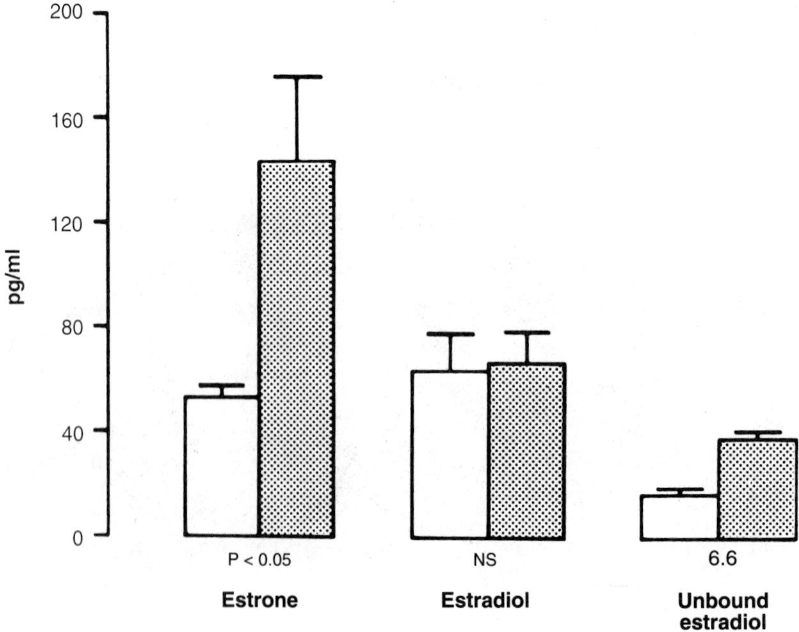

FIGURE 38-2.

producing hirsutism. In evaluating hirsute women, it is important to remember that serum levels of total testosterone may be similar in normal as well hirsute women but that there are significant differences in the amounts of non-SHBG bound testosterone as well as 3α-diol-G (a breakdown product of 5α-reductase). Thus, the clinician should remember there are three markers of androgen production in the serum, one for each compartment where androgens are produced: (1) ovary—testosterone; (2) adrenal gland—DHEA-S; (3) periphery—3α-diol-G.

4. **A,** Page 1174. Congenital adrenal hyperplasia is an inherited disorder caused by an enzymatic defect (usually 21-hydroxylase deficiency) or less often an 11 β-hydroxylase deficiency resulting in decreased cortisol biosynthesis. The increased production of C_{19} steroids are in turn peripherally converted to testosterone which produces signs of androgen excess. Because the enzymatic defects are congenital, the classic severe form (complete block) usually becomes manifest in fetal life and is the most common cause of sexual ambiguity in the newborn. The more attenuated (mild) block of 21-hydroxylase deficiency does not produce physical signs until after puberty making it a more common source of hirsutism and virilization in the second or early third decade of life.
5. **E,** Pages 1165-1169. The polycystic ovary syndrome is a relatively common endocrinologic disorder that begins soon after menarche and consists of a series of biochemical abnormalities, including an increased gonadotropin releasing hormone (GnRH) pulse amplitude and tonically elevated levels of luteinizing hormones (LH). Follicle stimulating hormone typically is not elevated in this disorder. In addition there are increased circulating levels of androgen produced by both the ovaries and the adrenal glands. It has been shown that the peripheral manifestations of hirsutism associated with this disorder are more likely related to the individual's ability to peripherally convert the increased androgen load by 5α-reductase. Thus, the hirsutism often found with this disorder is peripherally mediated. Interestingly, most patients with polycystic ovary syndrome have increased levels of biologically active (non-SHBG bound) estradiol although total circulating levels of estradiol are not increased.
6. **D,** Page 1169. Hyperinsulinemia occurs in women with polycystic ovary syndrome whether or not they are obese. Only obese women with polycystic ovary syndrome have impaired glucose tolerance however. Thus, the negative impact of obesity and polycystic ovary syndrome on insulin resistance is additive. Although the other endocrinopathies may occur with polycystic ovary syndrome they are not necessarily found in association with this disorder. Some investigators have suggested that hyperandrogenism causes insulin resistance while others have presented data indicating that the reverse is true: hyperinsulinemia produces hyperandrogenism in women with polycystic ovary syndrome. This relationship remains controversial.
7. **D,** Page 1158. There are two types of hair—vellous hair which is soft, fine and unpigmented and terminal hair. Terminal hair growth undergoes three phases; anagen which is the growth phase; a transitional phase called catagen; and a resting phase or telogen after which the hair sheds. Androgen is necessary to produce the development of terminal hair and the time spent in anagen is governed by circulating androgen levels. The level of activity of the enzyme 5α-reductase in the hair follicle influences the degree to androgenic activity. With elevated levels of androgen or increased activity of 5α-reductase, terminal hair appears where normally vellous hair is present. In this situation the length of anagen is prolonged. The presence of hirsutism, without other signs of virilization, is associated with relatively mild disorders of androgen production with circulating levels of testosterone either normal or mildly elevated (less than 1.5 ng/ml). Hirsutism usually has a gradual onset and is not caused by a severe enzymatic defect or neoplasm.
8. **D,** Page 1172. Stromal hyperthecosis is an uncommon benign ovarian disorder in which the ovaries are bilaterally enlarged and histologically have nests of luteinized theca cells within the stroma (Figure 38-18 in Herbst et al.). The size of the ovaries and capsular thickening are similar to those found in polycystic ovary syndrome. Anovulation is characteristic of both syndromes. This disorder is similar to polycystic ovary syndrome in that it is gradual and likely to be associated with amenorrhea and hirsutism. However, unlike polycystic ovary syndrome, with increasing age stromal hyperthecosis is associated with progressively increasing amounts of testosterone secretion. By the time a woman reaches her fourth decade of life the severity will have gradually progressed to cause virilization. Serum testosterone levels may reach those found usually in testosterone secreting tumors (>2 ng/ml).

9. **C,** Page 1164. Signs of androgen excess during this pregnancy is most likely caused by increased ovarian testosterone production. This is usually caused by either a luteoma of pregnancy orhyperreactio luteinalis. The former is a unilateral or bilateral solid ovarian enlargement whereas the later is bilateral cystic ovarian enlargement. After pregnancy the androgenic characteristics regress. Of significance is the acute onset and the marked degree of hirsutism.
10. **D,** Pages 1164-1165. Idiopathic hirsutism (a peripheral disorder of androgen metabolism) is the most common type of androgenic disorder. This usually occurs in regularly menstruating women and is associated with normal levels of serum testosterone and dehydroepiandrosterone sulfate (DHEA-S). It has recently been shown that nearly all of these individuals have increased levels of 3α-diol-G, indirectly indicating that the cause of hirsutism could be increased 5α-reductase activity, which converts normal levels of testosterone to increased amounts of biologically active androgens DHT and 3α-diol-G. If measured, serum androstenedione is usually normal. The other two androgens, androsterone and etiocholanolone, are both 17-ketosteroids and are the metabolic breakdown products of androstenedione.
11. **A,** Pages 1164-1165, 1181. Idiopathic hirsutism is related to abnormalities in the excessive peripheral production of 3α-diol-G and DHT. It has been shown that there is a localized increase in the activity of 5α-reductase. This is considered a condition of peripheral androgen metabolism in the pilosebaceous apparatus of the skin. Antiandrogens that block peripheral testosterone action or interfere with 5α-reductase activity are moderately effective therapeutic agents. The most widely used agent in this country is spironolactone. The other agents do not exert a direct end organ effect since they are not associated with appreciable changes in 5α-reductase activity. Electrolysis may improve the cosmetic appearance in select areas, but does not treat the underlying problem.
12. **D,** Pages 1165, 1169, 1171, 1174. Approximately half of the women with polycystic ovary syndrome have elevated levels of dehydroepiandrosterone sulfate (DHEA-S), with one-third of them having levels greater than 4 ng/ml. Although ACTH levels are normal in these women, infusions of ACTH produce an exaggerated response of DHEA-S, indicating that perhaps the adrenal gland in some patients with polycystic ovary syndrome has increased sensitivity to ACTH and that the adrenal gland may be involved in the pathogenesis of this syndrome. Cushing's disease is the result of excessive adrenal production of glucocorticoids due to increased secretion of ACTH. When the signs and symptoms are due to excessive glucocorticoids secondary to adrenal tumors, the problem is referred to as Cushing's syndrome. These disorders are best evaluated by studies of adrenal suppression such as the overnight dexamethasone suppression test. The findings of androgen excess and exaggerated androgen response in this patient are unrelated to the manifestations associated with acromegaly. Likewise, extremely high levels of DHEA sulfate found with rare adrenal carcinomas are relatively unaffected by the ACTH stimulation test. One would not expect to uncover an androgen-secreting ovarian tumor by this test since ACTH has no effect on the ovary.
13. **B,** Page 1174. Congenital adrenal hyperplasia involves an enzymatic defect of either 21-hydroxylase of 11 β-hydroxylase, resulting in decreased cortisone synthesis. ACTH production is thereby increased, and there is a progressive buildup of cortisol precursors, including 17-hydroxyprogesterone and 17-hydroxypregnenolone. These steroids are then converted to dehydroepiandrosterone (DHEA) and androstenedione, which in turn are peripherally converted to testosterone, causing hirsutism and/or virilization depending on the severity of the enzymatic block. Testosterone is normally not produced in high amounts directly from the adrenal gland and there is not an excessive amount of endogenously produced (adrenal) DHEA-S. The excessive amount of androstenedione produced is secondary to the enzymatic block and exerts its androgenic effect through peripheral conversion to testosterone.
14. **E,** Pages 1179-1180. The treatment of polycystic ovarian syndrome depends on which complaints are most bothersome to the patient. If hirsutism and irregular or infrequent bleeding are most bothersome and if the patient is not desirous of becoming pregnant, combination oral contraceptives using formulations that contain less than 50 mcg of estrogen and a progestin other than norgestrel are best. Norgestrel is not used because it is the most potent androgenic progestin in current use. Oral contraceptives are best because these agents inhibit LH secretion, decrease circulatingtestosterone levels, and increase the levels of sex hormone binding globulin (SHBG), thus binding and inactivating more

of the testosterone in circulation. Medroxyprogesterone acetate, conjugated estrogens, and norethindrone acetate do not inhibit LH or decrease circulating testosterone levels to the same extent that cyclic combination oral contraceptives do.

15. **B,** Pages 1164-1165, 1180. The case exemplifies a patient with idiopathic hirsutism. She has normal adrenal and ovarian androgen levels and is experiencing regular menstrual periods. Fertility has not been a concern. It can be assumed that this patient has increased peripheral androgen activity and if measured, would have a high 3α-diol-G value. This metabolite is not routinely measured since the presumptive diagnosis is one of exclusion made by excluding the other possibilities. This woman did not present with additional findings suggestive of Cushing's disease such as centripetal obesity, dorsal neck fat pads, abdominal striae, or muscle wasting and weakness. Likewise, she does not have the oligomenorrhea that most polycystic ovarian syndrome patients have and does not have the associated modestly elevated serum testosterone. Congenital adrenal hyperplasia is not suspect because of normal DHEA-S levels and an absence of menstrual irregularity and true virilization. Similarly, stromal cell hyperthecosis is ruled out by the lack of menstrual irregularity and a normal testosterone.
16. **E,** Pages 1165, 1180-1181. The best treatment for idiopathic hirsutism is an agent that inhibits peripheral androgen activity. Of the drugs approved for use in the United States, the most efficacious is Spironolactone. Cimetidine has also been used successfully. In Europe, cyproterone acetate has been used successfully, but is not available in the United States. It has been reported that hair shaft density and the rate of hair growth decreases after two months of Spironolactone therapy in doses in excess of 100 mg/day.
17. **A,** Page 1174. Patients with rapidly progressive signs of androgen excess, including virilization, who have modestly elevated testosterone values but markedly elevated DHEA-S values should be suspected of having an androgen-producing adrenal tumors. These tumors secrete a large amount of C_{19} steroids, which are normally produced by the adrenal gland, including DHEA-S, DHEA, and androstenedione. The peripheral conversion of these relatively weak androgens to testosterone produces the androgen stigmata. Because of the potential severity of this problem, patients with these laboratory findings and a history of rapid onset signs of androgen excess should undergo computerized tomography (CT) of the adrenal glands to confirm the diagnosis. An ACTH stimulation test would be of little value since one is not concerned with measuring cortisol precursors secondary to an enzymatic block. Similarly, dexamethasone suppression tests are not indicated since this patient did not present with the stigmata of Cushing's disease. Since the markedly excessive androgen in this case is of adrenal origin, and since the testosterone level is only mildly elevated, there should be little concern that there is a potential ovarian source, so laparoscopy is not indicated.
18. **D,** Page 1176. The diagnosis of congenital adrenal hyperplasia is established if serum levels of 17-hydroxyprogesterone are greater than 8 ng/ml. This test has replaced the less precise measurement of its metabolite, pregnanetriol. Since one is measuring metabolic products resulting from an enzymatic block, obtaining serum testosterone or DHEA-S will not reveal the source of the problem. Although urinary 17-ketosteroid levels may be elevated, this test is less specific, and awkward collection techniques make interpretation of test results difficult in the newborn.
19. **B,** Pages 1165-1168. Polycystic ovarian syndrome should be thought of as a disorder of hyperandrogenism with chronic anovulation. Serum testosterone levels and serum androstenedione levels are usually mildly to moderately elevated. In addition, about half of the women with this syndrome have elevated DHEA-S. It is estimated that approximately 30% of women of polycystic ovary syndrome do not have hirsutism even though nearly all of them have elevated circulating androgen levels. The presence or absence of hirsutism depends on whether those androgens are converted peripherally by 5α-reductase to the more potent androgens dihydrotestosterone and 3α-diol-G. This 5α-reductase activity is reflected by increased levels of 3α-diol-G. In this patient, with no hirsutism, it would be expected that her 3α-diol-G level would be normal. In the polycystic ovary syndrome, LH levels are tonically elevated, usually above 20 mIU/ml.
20. **A,** Pages 1174, 1175 (Table 38-7). Congenital adrenal hyperplasia is the most common cause of sexual ambiguity in the newborn. This is usually caused by a severe 21-hydroxylase block with a resultant increase in ACTH secretion and increased adrenal production of cortisol precursors proximal to the enzymatic block. These precursors include both 17-hy-

droxypregnenolone and 17-hydroxyprogesterone. These steroids are then converted to DHEA and androstenedione, which in turn are peripherally converted to testosterone, resulting in masculinization of the female external genitalia. The associated fluid and electrolyte changes occurring in these babies can be severe and lead to death. Cushing's syndrome results in excessive adrenal production of glucocorticoids due to increased ACTH secretion and is generally not manifest in the newborn. Likewise, androgen insensitivity syndrome and Turner's syndrome are generally disorders appreciated in girls at about the time of menarche or in their mid-adolescence because of their amenorrhea. Adrenal carcinoma is extremely rare in any age group and especially in the newborn. This would be suspected with markedly elevated levels of DHEA-S as opposed to the elevated levels of cortisol precursors one would find in congenital adrenal hyperplasia.

21. **D,** Page 1160. This patient's hirsutism has been partially investigated by the mildly elevated testosterone of 1.0 ng/ml. This is indicative of ovarian androgenic hyperfunction and may be the only source of hyperandrogenism in this patient. However, the other major source for androgen production, the adrenal gland, has not been investigated. The best test to measure the other major androgen source is to obtain a serum dehydroepiandrosterone sulfate (DHEA-S). This will give more complete information as to whether the patient has a combined source of androgen excess. This test is much better than urinary 17-ketosteroids because it gives a direct assessment of potential adrenal androgen excess. Androsterone and etiocholanolone are both17-ketosteroids and represent metabolic breakdown patterns of androstenedione. This in turn is produced in part from the metabolism of testosterone, which is not a 17-ketosteroid. Therefore, in investigating patients with complaints of hirsutism, the two basic tests of androgen hyperfunction should represent the two major sources for female androgen production, the adrenal gland and the ovary.

22. **B** (1, 2), Pages 1175-1176. Estimates by geneticists indicate that late onset 21-hydroxylase deficiency varies in incidence among different ethnic groups, but that overall it is probably the most frequent autosomal genetic disorder in humans. Both classic congenital adrenal hyperplasia and late onset 21-hydroxylase deficiency are transmitted in an autosomal recessive manner at the CYP21B locus. There are three possible manifestations of CYP21Y alleles (normal, mildly defective, or severely defective). Late onset 21-hydroxylase deficiency is a phenotype that is symptomatic after adolescence. Affected individuals may be homozygous for alleles yielding mildly abnormal enzymatic activity or compound heterozygotes with a combination of defective alleles.

    Patients with compound heterozygotes may have one mildly and one severely defective allele or they may be homozygous with two mildly defective alleles. If they were homozygous with two severely defective alleles, they would have been individuals with ambiguous genitalia at birth. The incidence of late onset 21-hydroxylase deficiency is highest in the Ashenazi Jewish population

23. **B** (1, 2), Page 1176. To differentiate late onset 21-hydroxylase deficiency from polycystic ovary syndrome, measurement of basal (early morning) serum 17-hydroxyprogesterone levels should be performed. This test has replaced less precise measurement of the urinary metabolite pregnanetriol. If basal levels of 17-hydroxyprogesterone are greater than 8 ng/ml, the diagnosis of late onset 21-hydroxylase deficiency is established. I17-hydroxyprogesterone is above normal (2.5-3.3 ng/ml) but less than 8 ng/ml, an ACTH stimulation test should be performed. After infusion of 25 mcgs of synthetic ACTH as a single bolus, a serum sample for 17-hydroxyprogesterone is obtained in one hour and if the level increases more than 10 ngs/ml the diagnosis of late onset 21-hydroxylase deficiency is established. 17-ketosteroids was formerly used to measure metabolites of androgen production but have largely been replaced by serum androgens or plasma androgens. Measurement of androgens is of more value in identifying cases of hirsutiŝm or virilism which are not associated with 21-hydroxylase enzymatic block.

24. **B** (1, 2), Page 1178. The three androgenic disorders most likely to be the source of this patient's problem are polycystic ovary syndrome, late onset 21-hydroxylase deficiency, and idiopathic hirsutism. They all may be associated with a similar history and physical findings. Menstrual irregularity is an uncommon finding in woman with idiopathic hirsutism. These women will have a normal testosterone and DHEA-S level. Patients with late onset 21-hydroxylase deficiency may have a history of prepubertal accelerated growth (ages 6 to 8 years) with later decreased growth and a short ultimate height. The age

TABLE 38-1. Genotypic Characterization of the Forms of 21-Hydroxylase Deficiency

Form of 21-Hydroxylase Deficiency	Clinical Phenotype	Hormonal Phenotype (in Response to ACTH)	Genotype
Classic (CAH)	Prenatal virilization, fully symptomatic	Marked elevation of precursors (serum 17-hydroxyprogesterone and Δ-androstenedione	21-OH-def^{severe} / 21-OH-def^{severe}
Nonclassic (LOHD)	Symptomatic: later development of virilization; milder symptoms Asymptomatic: no virilization or other symptoms	Moderate elevation of precursors	21-OH-def^{severe} / 21-OH-def^{mild} 21-OH-def^{mild} / 21-OH-def^{mild}
Carrier	Asymptomatic	Precursor level greater than normal	21-OH-def^{severe} / 21-OHase (normal) 21-OH-def^{mild} / 21-OHase (normal)
Normal	(Asymptomatic)	Lowest levels—some overlap seen with carriers	21-OHase (normal) / 21-OHase (normal)

From New MI, White PC, et al: The adrenal hyperplasias. In Scriver CR, Beaudet AL, Sly S, and Valle D: Metabolic basis of inherited diseases, ed 6, New York, 1989, McGraw-Hill Book Co.

at which hair growth became noticeable is not helpful in differentiating the source of the androgen. The rapidity with which the hirsutism appeared is pertinent. Tumors are associated with rapid onset.

25. **C** (2, 3), Pages 1178, 1181. After identifying the source of androgen excess in patients who are hirsute, an explanation about the likelihood of the success of the proposed treatment is appropriate. Because of the length of the hair growth cycle, response to treatment should not be expected within the first three months. Objective methods of assessing changes of hair growth, such as photographs, are useful. With the use of varying antiandrogenic agents (oral contraceptives, dexamethasone, spironolactone) successful response should occur in about 70% of patients within one year of treatment. The remaining excess hair can be removed by electrolysis. Treatment should be continued for two years and then stopped to determine if the hirsutism recurs and if so, therapy can be reinstated.

26. **A** (1, 2, 3) Pages 1165-1169 (Figure 38-1 from Wilroy RS Jr, Given JR, Wiser WL, Coleman SA, Anderson RN, Summitt RL: Hyperthecosis: An inheritable form of polycystic/ovarian disease. In Bergsma D (ed.): "Genetic Forms of Hypogonadism." Miami: Symposia Specialists for the National Foundation-March of Dimes, BD: OAS XI(4):81, 1975, with permission.). This photomicrograph depicts a histological picture typical of polycystic ovarian syndrome. There are characteristic multiple subcapsular cysts, and there are numerous premature atretic follicles. Biochemical associations with these findings include increased pulsatility of GnRH, which produces tonically elevated LH levels and increased ovarian androgen production. In addition, because of increased peripheral conversion of androstenedione to estrone in conjunction with decreased SHBG levels, there is tonic hyperestrogenism.

27. **B** (1, 2), Pages 1161-1162. Most testosterone in the circulation (about 85%) is tightly bound to sex hormone binding globulin (SHBG) and is believed to be biologically inactive. Only about 10 to 15% is loosely bound to albumin. About 1 to 2% is ***not*** bound to any protein, representing free testosterone. The measured concentration of free testosterone as a sample is generally reported only upon request. Serum testosterone can be measured in any of these forms. To exert a biologic effect, testosterone is metabolized peripherally in the target tissues to the more potent androgen, 5′-dihydrotestosterone (DHT). It has been shown that although serum levels of total testosterone are similar in normal and hirsute

women, there are significant differences in the amount of non-SHBG-bound testosterone, which is elevated in about 60-70% of hirsute women.

28. **B** (1, 2), Page 1169. Women with polycystic ovarian syndrome have increased levels of biologically active (non-sex hormone binding globulin, or non-SHBG) estradiol, although total circulating levels of estradiol are not increased. The increased amount of non-SHBG-bound estradiol is caused by a decrease in SHBG, which is produced primarily by increased levels of androgens and secondarily by the obesity present in many of these women. Even though the polycystic ovary does not secrete increased amounts of estrogen or estradiol, the increased levels of androstenedione are peripherally converted to estrone, causing increased circulating estrone levels. Appreciable amounts of estriol are present only in pregnancy as a function of the metabolism of the fetal placenta complex.
29. **C** (2, 3), Page 1169. In addition to increased levels of circulating androgens, women with polycystic ovary syndrome have increased levels of biologically active (non-SHBG bound) estradiol although total circulating levels of estradiol are not increased (Figure 38-2). The increased amount of non-SHBG bound estradiol is caused by a decrease in SHBG levels, which is produced primarily by the increased levels of androgens and secondarily by the obesity present in many of these women. Serum estrone is also increased, but is not as biologically active.

CHAPTER

39 Infertility

DIRECTIONS for questions 1 - 10: Select the one best answer or completion.

Questions 1-2

1. During the evaluation of an infertile couple, the husband's initial semen analysis is received. The report is shown below. The abnormal parameter is
   A. volume: 2.5 ml
   B. pH: 7.5
   C. sperm density: 15 million/ml
   D. sperm motility: 75% have good to excellent motility
   E. sperm morphology: 65% normal
2. Based on the previous semen analysis results, and assuming that the husband has a normal medical history, your recommendation would be to
   A. repeat the semen analysis immediately
   B. repeat the semen analysis in one month
   C. begin clomiphene citrate therapy
   D. begin tetracycline therapy
   E. have the man examined by a urologist
3. The only direct evidence of ovulation is
   A. a serum progesterone 10 ng/ml
   B. a history of regular menstrual cycles
   C. an endometrial biopsy revealing a secretory endometrium
   D. a biphasic basal body temperature chart
   E. pregnancy
4. A 25 year-old gravida 1, para 1, is undergoing laparoscopy for infertility of two years duration. You notice four 1 mm superficial implants of endometriosis on the left ovary and a few filmy adhesions around both ovaries. Assuming the rest of her work-up is normal, you should
   A. perform a laparotomy immediately
   B. perform laparotomy in 6 months
   C. begin danazol postoperatively
   D. recommend in vitro fertilization
   E. fulgurate and delay medical or other surgical intervention at least 12 months
5. The poorest prognosis for conception is associated with
   A. intrauterine adhesions
   B. leiomyomata
   C. a bicornuate uterus
   D. In utero DES exposure
   E. pelvic tuberculosis
6. A couple with primary infertility inquires about possible sexually-transmitted diseases associated with artificial insemination (AID). You should inform them that donors for AID must be screened for all of the following **EXCEPT**
   A. *Chlamydia trachomatis*
   B. Herpes simplex II
   C. *Neisseria gonorrhoeae*
   D. syphilis
   E. serum hepatitis B
7. A 28 year-old nulligravida is scheduled to begin clomiphene citrate treatment for anovulation. She should be informed that when compared with the general population, conception following clomiphene treatment is associated with an increased incidence of
   A. spontaneous abortion
   B. ectopic pregnancy
   C. multiple gestation
   D. congenital malformation
   E. intrauterine fetal death
8. A 23 year-old with a history of 2 years of infertility has had a hysterosalpingogram which is reproduced in figure 39-1. The most efficacious treatment for this problem would be
   A. transcervical balloon tuboplasty
   B. intrauterine insemination (IUI)
   C. gamete intrafallopian transfer (GIFT)
   D. tubal reanastomosis
   E. in vitro fertilization (IVF)
9. All of the following are indications for washed intrauterine insemination **EXCEPT**
   A. cervical stenosis
   B. oligospermia
   C. inadequate mucus
   D. small semen volume
   E. bilateral cornual obstruction
10. A 30 year-old gravida 1, para 1, is receiving clomiphene citrate 50 mg per day on

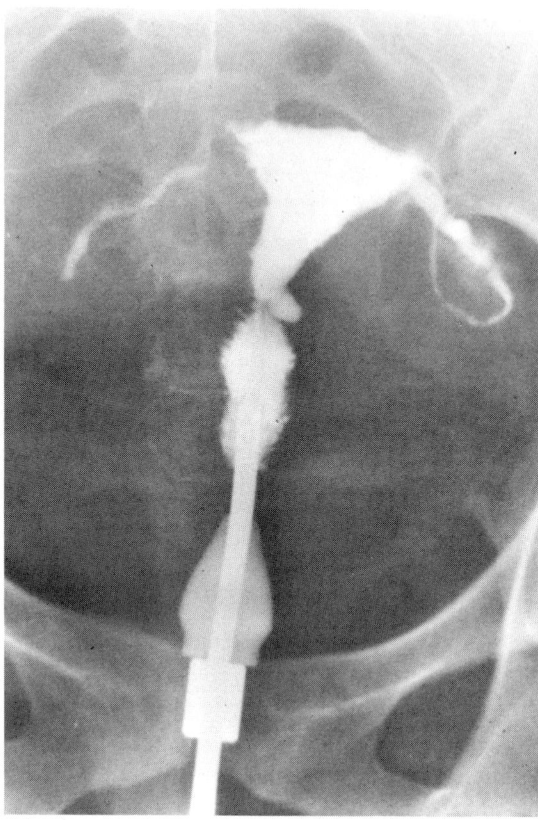

FIGURE 39-1.

days 5-9 of the cycle for the treatment of anovulation. A serum progesterone drawn on day 23 is 16 ng/ml. During the next cycle the dose of clomiphene prescribed per day on days 5-9 should be
A. 50 mg
B. 100 mg
C. 150 mg
D. 200 mg
E. 250 mg

DIRECTIONS for questions 11- 20: For each numbered item, select the one heading most closely associated with it. Each lettered heading may be used once, more than once, or not at all.

11-13. Match the medication best suited to correct the secondary infertility factors
(A) hyperprolactinemia
(B) luteal phase deficiency
(C) occult infection
(D) abnormality of sperm penetration
(E) sperm antibodies
11. bromocriptine
12. progesterone
13. corticosteroids

14-16. Match the infertility investigation with best menstrual cycle day to perform it
(A) 1
(B) 7
(C) 13
(D) 17
(E) 26
14. postcoital test
15. hysterosalpingogram
16. endometrial biopsy

17-20. Match the etiology with its reported frequency as a cause of infertility
(A) 5%
(B) 15%
(C) 35%
(D) 50%
(E) 75%
17. anovulation
18. abnormal semen
19. impairment of tubal motility
20. abnormal sperm transport through the cervix

DIRECTIONS: For each numbered item 21 - 26, indicate whether it is associated with
A only (A)
B only (B)
C both (A) and (B)
D neither (A) nor (B)

21-22. Match the tubal problem with therapeutic recommendations
(A) distal tubal disease
(B) proximal tubal blockage
(C) both
(D) neither
21. Use of microsurgery has improved subsequent pregnancy rates
22. Repeat surgical procedure recommended if occlusion reoccurs

23-26. Treatment for properly selected cases in which anovulation is the sole cause of infertility
(A) human menopausal gonadotrophin
(B) clomiphene citrate
(C) both
(D) neither
23. ovulatory rate >95%
24. pregnancy rate per cycle is 20%
25. ovarian enlargement in >5% of treatment cycles
26. overall conception rate ≤50%

DIRECTIONS for questions 27 - 32: For each of the questions below, ONE or MORE of the responses is correct. Select the best answer based on the following
A if 1, 2, and 3 are correct
B if only 1 and 2 are correct
C if only 2 and 3 are correct

D if only 1 is correct
E if only 3 is correct

27. Descriptors of an appropriately-timed postcoital test for a woman with an irregular cycle and for which a normal test is the finding of at least five motile sperm include that
    1. the mucus should be scanty and viscid
    2. the test should be scheduled on day 14 of the cycle
    3. the test should be performed 2-3 hours after coitus
28. In informing a candidate for in vitro fertilization (IVF) on human menopausal gonadotrophin about different aspects of the procedure, one should mention the
    1. need for midcycle daily ultrasound
    2. possibility of ovarian hyperstimulation
    3. need for midcycle laparoscopy
29. A 32 year-old female medical student and her 34 year-old accountant husband seek advice regarding the possibility of needing an infertility work-up. Neither has been married previously and they have been trying to conceive for three months. Both are healthy, with no significant past medical history. You would mention to them that
    1. up to 15% of married couples in the U.S. are infertile
    2. the incidence of infertility increases with increasing age of the woman
    3. in 50% of infertile couples, the only abnormal factor found is in the semen
30. A hysterosalpingogram is interpreted as normal. It would be correct to inform the patient that
    1. there are no pelvic adhesions
    2. there is no evidence of salpingitis isthmica nodosa
    3. both fallopian tubes are patent
31. A 25 year-old patient has undergone an infertility investigation, including serum progesterone, semen analysis, postcoital test, and hysterosalpingogram. All tests were normal. A diagnostic laparoscopy is now scheduled. Tests performed at the time of laparoscopy that would likely provide additional information as to the etiology of infertility include
    1. hysteroscopy
    2. a cervical culture
    3. transcervical insufflation with indigo carmine
32. A recently married, healthy 23 year-old patient comes to your office inquiring how she and her husband might maximize their chance of conception as soon as possible. Assuming that she and her husband are both normal, reassurance can be provided by telling her
    1. that among fertile couples who have coitus just before ovulation, there is only a 20% chance of achieving a clinical pregnancy in each ovulatory cycle
    2. to try to have intercourse for 3 consecutive days at midcycle
    3. the basal body temperature chart is prospectively useful to predict the time of ovulation

ANSWERS

1. **C**, Pages 1196, 1197. Although there are no absolute standards for a normal semen sample, there are some recommended guidelines.

TABLE 39-1. Recommended Standards for Semen Analysis

Parameter	Recommended Normal Value
Volume	2-6 ml
Viscosity	Full liquefaction within 60 minutes
Sperm density	20-250 million/ml*
Sperm motility	
Progressive	Good to very good‡
Quantitation	First hour ≥60%, 2-3 h ≥50%
Vital Staining	≤35% dead cells
Sperm morphology	≥60% within normal configuration

Modified from Eliasson R: Parameters of male fertility. In Hafez ESE, Evans TN, eds: Human reproduction. New York, Harper & Row, Publishers, 1973.
*20 million/ is low normal, in contrast to 40 million/ml, International Society of Andrology.
‡3 to 4 + quality.

2. **B**, Page 1197. Given a semen sample that shows normal parameters except for a low count, this specimen might merely reflect one extreme in the wide variability normally seen in a man's semen sample. Repeating the test in one month with an appropriate abstinence period of 2-3 days preceding collection would be the appropriate next step. Immediately repeating the test might be stressful or provide an abnormally low value. It should be recalled that it takes 74 days for germ cells to become mature sperm. Therefore, the

appropriate timing of a repeat semen analysis is important. Clomiphene citrate and tetracycline therapy would be inappropriate until a specific diagnosis is made. A physical examination by a qualified urologist or reproductive gynecologist is a part of the work-up of a male with a semen abnormality, but at this point there is no evidence that it is needed.

3. **E,** Page 1194. The first diagnostic step in the evaluation of infertility is to obtain presumptive evidence that the woman is ovulating. A history of regular menses constitutes presumptive evidence of ovulation, and a midluteal serum progesterone above 10 ng/ml is also indirect evidence of adequate ovulation. Both endometrial biopsy and basal body temperature charts reflect response to progesterone but are not direct evidence of ovulation. The only direct evidence of ovulation is pregnancy.
4. **E,** Pages 1222-1224, Figure 39-26. Based on the American Fertility Society classification of endometriosis, the patient has minimal endometriosis (Stage I). No therapy, either medical or surgical, has been shown to be efficacious in patients with less than moderate endometriosis (Stage III). Since no other cause of infertility has been identified, it is advisable to delay medical or surgical intervention for at least 12 months. In all likelihood, at the time of laparoscopy, the laparoscopist would fulgurate the implants and lyse the adhesions.
5. **E,** Page 1214. Women with pelvic tuberculosis should be considered "sterile" because pregnancies after chemotherapy are rare. On the other hand, if intrauterine adhesions are the sole abnormality and not overly extensive, prognosis for conception after lysis of adhesions is good. Congenital uterine defects such as a bicornuate uterus are a cause of infertility but these patients are not sterile. Maternal ingestion of DES has not been clearly shown to be a cause of infertility. There are fairly uncommon circumstances in which leiomyomata can be associated with infertility. In selected cases, myomectomy has been reported to achieve pregnancy rates as high was 50%.
6. **B,** Page 1213. Donors for AID should be carefully screened to ascertain that they are in good health, do not have a potentially inheritable disorder, and will not transmit an infectious agent in the semen. Screening must be performed to rule out hepatitis B, syphilis, *Neisseria gonorrhoeae*, and *Chlamydia trachomatis*. Since cultures for the human immunodeficiency virus (HIV) may not turn positive for several months after the disease is acquired, it is suggested that only frozen semen of over six months' storage be used. The donor is then tested for HIV after the six months storage period.
7. **C,** Page 1207. When conception occurs after ovulation has been induced with clomiphene, the incidence of multiple gestation increases to 5%. The rates of spontaneous abortion, ectopic gestation, intrauterine fetal death, and congenital malformation are not significantly increased over the general population.
8. **E,** Page 1218 Figure 39-1 from Infertility, contraception and reproductive endocrinology, 2nd ed, by Daniel R. Mishell, Jr., M.D., and Val Davajan, M.D. Copyright 1986 Medical Economics Books, Oradell, N.J. 07649. All rights reserved. The hysterosalpingogram shown demonstrates bilateral hydrosalpinges with dilation, clubbing and obstruction at the fimbriated ends. Since the prognosis for a term pregnancy after repair of this disease is poor, the patient would best be advised to consider in vitro fertilization. Transcervical balloon tuboplasty is reserved only for proximal tubal disease. Intrauterine insemination would be inappropriate because with extensive tubal disease sperm would still not have to access to the egg. Gamete intrafallopian transfer (GIFT) is inappropriate because of the extensive tubal disease. Tubal reanastomosis is only suitable in cases where previous surgical sterilization of the tubes has occurred. The anatomy should otherwise be normal.
9. **E,** Page 1210. Washed intrauterine insemination (IUI) is a technique in which sperm are inseminated into the uterus after they have been separated from the semen by centrifugation. It is used in several different circumstances: if the amount of mucus is small or the mucus is not thin and watery with good spinnbarkeit; if the patient has undergone conization with resultant scant mucus; if the male is oligospermic; if the semen volume is small (less than 2 ml) or large (greater than 8 ml); or if the semen is of high viscosity. Insemination of sperm into the uterus is of no benefit if there is no access to the egg. There is, therefore, no role for IUI in the treatment of bilateral cornual obstruction.

10. **A**, Pages 1204-1207. Serum levels of progesterone in patients in whom ovulation is induced by clomiphene citrate are consistently above 15 ng/ml. These levels are higher than the 10 ng/ml seen in spontaneous ovulatory cycles because clomiphene induces more than one follicle to mature and luteinize. As this patient demonstrates a sufficient response on 50 mg per day, clomiphene should be continued at the same dose in the next cycle.

11-13. 11, **A**; 12, **B**; 13, **E**; Pages 1227-1229. There is no evidence that treatment of secondary infertility factors significantly improves pregnancy rates when compared with withholding therapy. Nevertheless, if hyperprolactinemia is discovered, it would be reasonable to begin bromocriptine, anticipating good results. Both clomiphene citrate and progesterone are advocated for the treatment of luteal phase defects. Antisperm antibodies can be treated with condoms to prevent the woman's exposure to sperm or corticosteroid immunosuppressive therapy with variable results.

14-16. 14, **C**; 15, **B**; 16, **E**; Pages 1198, 1199, 1227-1228. Certain infertility tests should be performed at specific times of the cycle in order to avoid potential complications and to maximize the information obtained. The postcoital test is best performed on the day prior to ovulation (day 13) in order to assess maximal estrogen effect on cervical mucus. The hysterosalpingogram should be performed during the week after menses in order to avoid either irradiating a possible pregnancy or inducing iatrogenic endometriosis. An endometrial biopsy late in the luteal phase will reflect the maximal effect from the sex steroids produced by the corpus luteum.

17-20. 17, **B**; 18, **C**; 19, **C**; 20, **B**; Page 1193. Currently, available techniques are able to identify the etiology of infertility in 85-90% of couples. In the United States, 10-15% of cases are due to anovulation, 30-40% to an abnormality of the semen, 30-40% to pelvic disease interfering with normal tubal motility, and 10-15% to abnormalities of sperm transport through the cervical canal.

21-22. 21, **B**; 22, **D**; Pages 1214-1221. The prognosis for fertility after tubal reconstruction depends on the extent of damage to the tube as well as the location of the obstruction. If both proximal and distal obstructions exist, operative repair should not be undertaken. Similarly, if obstruction reoccurs, a second procedure is not advised because subsequent pregnancy rates are less than 10%. Rates for conception after initial salpingostomy are about 30%, whereas after salpingolysis and fimbrioplasty for only partial obstruction they are 65%. Unlike results for distal disease, the use of microsurgery has improved pregnancy rates for proximal tubal obstruction. Term pregnancy rates of 50% have been reported after tubocornual reanastomosis for proximal blockage. Recently, several investigations have reported successful treatment of proximal tubal obstruction with the use of transcervical balloons and catheters.

23-26. 23, **A**; 24, **C**; 25, **A**; 26, **D**; Pages 1204-1208. Both clomiphene citrate and human menopausal gonadotrophin (HMG) are used to induce ovulation. Typically, HMG is withheld unless the patient fails to respond to clomiphene or she is amenorrheic with low estrogen levels. The ovulatory rate with HMG approaches 100%. With clomiphene, 90% of women with oligomenorrhea and 66% with secondary amenorrhea have presumptive evidence of ovulation. Both drugs achieve a pregnancy rate per cycle of approximately 22%. Ovarian enlargement is detectable in 1% of clomiphene cycles and up to 10% of HMG treatment cycles. Overall, conception rates are 60% for HMG and up to 85% with clomiphene. Pregnancy and conception rates are important, but the patient should also be aware of the percent of live births following treatment. This is the most important figure.

27. **E** (3 only), Pages 1198-1199. The postcoital test (PCT) is the only in vivo test that provides information about both partners in an infertility work-up. Ideally the test is performed on the day prior to ovulation, when there is maximal estrogen stimulation. The exact day of ovulation is anticipated, not known. Realistically a PCT is scheduled properly if the mucus has a good estrogen effect. This means a clear, watery cervical mucus with a spinnbarkeit of at least 6 cm. If the mucus is cloudy and thick, either the timing of the test was poor or the woman has a cervical problem. For a PCT to be normal, at least five motile sperm should be seen in each high-powered field. The number of motile sperm seen is directly related to the time interval between the test and coitus. Thus, a standard different from the one

stated should be used if the test is more than 2-3 hours after coitus.

28. **B** (1, 2), Page 1232. Although in vitro fertilization (IVF) was originally intended for women with severe tubal disease, it is now being used for women with severe endometriosis and couples with male factor or unexplained infertility. Nearly all centers utilize some type of ovarian hyperstimulation because the rate of pregnancy is related to the number of embryos placed in the uterine cavity. Because of the use of hyperstimulation, daily midcycle ultrasound and estrogen measurements must be done. The widespread use of hyperstimulation may change, however, because of the recent reports citing good success rates achieved after unstimulated cycles. The latter avoids the cost of human menopausal gonadotrophin treatment as well as the attendant monitoring. It also allows for more aspiration cycles in a given time period. Originally, oocyte retrieval was accomplished with laparoscopy. With the development of high resolution ultrasound, oocyte retrieval can be accomplished either transvaginally or transabdominally.
29. **B** (1, 2), Pages 1190-1191 . The inability to conceive is one of the most common problems for which women seek gynecologic care. It is estimated that 10-15% of married couples in the United States are infertile (usually defined as the inability to conceive within 1 year). The incidence of infertility increases with the increasing age of the woman. For example, in the 20-24 year-old age group, 80% of nonsterile married women will conceive within 12 months of unprotected intercourse, whereas the percentage drops to 63% for the 30-34 year-old age group. An abnormality in semen production is identifiable in 30-40% of infertile couples. In up to 10% of cases, the etiology of infertility cannot be determined by currently available techniques.
30. **C** (2, 3), Page 1200. A normal hysterosalpingogram (HSG) demonstrates bilateral tubal patency and thus excludes the presence of salpingitis isthmica nodosa (diverticula of the endosalpinx into the muscularis of the isthmic portion of the tube). Although tubal patency is documented, the presence of peritubal pelvic adhesions cannot be completely ruled out by HSG alone. Laparoscopy would be necessary to rule out pelvic adhesions.
31. **E** (3 only), Page 1200. When performing diagnostic laparoscopy for infertility, indigo carmine should be introduced through the cervix to confirm tubal patency. If the hysterosalpingogram were normal, hysteroscopy is not indicated. A cervical culture should have been performed earlier in the work-up had there been any suspicion of cervical infection. A normal postcoital test in which no white cells were seen and there are an ample number of motile sperm, negates the need for a cervical culture.
32. **B** (1, 2), Pages 1193-1194. Often a young, healthy couple requires only education and specific instruction rather than a costly medical evaluation in order to achieve pregnancy. Unless the husband has oligospermia, daily intercourse for three consecutive days at midcycle should be encouraged, because sperm are capable of fertilization for 1-2 days after coitus. The egg probably degenerates a few hours after it reaches the ampulla of the oviduct if fertilization does not occur. Ovulation cannot be predicted in a current cycle by use of a basal body temperature chart since it demonstrates a biphasic temperature shift only after levels of progesterone have increased. Reassurance that a fertile couple has only a 20% chance of getting pregnant each ovulatory cycle may help relieve patient anxiety. In telling the patient to have coitus at the time of ovulation, one should not neglect the marital aspects of the act by focusing only on conception.

Menopause

DIRECTION for questions 1 - 22: Select the one best answer or completion.

1. A 45-year-old diabetic, hypertensive patient complains of severe hot flushes following a recent hysterectomy and bilateral salpingo-oophorectomy for large uterine leiomyomata. Without medication, the patient's blood pressure is 145/95. This woman has a past history of thrombophlebitis at age 30 and a myocardial infarction at age 44. Before surgery, blood lipids were measured. This woman's LDL cholesterol was high, and her HDL cholesterol low. You would
   A. prescribe estrogen
   B. prescribe a regimen of estrogen and progesterone
   C. not prescribe estrogen because of her blood lipid profile
   D. not prescribe estrogen because of her past history of thrombophlebitis
   E. not prescribe estrogen because of her hypertension
2. The increase in facial hair noted in postmenopausal women is a direct consequence of
   A. increased levels of testosterone
   B. increased levels of androstenedione
   C. increased sensitivity of the hair follicles
   D. increased luteinizing hormone (LH)
   E. a decrease in the estrogen-androgen ratio
3. See above, right.
3. A 53-year-old white, type II diabetic has been on hormonal replacement for her hot flashes. These are unbearable unless she takes at least 1.25 mg per day of conjugated equine estrogen. Previously the patient had not been on a progestin. She would prefer not to have withdrawal bleeding. Of the regimens listed at the bottom of the page, the one that will most likely meet her request and still provide the protection to the endometrium is
4. A 67-year-old gravida 5 para 5 has urgency, urge incontinence, and stress incontinence. The stress incontinence is confirmed by urodynamic testing. Urinalysis is normal, and the urine culture is negative. She has a pale atrophic vagina. The patient takes no medication, or vitamin supplementation, and otherwise feels well. At this point you should
   A. do a retropubic suspension
   B. do a vaginal hysterectomy and anterior colporrhaphy
   C. start a beta-adrenergic
   D. start an anticholinergic
   E. start vaginal estrogen
5. The mean age for the menopause is
   A. 45
   B. 47
   C. 49
   D. 51
   E. 53
6. In a patient whose major complaint is hot

	Estrogen & amount	Number of Estrogen days/month	Progestin & amount	Number of Progestin days/month
A.	conjugated equine estrogen 0.625 mg	first 25	medroxyprogesterone 2.5 mg	first 10
B.	estrone sulfate 0.625 mg	first 25	medroxyprogesterone 5 mg	last 10
C.	estrone sulfate 1.25 mg	first 21	medroxyprogesterone 10 mg	last 14
D.	micronized estradiol 2 mg	continuous	medroxyprogesterone 5 mg	first 12
E.	esterified estrogen 1.25 mg	continuous	methyltestosterone 2.5 mg	continuous

flushes that greatly interfere with her daily life, you would expect to find all of the following **EXCEPT**
   A. less than ideal body weight
   B. decreased estrone
   C. decreased estradiol
   D. increased sex hormone binding globulin (SHBG) bound estradiol
   E. increased FSH
7. In those women at risk for the development of osteoporosis who are not properly treated, the percent loss of bone mass each year after the menopause is
   A. 0.25-0.75
   B. 1.00-1.50
   C. 2.00-2.50
   D. 3.00-3.50
   E. 4.50-5.00
8. Estrogen replacement therapy **CAUSES**
   A. adenocarcinoma of the endometrium
   B. hypertension
   C. thrombosis
   D. a thickened vaginal epithelium
   E. ductal carcinoma of the breast
9. There are multiple prospective and retrospective studies that look at the likelihood of developing cancer if the woman has been on estrogen replacement. The conclusions reached are that postmenopausal estrogen is associated with
   A. an endometrial adenocarcinoma that is relatively undifferentiated
   B. a relative risk of more than 5.0 of developing adenocarcinoma of the endometrium
   C. a risk of adenocarcinoma of the endometrium that has no correlation with the length of therapy
   D. a risk of adenocarcinoma of the endometrium that has no correlation with the dose of estrogen prescribed
   E. a higher risk in those women who have taken oral contraceptives prior to the menopause
10. A 42-year-old woman complains of hot flushes. Her periods are fairly regular every 26 to 30 days. Flow lasts 3 to 7 days. In the past, periods were exactly 28 to 29 days, and flow lasted 3 to 4 days. A serum FSH was elevated and the serum progesterone was 10 ng/ml. Your advice would be that this patient should
   A. stop worrying about contraception
   B. use progestin supplementation
   C. consider herself menopausal
   D. have a LH determination
   E. take estrogen
11. Of the several women listed below, who is **unlikely** to experience hot flushes?
   A. a 50-year-old 45, X who had been taking 1 mg of micronized estradiol until 3 months ago
   B. a 55-year-old white, 5 feet 2 inch tall, 100 pound woman
   C. a 50-year-old 5 foot, 85 pound Asian woman
   D. a 38-year-old white, 5 feet 4 inch tall, 180 pound woman who has just undergone a total abdominal hysterectomy, bilateral salpingo-oophorectomy
   E. an 18-year-old woman who has pure gonadal dysgenesis who has just undergone a total abdominal hysterectomy, bilateral salpingo-oophorectomy
12. Postmenopausal serum levels of
   A. calcium are decreased
   B. phosphorus are decreased
   C. calcitonin are decreased
   D. parathyroid hormone are increased
   E. 1,25-dihydroxyvitamin D are increased
13. The histologic appearance of the ovaries of a woman 49 years of age who had her last normal menstrual period 1 year ago would reveal
   A. lack of ovarian follicles
   B. proliferation of the theca
   C. proliferation of the granulosa
   D. degeneration of the stroma
   E. absence of surface epithelial cysts
14. A typical 55-year-old woman who has hot flushes describes them to you. She is likely to tell you that hot flushes
   A. have interfered with her activities for 6-7 years
   B. are occasionally followed by profuse perspiration
   C. come on gradually over a 15 minute period
   D. rarely occur more than once in 24 hours
   E. last 10 to 15 minutes
15. The diagnosis of osteoporosis in trabecular bone can be accomplished by all of the following **EXCEPT**
   A. computerized tomography (CT) scans
   B. single photon absorptiometry
   C. dual photon absorptiometry
   D. X-ray
   E. dual-energy x-ray absorptiometry
16. The **parenteral** administration of estrogen to post-menopausal women
   A. increases serum triglyceride
   B. significantly lowers total cholesterol
   C. decreases low-density lipoprotein (LDL)cholesterol

D. increases high-density lipoprotein (HDL) cholesterol
E. none of the above

17. The addition of 10 to 12 days of a synthetic progestin to a cyclic postmenopausal estrogen regimen
A. renders it less effective in the prevention of hot flushes
B. negates the beneficial effect that estrogen has on bone density
C. enhances the beneficial effect that estrogen has on serum lipids
D. may cause mild depression and irritability
E. prevents vaginal atrophy

18. A factor that appears to affect the age of a woman's menopause is
A. weight
B. use of oral contraceptives
C. number of term pregnancies
D. smoking
E. age at menarche

19. Follicle-stimulating hormone (FSH) is elevated in the postmenopausal woman because of decreased levels of
A. estradiol
B. estrone
C. prolactin
D. inhibin
E. luteinizing hormone (LH)

20. A hot flush is **followed** by
A. increases in digital perfusion
B. increases in peripheral skin temperature
C. decreases in luteinizing hormone (LH)
D. decreases in heart rate
E. decreases in cortisol

21. A number of complaints such as anxiety and worry about self have been attributed to the menopause. Recent studies suggest that postmenopausal patients who receive exogenous estrogen improve because the estrogen
A. increases prolactin
B. decreases testosterone
C. increases plasma β-endorphin
D. increases estrogen receptors
E. decreases luteinizing hormone (LH)

22. The postmenopausal patient who uses estrogen without progestin has an increased risk of
A. hypertension
B. a decrease in glucose tolerance
C. thrombophlebitis
D. thromboembolism
E. none of the above

DIRECTIONS for questions 23 - 27: For each numbered item, select the one heading most closely associated with it. Each lettered heading may be used once, more than once, or not at all.

23-25. Percent effected without hormonal replacement
(A) 5%
(B) 10%
(C) 15%
(D) 20%
(E) 25%

23. percent of Caucasian or Asian women who develop spinal compression fractures by age 60
24. percent of 80-year-old women with a hip fracture who die from the hip fracture or its complications within 6 months
25. percent of 80-year-old white women who will develop hip fractures

26-27. Daily dose
(A) 0.3 mg
(B) 0.625 mg
(C) 2.5 mg
(D) 1.0 g
(E) none

26. the minimum amount of conjugated equine estrogen that will prevent osteoporosis in patients who ingest an adequate amount of calcium in their diet or with the addition of a calcium supplement
27. the minimum recommended amount of daily supplemental vitamin D necessary to retard osteoporosis

DIRECTIONS: For each numbered item 28 - 33, indicate whether it is associated with
A only (A)
B only (B)
C both (A) and (B)
D neither (A) nor (B)

28-30. Studies support the effect listed below
(A) diminishes severity of hot flushes
(B) prophylaxis against osteoporosis
(C) both
(D) neither

28. conjugated equine estrogens
29. intramuscular medroxyprogesterone acetate
30. clonidine

31-33. Physiologic activity
(A) estrogen
(B) progesterone
(C) both
(D) neither

31. increases the synthesis of estrogen receptors
32. increases the synthesis of progesterone receptors
33. decreases the synthesis of progesterone receptors

DIRECTIONS for questions 34 - 35: For each of the questions below, ONE or MORE of the responses is correct. Select the best answer based on the following

A if 1, 2, and 3 are correct
B if only 1 and 2 are correct
C if only 2 and 3 are correct
D if only 1 is correct
E if only 3 is correct

34. Factors known to increase the risk of osteoporosis include
    1. diet high in alcohol
    2. early spontaneous menopause
    3. cigarette smoking
35. In the postmenopausal woman androstenedione is
    1. secreted primarily by the ovary
    2. secreted by the adrenal
    3. converted to estrone in peripheral body fat

ANSWERS

1. **A,** Pages 1264-1270, 1273. This patient's hot flushes are an indication for estrogen replacement. There is no contraindication given in the history to its application. Although the use of oral contraceptive agents has been associated with the development of hypertension and thrombophlebitis, postmenopausal estrogen therapy has not. This is due in part to the potency and formulation of the estrogens involved. Studies demonstrate that postmenopausal estrogen users have improved lipid profiles. Both retrospective and prospective cohort studies have shown that postmenopausal estrogen users have a decreased likelihood of death due to myocardial infarction. In fact, the age-adjusted all-cause mortality rate is lower in estrogen users. There is evidence that use of progestin lowers the chances of postmenopausal estrogen users' developing endometrial cancer. Depending upon the formulation it may have an adverse effect on serum lipids. In vitro studies demonstrate increased mitotic activity in breast tissue with progestin exposure. This suggests a potential deleterious effect on the human breasts. Until additional studies are available, it appears prudent not to add a progestin to the postmenopausal hormonal therapy ofa patient who has had a hysterectomy.
2. **E,** Page 1248. The postmenopausal levels of testosterone and androstenedione are not elevated. Although luteinizing hormone (LH) is increased in the postmenopausal woman, it is not directly associated with hirsutism. The physiologic process of a decrease in the estrogen-androgen ratio is the cause of the increased facial hair growth that frequently occurs after menopause.
3. **D,** Pages 1251-1254, 1259, 1273, Figure 40-30 (Herbst et al) [Weinstein L, Bewtra C, Gallagher JC. Evaluation of a continuous combined low-dose regimen of estrogen-progestin for treatment of the menopausal patient. Am J Obstet Gynecol 1990;162(6):1534-9]. The patient has demonstrated that she currently requires 1.25 mg per day of conjugated equine estrogen to control adequately her hot flashes. Later one will be able to reduce this to 0.625 mg per day. The 0.625 mg per day dose is the amount necessary to retard development of osteoporosis. Two milligrams per day of micronized estradiol is equivalent in the control of hot flashes to 1.25 mg/day of conjugated equine estrogen or 1.25 mg/day of estrone sulfate. It has been demonstrated that for postmenopausal women receiving 0.625 mg of conjugated equine estrogen 2.5 mg of medroxyprogesterone reduced nuclear and cytosol estrogen receptor levels to those found before estrogen administration. With a daily dose of 1.25 of conjugated equine estrogen, 5 mg of medroxyprogesterone was necessary to decrease the receptor synthesis to the same degree. Estrogen may be given every day of the month in a continuous fashion and the progestin given daily for the first 10 to 13 days of the month with the combined regimen. The continuous estrogen regimen frequently results in breakthrough bleeding during the first 6 months, but with longer use nearly all women remain amenorrheic. Given this patient's request, this would appear to be the appropriate approach at this time. Another approach suggested by Weinstein et al would be both continuous estrogen and progestin. The combination of 1.25 mg esterified estrogen and 2.5 mg of methyltestosterone is distributed under the trade name Estratest. The addition of testosterone has been advocated to increase libido. There is concern that its use will have a deleterious effect on lipid metabolism and possibly cause hirsutism.
4. **E,** Page 1248. The trigone of the bladder and the urethra are embryologically derived from estrogen-dependent tissue, and

estrogen deficiency can lead to their atrophy, producing symptoms of urinary urge incontinence, dysuria, and urinary frequency. With a decrease of elastic tissue around the vagina, due to estrogen deficiency, a urethrocele may develop. Although surgery may ultimately be needed, local estrogen should be tried first since it may relieve the symptoms. It should be given before surgery to thicken the vaginal mucosa. This patient might also benefit from Kegel exercises. Because vaginal administration of estrogen results in irregular systemic absorption, for long-term prevention of vaginal atrophy as well as osteoporosis and atherosclerosis, the patient is best treated with oral or transdermal estrogen after 2-3 weeks of vaginal estrogen.

5. **D,** Pages 1245-1246. The mean age of menopause is 51.4 years. The 95% confidence limits are between ages 45 and 55 years. Menopause is defined as the cessation of menstruation for at least 6 months due to depletion of ovarian follicles.
6. **D,** Page 1249. Postmenopausal women with hot flushes have lower circulating estrone and estradiol levels, less total body weight, and a lower percentage of ideal body weight as compared to those without hot flushes. They also have less sex hormone binding globulin (SHBG) bound estradiol.
7. **B,** Page 1255. In short, frail, thin-skinned, sedentary women who do not receive hormonal therapy about 1% to 1.5% of bone mass is lost each year after the menopause.
8. **D** (4), Pages 1251, 1268-1269. An association between the use of estrogen and adenocarcinoma of the endometrium, hypertension, and thrombosis has been established. The association with breast cancer is much more controversial. An association is not the same as cause and effect. Furthermore, the development of these complications is highly dependent on the dosage, mode of administration, length of treatment, and type of estrogen. For example, 2.5 mg of conjugated equine estrogen causes less of an increase in the liver's production of binding globulin than does 30 μg of ethinyl estradiol, the estrogen used in many contraceptive pills. One such globulin is angiotensinogen, which when converted to angiotensin is associated with an increase in blood pressure. Probably patient predisposition is also a factor in the development of these complications. The potency of an estrogen depends upon the effect used to measure potency, that is, vaginal thickness, lipid concentration, etcetera. Estrogen does thicken the vaginal epithelium.
9. **B,** Pages 1270-1271. Since 1975, many studies have addressed the question of the relative risk of estrogen users developing adenocarcinoma. These have been both prospective and retrospective investigations. There are several reviews that critique these studies. Given all of this, it would appear that the relative risk for patients who have taken an estrogen without a progestin is 3 to 7. The endometrial cancer that develops in estrogen users is nearly always well differentiated and is usually cured by performing a simple hysterectomy. The risk increases with increasing duration of use of estrogen as well as with increased dosage. It has been reported that prior oral contraceptive use of 1 year or longer negated the increased risk of endometrial cancer in postmenopausal women who were receiving only estrogen.
10. **E,** Pages 1246-1248. About 5 years before the actual menopause, FSH is elevated because of lack of negative feedback because although a serum estradiol may be in the normal range, the total estrogens from cycle to cycle are decreased. The low estrogen is responsible for this patient's hot flushes. Since her progesterone is normal, this patient is still ovulating, and although unlikely, she can still become pregnant. Obtaining a serum LH would not be cost-effective. Given the FSH, it is predictable. This woman would benefit from low dose estrogen supplementation, 0.3 mg of conjugated equine estrogen, 0.3 mg of estrone sulfate, or 0.5 mg of micronized estradiol from the fifth day after menstruation begins until the onset of the next menses.
11. **E,** Page 1249. A woman who has had low estrogen levels throughout her life, such as an 18-year-old with pure gonadal dysgenesis, will not have hot flushes. This is true even if she has her gonads removed. If a woman without any ovaries, the 50-year-old 45, X were to receive estrogen, she would probably experience hot flushes when the estrogen is stopped. The change in estrogen levels leads to alterations in the hypothalamus that are probably mediated through the central nervous system.

Hot flushes do not persist in most women for more than 2 to 3 years, and it is uncommon for a woman to have hot flushes that last more than 5 years after the menopause. Ninety-five percent of women will be menopausal by the age of 55 years. When the change in estrogen levels is not gradual but sudden, such as occurs after castration, the individual is more likely to develop symptomatic hot flushes. Postmenopausal women with hot flushes have lower circulating estrone and estradiol levels, less total body weight, and a lower percentage of ideal body weight when compared to those without hot flushes.

12. **C,** Pages 1256-1258. Although the mechanism whereby estrogen prevents a decrease in bone density is not precisely known, it has been determined that postmenopausal serum levels of calcium and phosphorus are slightly increased. Serum levels of parathyroid hormone and the active form of vitamin D (1,25-dihydroxyvitamin D) are decreased, as is calcium absorption. In addition, calcitonin levels are lowered. Serum calcium levels are maintained within a fairly narrow range and regulated in part by parathyroid hormone production. Parathyroid hormone increases serum calcium levels by three mechanisms: bone resorption, tubal resorption of calcium in the kidney, and production of an enzyme (1-alpha-hydroxylase) that changes vitamin D from its inactive form to its active form and thereby increases calcium absorption from the gut. It has been postulated that estrogen, androgens, and progestins block the action of parathyroid hormone on bone resorption, reducing the amount of calcium reabsorbed from the bone. Estrogen increases calcitonin levels, and calcitonin prevents bone resorption. Human osteoblast cells have estrogen receptors, and it may be through a receptor phenomenon that estrogen therapy decreases bone loss. Bone formation in women with osteoporosis is normal.
13. **A,** Pages 1246-1247 [Nicosia SV. The aging ovary. Med Clin North Am 1987; 71(1):1-9]. The basic feature of the menopause is depletion of ovarian follicles with degeneration of the granulosa and theca cells. As theca cells degenerate, they fail to react to endogenous gonadotrophins. As a result, less estrogen is produced, and there is a decrease in the negative feedback on the hypothalamic-pituitary axis. In contrast to the follicular cells, the stroma cells of the ovary continue to function and are the major source of androgens. Other structural features of the "aged" ovary are obliterative arteriolar sclerosis and surface epithelial cysts.
14. **B,** Pages 1249-1251. Hot flushes do not persist in most women for more than 2 to 3 years, and it is uncommon for a woman to have hot flushes that last more than 5 years after the menopause. About one-half of women with flushes have at least one a day, and about 20% have more than one a day. These flushes frequently occur at night, awaken the individual and then produce insomnia. A hot flush is a sudden explosive systemic physiologic phenomenon that takes place over a period of 30 seconds to 5 minutes. The flush is preceded by an increase in digital perfusion, which is followed by increases in peripheral skin temperature, which sometimes includes profuse perspiration.
15. **B,** Page 1255. At least 25% of the bone needs to be lost before osteoporosis is diagnosed by routine X-ray examination. Dual photon absorptiometry and computerized tomography (CT) scans effectively measure bone density in trabecular bone. Dual-energy x-ray absorptiometry (DEXA) is a new method of measuring bone density that has precision and can be completed in a short time. Because an anteroposterior projection is used, dual photon absorptiometry measures not only the mainly trabecular bone of the vertebral body but also the cortical bone of the posterior processes, which does not contribute to the development of osteoporotic fractures. DEXA is based on a lateral projection technique. The technique of single photon absorptiometry can only be used to measure the density of structures composed primarily of cortical bone—bones in the axial skeleton such as the radius, femur, or os calcis. Since postmenopausal osteoporosis affects trabecular bone more rapidly than it does cortical bone, utilization of single photon absorptiometry on bones in the limbs can fail to detect the presence of loss of trabecular bone in the thoracic spine because the density of the bone being measured may remain within the normal range.
16. **E,** Pages 1264-1265. Numerous studies have shown that the administration of oral conjugated equine estrogens as well as

other oral estrogens raises triglyceride and serum high-density lipoprotein (HDL) cholesterol levels and lowers low-density lipoprotein (LDL) cholesterol levels, with minimal changes in total cholesterol levels. Data regarding parenteral administration of estrogen fail to show similar consistent significant lipid changes. This indicates the first pass of the oral estrogen through the liver has a major influence on lipid metabolism.

17. **D,** Page 1273. The addition of a progestin to estrogen therapy does not appear to cause an increase of any other systemic disease and acts synergistically with estrogen to cause a slight increase in bone density. The use of synthetic progestins may reverse the beneficial effect of estrogen upon serum lipids. This effect on lipids is most pronounced with 19 nor-progestins. The epidemiologic data showing a reduction in heart attacks in estrogen users were derived from women taking estrogen without a progestin. Whether the addition of a progestin to the regimen will reverse the beneficial action of estrogen upon cardiovascular disease remains to be determined. Progestin is active alone in the treatment of hot flushes. Estrogen and progestin together do not cancel each other and constitute effective treatment for hot flushes. A progestin may have an adverse effect on the vaginal and urethral mucosa and may produce undesired central nervous system symptoms and adversely affect mood and the sense of well-being. Some patients on norethindrone have reported depression, anxiety, and irritability.
18. **D,** Page 1245. The age at which the menopause occurs is genetically predetermined. It is not related to the number of prior ovulations; it is not affected by pregnancy, lactation, use of oral contraceptives, or failure to ovulate spontaneously. It is also not related to race, socioeconomic conditions, education, height, weight, age at menarche, or age at the last pregnancy. The age of menopause may be affected by smoking, as it has been reported that cigarette smokers experience an earlier spontaneous menopause than do nonsmokers.
19. **D,** Pages 1246-1247. After menopause circulating estradiol levels are generally less than 15 pg, whereas follicle-stimulating hormone (FSH) levels are greater than 40 mIU/ml and luteinizing hormone (LH) levels are also increased. Administration of large amounts of oral or parenteral estrogen will not cause FSH levels to return to premenopausal concentrations, since FSH release is mainly controlled by circulating inhibin levels. Since inhibin levels decline with absent ovarian follicular activity, FSH will remain elevated even when estrogen replacement is given.
20. **B,** Page 1251. A hot flush is preceded by an increase in digital perfusion, which is **followed** by increases in peripheral skin temperature, circulating norepinephrine and luteinizing hormone (LH) levels, and heart rate. With each flush there are increases in LH, adrenocorticotropic hormone, and cortisol but not follicle-stimulating hormone (FSH) or estradiol. The LH increase is an effect of the change in the hypothalamic-pituitary axis and not a cause of the hot flush, because patients without a pituitary gland also have hot flushes. Infusing a patient with LH will not cause a hot flush.
21. **C,** Page 1254. The following symptoms improve in women who receive postmenopausal estrogen: vaginal dryness, poor memory, anxiety, and worry about self. In addition there was an increase in optimism and good spirits with psychologic testing. Thus, estrogen improves many psychologic symptoms in addition to relieving the hot flush and allowing the patient to sleep better. Postmenopausal women have lower levels of plasma β-endorphin (β-EP) and β-lipotrophin (β-LPH) than women of reproductive age. Estrogen administration to postmenopausal women increases plasma β-EP and β-LPH to normal levels. The modulation of these peptide levels by estrogen may be one mechanism whereby estrogen replacement therapy improves the woman's mood and sense of well-being, since lowered endorphin levels have been associated with symptoms of depression.
22. **E,** Pages 1266, 1268-1269. Metabolic changes are related to the dosage and type of estrogen administered. The doses and type of estrogen given for postmenopausal hormone replacement therapy are much less potent than those used in oral contraceptives. In contrast to the increase in blood pressure that has been reported in some women using oral contraceptives, no such increase has been observed with use of estrogen replacement therapy. There is no epidemiologic evidence of an increased

incidence of thrombophlebitis or thromboembolism in postmenopausal estrogen users as compared with control subjects. Estrogen appears to have little effect on glucose metabolism. Recent studies have failed to show a decrease in glucose tolerance in patients treated with doses of estrogen equivalent to 1.25 mg of conjugated equine estrogen.

23-25. 23, **E**; 24, **C**; 25, **D**; Page 1255. By age 60, 25% of Caucasian and Asian women develop spinal compression fractures. Loss of bone mass in cortical bone occurs at a much slower rate than in trabecular bone. Thus, osteoporotic fractures of the femur usually do not begin to occur until about age 70 or 75. By age 80, 20% of all Caucasian women will develop hip fractures, and of these about 15% will die from the fracture itself or from complications within 6 months.

26-27. 26, **B**; 27, **E**; Pages 1257, 1260-1261. The minimum dosage of estrogen needed to prevent osteoporosis is 0.625 mg of conjugated equine estrogen. In addition to estrogen replacement, calcium supplementation and weight-bearing exercises are of ancillary benefit in preventing postmenopausal osteoporosis. The addition of Vitamin D has not been shown to be useful in the prevention of osteoporosis.

28-30. 28, **C**; 29, **C**; 30, **A**; Pages 1251-1254. The most effective treatment for the hot flush is estrogen, and conjugated equine estrogens are the most frequently prescribed estrogen for the menopausal population. Its use appears to retard the development of osteoporosis. Depomedroxyprogesterone acetate has been compared with conjugated equine estrogens in the treatment of hot flushes and was as effective as estrogens in relieving the symptoms of the hot flush. Depomedroxyprogesterone acetate decreases markers of bone resorption—urinary calcium and hydroxyproline urinary excretion—to an extentsimilar to that of 0.625 mg of conjugated equine estrogen. Other agents shown to reduce hot flushes include clonidine, naloxone, and methyldopa (Aldomet) but these drugs are not usually prescribed for this purpose.

31-33. 31, **A**; 32, **A**; 33, **B**; Pages 1270-1272. Estrogen increases the synthesis of both estrogen and progesterone receptors in the endometrium; progesterone and synthetic progestins decrease the synthesis of both these receptors and thus have an antiproliferative action.

34. **A** (1, 2, 3), Page 1255. Factors known to increase the risk of osteoporosis include
    A. Race:white or Asian
    B. Reduced weight for height
    C. Early spontaneous menopause
    D. Early surgical menopause
    E. Family history of osteoporosis
    F. Diet: low calcium intake, low vitamin D intake, high caffeine intake, high alcohol intake, and high protein intake
    G. Cigarette smoking
    H. Endocrine disorders such as diabetes mellitus, hyperthyroidism, and Cushing's disease
    I. Sedentary life-style

35. **C** (2, 3), Page 1248. Ninety-five percent of postmenopausal androstenedione is produced by the adrenal while 5% comes from the ovary. Androstenedione is an androgen and is converted in the peripheral body fat to estrone. This rate of conversion increases as individuals age.

Notes

Notes

Notes

Notes

Notes

Notes

Notes